Bile Acids: Biological Actions and Clinical Relevance

FALK SYMPOSIUM 155

Bile Acids: Biological Actions and Clinical Relevance

Edited by

D. Keppler
German Cancer Research Center
Heidelberg
Germany

U. Beuers
University of Amsterdam
Amsterdam
The Netherlands

U. Leuschner
Johann Wolfgang Goethe University
Frankfurt
Germany

A. Stiehl
University Clinic
Heidelberg
Germany

M. Trauner
Medical Clinic University Graz
Graz
Austria

G Paumgartner
University Clinic
Munich
Germany

Proceedings of the Falk Symposium 155 held in Freiberg, Germany,
October 6–7, 2006

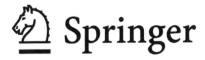 Springer

Library of Congress Cataloging-in-Publication Data is available.

ISBN-13 978-1-4020-6251-3

Published by Springer,
PO Box 17, 3300 AA Dordrecht, The Netherlands

Sold and distributed in North, Central and South America
by Springer,
101 Philip Drive, Norwell, MA 02061 USA

In all other countries, sold and distributed
by Springer,
PO Box 322, 3300 AH Dordrecht, The Netherlands

Printed on acid-free paper

Contents

CONTENTS

SECTION V: BILE ACIDS, CELLULAR INJURY, AND DISEASE MECHANISMS
Chair: M Trauner, U Beuers

SECTION VI: BILE ACIDS, CELLULAR INJURY, AND HEPATIC FIBROSIS
Chair: D Häussinger, PLM Jansen

SECTION VII: BILE ACIDS AS THERAPEUTIC AGENTS: MECHANISMS AND ACTIONS
Chair: GP van Berge Henegouwen, A Stiehl

CONTENTS

SECTION VIII: BILE ACIDS IN THE TREATMENT OF CHOLESTATIC LIVER DISEASE
Chair: H-U Marschall, U Leuschner

List of principal contributors

MS Anwer
Department of Biomedical Sciences
Tufts Cummings School of
   Veterinary Medicine
200 Westboro Road
North Grafton, MA 01536
USA

U Beuers
Department of Gastroenterology and
   Hepatology, AMC
University of Amsterdam B1-244.2
Meibergdreef 9
NL-1105 AZ Amsterdam
The Netherlands

I Björkhem
Karolinska Institute
Department of Clinical Chemistry
Huddinge University Hospital
S-14186 Huddinge
Sweden

JL Boyer
Liver Center
Yale University School of Medicine
333 Cedar Street
PO Box 208019
New Haven, CT 06520-8019
USA

RW Chapman
Department of Hepatology and
   Gastroenterology
Oxford Radcliffe Hospital
Oxford, OX3 9DU
UK

JYL Chiang
Department of Microbiology,
   Immunology and Biochemistry
Northeastern Ohio Universities
   College of Medicine
4209 State Route 44
Rootstown, OH 44272
USA

PA Dawson
Department of Internal Medicine
Section of Gastroenterology
Wake Forest University School of
   Medicine
Medical Center Blvd
Winston-Salem, NC 27157-1048
USA

P Fickert
Laboratory of Experimental and
   Molecular Hepatology
Division of Gastroenterology and
   Hepatology
Department of Internal Medicine
Medical University of Graz
Auenbruggerplatz 15
A-8036 Graz
Austria

D Häussinger
Universitätsklinikum Düsseldorf
Klinik für Gastroenterologie,
   Hepatologie und Infektiologie
Moorenstrasse 5
D-40225 Düsseldorf
Germany

PB Hylemon
Department of Microbiology and
   Immunology
VCU Medical Center
PO Box 980678
Richmond, VA 23298-0678
USA

T Ikegami
Division of Gastroenterology and
  Hepatology
Tokyo Medical University
  Kasumigaura Hospital
3-20-6 Chuo, Ami-Town
Inashika-gun
Ibaraki 300-0395
Japan

TH Karlsen
Medical Department
Rikshospitalet-Radiumhospitalet
  Medical Center
N-0027 Oslo
Norway

V Keitel
Klinik für Gastroenterologie,
  Hepatologie und Infektiologie
Universitätsklinikum Düsseldorf
Moorenstr. 5
D-40225 Düsseldorf
Germany

D Keppler
Division of Tumor Biochemistry
German Cancer Research Center
Im Neuenheimer Feld 280
D-69120 Heidelberg
Germany

SA Kliewer
Departments of Molecular Biology
  and Pharmacology
University of Texas Southwestern
  Medical Center
Dallas, TX 75390-9041
USA

R Kubitz
Gastroenterologie/Hepatologie
Universitätsklinikum Düsseldorf
Moorenstr. 5
D-40225 Düsseldorf
Germany

GA Kullak-Ublick
Division of Clinical Pharmacology
  and Toxicology
University Hospital Zurich
Ramistrasse 100
CH-8091 Zurich
Switzerland

G LeSage
University of Texas Houston Medical
  School
6431 Fannin Street, MSB 4.234
Houston, TX 77030
USA

KD Lindor
Mayo Clinic
200 First Street, SW
Rochester, MN 55905
USA

K Maeda
Department of Molecular
  Pharmacokinetics
Graduate School of Pharmaceutical
  Sciences
University of Tokyo
7-3-1 Hongo, Bunkyo-ku
Tokyo 113-0033
Japan

DJ Mangelsdorf
Howard Hughes Medical Institute
Department of Pharmacology
University of Texas Southwestern
  Medical Center
Dallas, TX 75390
USA

H-U Marschall
Karolinska University Hospital
  Huddinge K63
S-14186 Stockholm
Sweden

H Moshage
Department of Gastroenterology and
  Hepatology
University Medical Center
  Groningen
NL-9700 RB Groningen
The Netherlands

R Poupon
Service d'Hepato-Gastro-
  Enterologie
Hôpital Saint-Antoine
184, rue du Faubourg St Antoine
F-75571 Paris
France

S Ren
Veterans Affairs Medical Center
Research 151
1201 Broad Rock Blvd
Richmond, VA 23249
USA

M Rudling
Department of Medicine
Molecular Nutrition Unit
Center of Nutrition and Toxicology
Karolinska Institute
Karolinska University Hospital
  Huddinge
S-14186 Stockholm
Sweden

DW Russell
Department of Molecular Genetics
University of Texas Southwestern
  Medical Center
5323 Harry Hines Boulevard
Dallas, TX 75390-9046
USA

C Rust
Department of Medicine II -
  Grosshadern
University of Munich
Marchioninistrasse 15
D-81377 Munich
Germany

KDR Setchell
Department of Pathology and
  Laboratory Medicine
Cincinnati Children's Hospital
  Medical Center
3333 Burnet Avenue
Cincinnati, Ohio 45229-3039
USA

BL Shneider
Children's Hospital of Pittsburgh
Pediatric Gastroenterology
3705 Fifth Avenue
Pittsburgh, PA 15213
USA

A Stiehl
Medizinische Universitätsklinikum
Im Neuenheimer Feld 410
D-69120 Heidelberg
Germany

M Trauner
Laboratory for Experimental and
  Molecular Hepatology
Division of Gastroenterology and
  Hepatology
Department of Medicine
Medical University of Graz
Auenbruggerplatz 15
A-8036 Graz
Austria

DQ-H Wang
Gastroenterology Division
Beth Israel Deaconess Medical
  Center
Harvard Medical School
330 Brookline Avenue, DA 601
Boston, MA 02215
USA

List of chairpersons

GP van Berge Henegouwen
Department of Gastroenterology,
   F02.618
University Hospital Utrecht
Academisch Ziekenhuis
NL 3508 GA Utrecht
The Netherlands

JL Boyer
Liver Center
Yale University School of Medicine
333 Cedar Street
PO Box 208019
New Haven, CT 06520-8019
USA

U Beuers
Department of Gastroenterology and
   Hepatology, AMC
University of Amsterdam B1-244.2
Meibergdreef 9
NL-1105 AZ Amsterdam
The Netherlands

D Häussinger
Universitätsklinikum Düsseldorf
Klinik für Gastroenterologie,
   Hepatologie und Infektiologie
Moorenstrasse 5
D-40225 Düsseldorf
Germany

AF Hofmann
Department of Medicine, MC-0813
University of California, San Diego
9500 Gilman Drive
La Jolla, CA 92093-0813
USA

PLM Jansen
Division of Gastroenterology/
   Hepatology
University of Amsterdam, AMC
Meibergdreef 9
NL 1105 AZ Amsterdam
The Netherlands

W Kramer
Sanofi-Aventis Deutschland GmbH
Industriepark Höchst, Gebaude G879
D-65926 Frankfurt/Main
Germany

U Leuschner
Medizinische Klinik
Johann Wolfgang Goethe Universität
D-60596 Frankfurt
Germany

DJ Mangelsdorf
Howard Hughes Medical Institute
Department of Pharmacology
University of Texas Southwestern
   Medical Center
Dallas, TX 75390
USA

H-U Marschall
Karolinska University Hospital
   Huddinge K63
S-14186 Stockholm
Sweden

PJ Meier-Abt
University of Basel
Petersgraben 35
CH 4003 Basel
Switzerland

DW Russell
Department of Molecular Genetics
University of Texas Southwestern
  Medical Center
5323 Harry Hines Boulevard
Dallas, TX 75390-9046
USA

J Sjövall
Department of Medical Biochemistry
  and Biophysics
Karolinska Institute
S-17177 Stockholm
Sweden

A Stiehl
Medizinische Universitätsklinikum
Im Neuenheimer Feld 410
D-69120 Heidelberg
Germany

FJ Suchy
Department of Pediatrics, Box 1198
Mount Sinai School of Medicine
One Gustave L. Levy Place
New York, NY 10029-6574
USA

M Trauner
Laboratory for Experimental and
  Molecular Hepatology
Division of Gastroenterology and
  Hepatology
Department of Medicine
Medical University of Graz
Auenbruggerplatz 15
A-8036 Graz
Austria

Preface

This volume contains the contributions of the speakers at the 19th International Bile Acid Meeting, which was held in Freiburg, Germany, from October 6th to 7th 2006 with Gustav Paumgartner as president. As in previous Bile Acid Meetings, this symposium attracted a large number of basic scientists and clinical hepatologists from all over the world. The International Bile Acid Meetings have been held biannually since 1970 when Herbert Falk and the Falk Foundation started to sponsor these events and thereby contributed successfully to the bridging of basic science and clinical hepatology in the field of bile acids.

The scientific organizers and editors of this volume have assembled contributions reflecting the recent progress in bile acid metabolism and transport, nuclear receptor regulation and signalling by bile acids, as well as mechanisms of bile acid-induced cellular injury. Bile acids as therapeutic agents, particularly for the treatment of cholestatic liver diseases, were in the focus of several clinically oriented contributions.

A high-light of the 19th International Bile Acid Symposium was the presentation of the Adolf Windaus Prize, sponsored by the Falk Foundation, to Raoul Poupon from Paris. He summarizes in this volume his work on 'Primary biliary cirrhosis: from ursodeoxycholic acid towards targeting strategies for therapy'.

The editors are grateful to the contributors to this volume, to Dr. Martin Falk, Ursula Falk, and Dr. Herbert Falk for their generous sponsorship of the 19th International Bile Acid Meeting, to Silvia Maresch for her perfect organizational support, and to Lancaster Publishing Services for their excellent cooperation in publishing these proceedings.

Dietrich Keppler

Section I
Metabolism of bile acids

Chair: AF HOFMANN and J SJÖVALL

1
Analysis of mice deficient in the bile acid biosynthetic enzyme 3β-hydroxy-Δ^5-C$_{27}$-steroid oxidoreductase (HSD3B7)

H. C. SHEA, K. D. R. SETCHELL and D. W. RUSSELL

INTRODUCTION

The conversion of cholesterol into bile acids is essential for the maintenance of cholesterol homeostasis, the regulation of hepatic function, and the absorption of fats and fat-soluble vitamins from the gastrointestinal tract. Inherited mutations that decrease the synthesis of bile acids or their transport cause a disorder beginning in infants and consisting of impairment of liver function due to decreased bile flow (neonatal cholestasis) and lipid and vitamin malabsorption. Research over the past three decades has led to the annotation of the pathways by which cholesterol is converted into conjugated bile acids in the liver[1]. At least 16 enzymes that catalyse 17 different reactions participate in these metabolic pathways.

The genetic basis of neonatal cholestasis is heterogeneous. Mutations in four genes encoding bile acid biosynthetic enzymes have so far been identified as causes of this disease. These include the oxysterol 7α-hydroxylase gene (*CYP7B1*)[2], the 3-oxo-Δ^4-steroid 5β-reductase gene (*AKR1D1*)[3], the 2-methylacyl-coenzyme A racemase gene (*AMACR*)[4], and the 3β-hydroxy-Δ^5-C$_{27}$-steroid oxidoreductase (C$_{27}$ 3β-HSD) gene (*HSD3B7*)[5]. Each of the encoded enzymes catalyses an important step in the biosynthetic pathway; consequently, their loss prevents the synthesis of adequate levels of primary bile acids required for the promotion of bile secretion and intralumenal fat absorption. Deficiencies in bile acid transport also cause neonatal cholestasis, and these have been traced to mutations in three genes, i.e. *FIC1*, *ABCB11*, and *ABCB4*[6].

Although neonatal cholestasis is genetically heterogeneous, the manifestations of loss of either a biosynthetic enzyme or a transport protein are similar. Affected individuals present at birth or in early childhood with cholestatic jaundice, fat-soluble vitamin deficiency, and acholic or fatty stools (steatorrhoea). Serum transaminases are usually elevated, and a conjugated hyperbilirubinaemia is often present. Liver biopsies may reveal non-specific changes, but giant cell transformation of hepatocytes, inflammation, fibrosis, and canalicular and hepatocyte cholestasis are usual[7]. Chemical analysis of body fluids reveals an accumulation of atypical bile acids and sterol intermediates. Bile acid biosynthetic defects, in particular C_{27} 3β-HSD deficiency, may also cause late-onset chronic cholestasis, and in these individuals the clinical history generally reveals a pattern of mildly elevated transaminases in infancy that often resolves only to re-emerge later, and an early onset of vitamin D-deficient rickets[8].

Despite a shared clinical presentation the various genetic forms of neonatal cholestasis require different treatments. Loss of either the C_{27} 3β-HSD or the 3-oxo-Δ^4-steroid 5β-reductase enzyme is treated by oral administration of bile acids[9]. In contrast, loss of the oxysterol 7α-hydroxylase enzyme[2], or of the various bile acid transporters[10], requires liver transplantation. The marked differences in the treatment regimens for the various forms of inherited neonatal cholestasis underscore the importance of defining the molecular basis of the disease in individual patients.

The study of neonatal cholestasis would be facilitated by the availability of an animal model in which the symptoms of the disease are faithfully reproduced. To this end mice deficient in the CYP7B1 oxysterol 7-hydroxylase gene were produced and their phenotype characterized[11]. Although these animals exhibited some of the expected features arising from a deficiency of this bile acid biosynthetic enzyme, they failed to develop liver disease, presumably due to the presence of other enzymes that compensated for the loss of CYP7B1. An examination of the bile acid pathway suggested that a better target for the generation of a mouse model of cholestasis might be the C_{27} 3β-HSD enzyme. This membrane-bound enzyme acts on all intermediates in the bile acid biosynthetic pathway (Figure 1), and is thought to be the only enzyme that catalyses these essential reactions.

RESULTS

Mice lacking the C_{27} 3β-HSD gene were produced by homologous recombination in embryonic stem cells. The targeting vector was designed to remove exons 1–6 of the *Hsd3b7* gene. Electroporation of the linearized targeting vector into the AB-1 line of 129S6/SvEv embryonic stem cells, followed by selection and screening, identified 132 independent clones out of 384 with the desired homologous recombination event. Injection of four of these clones into C57Bl/6J blastocysts produced 24 chimeric males that had contributions from the embryonic stem cells ranging from 50% to 80% based on the amount of *agouti* colour in the animal's fur. Of these mice, six transmitted the disrupted gene through the germline. The mutant allele was inherited in Mendelian fashion and expected numbers of wild-type, heterozygous, and homozygous offspring were born. Equal numbers of male and female pups were obtained in crosses between heterozygous carriers of the mutant C_{27} 3β-HSD gene. Fertility and fecundity were normal in mice heterozygous and homozygous for the introduced mutation.

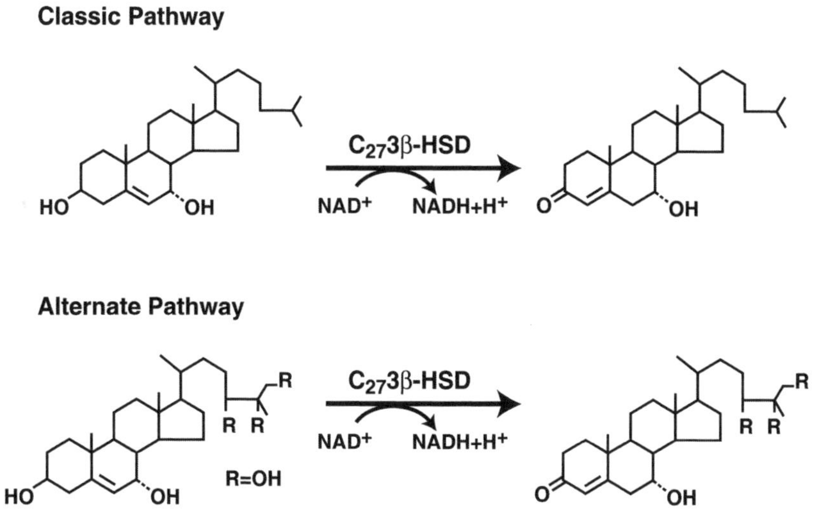

Classic Pathway

Alternate Pathway

Figure 1 Reactions catalysed by the C_{27} 3β-HSD enzyme in bile acid biosynthesis

The effect of the mutation on the expression of the C_{27} 3β-HSD was determined by real-time PCR measurement of RNA and immunoblotting of protein. A high level of C_{27} 3β-HSD mRNA was detected in the liver of wild-type mice, and the level of this mRNA was reduced by half in heterozygous mice and to undetectable levels in homozygous mice. The C_{27} 3β-HSD protein migrated with an apparent molecular weight of $\sim 40\,000$. The amount of this protein was reduced by half in mice heterozygous for the disrupted gene and was undetectable in animals homozygous for the mutant allele. Together, these data indicated that the introduced mutation eliminated expression of the C_{27} 3β-HSD mRNA and protein.

Mice lacking C_{27} 3β-HSD were outwardly normal at birth but a majority died within the first 18 days of postnatal life. Death occurred in two waves, with $\sim 45\%$ of the homozygous animals dying in the first 4 days of life and another 45% dying between days 8 and 18. Only a few animals survived beyond weaning (postnatal day 21). Dietary supplementation with cholic acid during gestation (from day 12 of pregnancy onwards) and suckling stages prevented the death of most ($>90\%$) but not all homozygous animals.

Immunohistochemical analysis of adult liver from the few surviving homozygous mice maintained on normal chow revealed little evidence of cholestasis. Lymphocyte infiltration was not significantly different from that of wild-type controls and marked fibrosis was not present.

Analysis of bile acids by mass spectrometry revealed an altered composition of bile, including the presence of atypical bile acids. Levels of cholic acid were reduced and, in agreement with this observation, expression of CYP7A1 cholesterol 7α-hydroxylase mRNA and protein were elevated. The altered composition of the bile acid pool led to a reduction in cholesterol absorption by the small intestine and a compensatory increase in hepatic cholesterol synthesis.

DISCUSSION

The analysis of mice deficient in C_{27} 3β-HSD reveals expected and unexpected phenotypes. The loss of this enzyme was predicted to disrupt bile acid synthesis and, along this line, the normal complement of bile acids was not made in the knockout mice. In human subjects who inherit mutations in the *HSD3B7* gene, two intermediates in the bile acid pathway accumulate in the urine and plasma, 3β,7α-dihydroxy-5-cholenoic acid and 3β,7α,12α-trihydroxy-5-cholenoic acid[12]; however, these C_{27} steroids did not accumulate in the mouse. This unexpected finding suggests that mice may utilize alternative pathways of bile acid synthesis to ensure that these otherwise hepatotoxic intermediates do not build up when the C_{27} 3β-HSD enzyme is impaired.

A majority of the mutant mice die in the first 3 weeks of postnatal life for as-yet-undetermined reasons. The temporal pattern of death and the ability of oral bile acids to prevent it are outcomes similar to those observed in mice lacking CYP7A1 cholesterol 7α-hydroxylase[13], and in which death is attributed to the accumulation of monohydroxy bile acids and associated cholestasis[14]. It remains to be determined which if any of the atypical bile acids observed in the C_{27} 3β-HSD deficient animals causes death.

SUMMARY

The loss of the C_{27} 3β-HSD enzyme in humans causes neonatal cholestasis, and a preliminary characterization of mice with an induced mutation in the encoding gene suggests that similar symptoms are present in this species. Experiments to determine the mechanism causing death, the ability of dietary cholic acid to rescue the mutant animals, and the changes that occur in hepatic gene expression in the presence and absence of bile acids are ongoing.

Acknowledgements

We thank Daphne L. Head and Pinky Jha for excellent technical assistance, Drs Wenling Chen and Steven Turley for helpful advice, and the National Institutes of Health and the Robert A. Welch Foundation for research support (grants HL20948 and I-0971, respectively).

References

1. Russell DW. The enzymes, regulation, and genetics of bile acid synthesis. Annu Rev Biochem. 2003;72:137–74.
2. Setchell KDR, Schwarz M, O'Connell NC et al. Identification of a new inborn error in bile acid synthesis: mutation of the oxysterol 7α-hydroxylase gene causes severe neonatal liver disease. J Clin Invest. 1998;102:1690–703.

3. Setchell KD, Suchy FJ, Welsh MB, Zimmer-Nechemias L, Heubi J, Balistreri WF. Δ^4-3-Oxosteroid 5β-reductase deficiency described in identical twins with neonatal hepatitis. A new inborn error in bile acid synthesis. J Clin Invest. 1988;82:2148–57.

4. Setchell KDR, Heubi JE, Bove KE et al. Liver disease caused by failure to racemize trihydroxycholestanoic acid: gene mutation and effect of bile acid therapy. Gastroenterology. 2003;124:217–32.

5. Schwarz M, Wright AC, Davis DL, Nazer H, Bjorkhem I, Russell DW. Expression cloning of 3β-hydroxy-Δ^5-C_{27}-steroid oxidoreductase gene of bile acid synthesis and its mutation in progressive intrahepatic cholestasis. J Clin Invest. 2000;106:1175–84.

6. Kullak-Ublick GA, Stieger B, Meier PJ. Enterohepatic bile salt transporters in normal physiology and liver disease. Gastroenterology. 2004;126:322–42.

7. Bove K, Daugherty CC, Tyson W, Heubi JE, Balistreri WF, Setchell KDR. Bile acid synthetic defects and liver disease. Pediatr Dev Pathol. 2000;3:1–16.

8. Setchell KDR, O'Connell NC. Disorders of bile acid synthesis and metabolism: a metabolic basis for liver disease. In: Suchy FJ, Sokol RJ, Balistreri WF, editors. Liver Disease in Children. Philadelphia: Lippincott Williams & Wilkins; 2001:701–34.

9. Daugherty CC, Setchell KDR, Heubi JE, Balistreri WF. Resolution of liver biopsy alterations in three siblings with bile acid treatment of an inborn error of bile acid metabolism (Δ^4-3-oxosteroid 5β-reductase deficiency). Hepatology. 1993;18:1096–101.

10. Trauner M, Meier PJM, Boyer JL. Molecular pathogenesis of cholestasis. N Engl J Med. 1998;339:1217–27.

11. Li-Hawkins J, Lund EG, Turley SD, Russell DW. Disruption of the oxysterol 7α-hydroxylase gene in mice. J Biol Chem. 2000;275:16536–42.

12. Clayton PT, Leonard JV, Lawson AM et al. Familial giant cell hepatitis associated with synthesis of 3α,7α-dihydroxy- and 3β,7α,12α-trihydroxy-5-cholenoic acids. J Clin Invest. 1987;79:1031–8.

13. Ishibashi S, Schwarz M, Frykman PK, Herz J, Russell DW. Disruption of cholesterol 7α-hydroxylase gene in mice. J Biol Chem. 1996;271:18017–23.

14. Arnon R, Yoshimura T, Reiss A, Budai K, Lefkowitch JH, Javitt NB. Cholesterol 7α-hydroxylase knockout mouse: a model for monohydroxy bile acid-related cholestasis. Gastroenterology. 1998;115:1223–8.

2
Role of oxysterols and cholestenoic acids in a crosstalk between the brain and the liver

I. BJÖRKHEM, S. MEANEY, M. HEVERIN, U. ANDERSSON, M. AXELSSON, U. PANZENBOECK and W. SATTLER

Almost all cholesterol in the brain is a product of local synthesis with the blood–brain barrier efficiently protecting from exchange with lipoprotein cholesterol in the circulation. Although the blood–brain barrier appears to be completely impermeable to cholesterol it allows passage of some side-chain oxidized metabolites of cholesterol, metabolites that are also precursors to bile acids. We and others have shown that about two-thirds of the *de-novo* synthesis of cholesterol in the brain of experimental animals is balanced by excretion of 24S-hydroxycholesterol, an oxysterol generated by a brain-specific species of cytochrome P450 (for a review see ref. 1). In contrast to cholesterol, 24S-hydroxycholesterol is able to traverse the blood–brain barrier. The fact that the 24S-hydroxylase mechanism does not balance all cholesterol synthesis is consistent with presence of at least one additional pathway for elimination of cholesterol from the brain.

Recently we showed that another side-chain oxidized oxysterol, 27-hydroxycholesterol, is taken up by the brain from the circulation[2]. In cultured neurogenic cells of human origin this oxysterol was found to be metabolized into a C27 steroid acid, 7α-hydroxy-3-oxo-4-cholestenoic acid[3]. In catheterization experiments on healthy volunteers, measurement of the concentration of the acid in the internal jugular vein and an artery revealed a significant net excretion of 7α-hydroxy-3-oxo-4-cholestenoic acid from the brain. In an *in-vitro* model for the blood–brain barrier, utilizing cultured porcine brain endothelial cells, there was an efficient transfer of 7α-hydroxy-3-oxo-4-cholestenoic acid. The cytochrome P450 species CYP7B1, appeared to catalyse the rate-limiting step in the overall conversion of 27-hydroxycholesterol into 7α-hydroxy-3-oxo-4-cholestenoic acid.

Figure 1 summarizes the different fluxes of oxysterols over the blood–brain barrier. The flux of 24S-hydroxycholesterol from the human brain to the circulation is the most prominent transport[1], corresponding to about

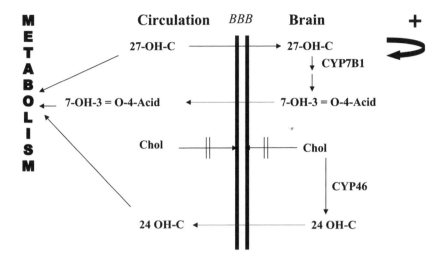

Figure 1 Crosstalk of steroids between the brain and the liver

6 mg/24 h. According to our catheterization experiments in healthy volunteers[2] the flux of 27-hydroxycholesterol from the circulation into the brain corresponds to about 5 mg/24 h. The flux of 7α-hydroxy-3-oxo-4-cholestenoic acid from the brain into the circulation[3] corresponds to about 2 mg/24 h.

It is notable that the latter acid is taken up very efficiently by the liver, with an apparent extraction of about 40% in a single pass[4]. It is evident thar 7α-hydroxy-3-oxo-4-cholestenoic acid is a steroid that is well adapted to fulfil a role as a transport form of a steroid from the brain to the liver.

The critical enzyme in the metabolism of 27-hydroxycholesterol in the brain seems to be the oxysterol 7α-hydroxylase (CYPB1). In our experiments this enzyme was found in cells of neurogenic origin only. According to results of preliminary experiments there is a significant positive correlation between the levels of CYP7B1 as measured by Western blotting and levels of 27-hydroxycholesterol in the human brain, suggesting a regulatory effect of 27-hydroxycholesterol on CYP7B1 (Figure 1). The regulatory mechanism behind this remains to be established, however, and attempts to demonstrate an effect of 27-hydroxycholesterol on the transcription rate of the CYP7B1 gene have failed thus far.

Our studies identify a novel metabolic circuit over the blood–brain barrier in which the oxysterol 27-hydroxycholesterol is a link between the extracerebral and intracerebral pools of cholesterol. It should be noted that there is a good correlation between the levels of cholesterol and 27-hydroxycholesterol in the circulation, and thus it is likely that hypercholesterolaemia is associated with an increased flux of cholesterol into the brain.

In view of the marked effects of 27-hydroxycholesterol on critical enzymes in cholesterol homeostasis, the mechanism may be regarded as a detoxification. Since 27-hydroxycholesterol may be formed from cholesterol in the brain, the mechanism may also be an alternative pathway for elimination. The absence of this cholesterol-removing mechanism in patients with cerebrotendinous xanthomatosis, lacking the sterol 27-hydroxylase, may be part of the explanation for the development of brain xanthomas in this disease.

In view of the effects of side-chain oxidized oxysterols on the generation of amyloid[5], we have suggested that the flux of 27-hydroxycholesterol may be the missing link between hypercholesterolaemia and Alzheimer's disease[6].

References

1. Björkhem I, Meaney S. Brain cholesterol: long secret life behind a barrier. Arterioscler Thromb Vasc Biol. 2004;24:806–15.
2. Heverin M, Meaney S, Lutjohann D, Diczfalusy U, Wahren J, Björkhem I. Crossing the barrier: net flux of 27-hydroxycholesterol into the human brain. J Lipid Res. 2005;46:1047–52.
3. Meaney S, Heverin M, Panzenboeck U et al. A novel route for the elimination of brain oxysterols: elimination of 27-hydroxycholesterol via conversion to 7alpha-hydroxy-3-oxo-4-cholestenoic acid. J Lipid Res. 2007 [Epub ahead of print].
4. Lund E, Andersson O, Zhang J et al. Importance of a novel oxidative mechanism for elimination of intracellular cholesterol in humans. Arterioscler Thromb Vasc Biol. 1996;16: 208–12.
5. Brown J, Theisler C, Silberman S et al. Differential expression of cholesterol hydroxylases in Alzheimer's disease. J Biol Chem. 2004;279:34674–81.
6. Björkhem I, Heverin M, Leoni V, Meaney S, Diczfalusy U. Oxysterols and Alzheimer's disease. Acta Neurol Scand Suppl. 2006;185:43–9.

3
Activation of a G-protein coupled receptor by conjugated bile acids in primary hepatocytes and liver: effects on glucose metabolism

P. B. HYLEMON, Y. FANG, E. STUDER, W. M. PANDAK and
P. DENT

INTRODUCTION

Bile acids are synthesized in the liver from cholesterol, conjugated to either glycine or taurine, actively secreted into bile and stored in the gallbladder. Following a meal, the gallbladder is stimulated to contract, releasing its contents into the small intestine. Bile acids, acting as detergent molecules, play an important role in the solubilization and absorption of cholesterol, fats and fat-soluble vitamins. Bile acids are efficiently (>95%) recovered from the intestine by a sodium-dependent active transporter expressed in epithelial cells in the ileum[1]. Bile acids are returned to the liver via the portal blood where they are actively transported back into the liver hepatocytes and again secreted. This process is termed enterohepatic circulation.

In the past few years it has become clear that bile acids also function as regulatory molecules helping to coordinately regulate various metabolic pathways in the liver[2,3]. Bile acids act as regulatory molecules through their ability to activate specific nuclear receptors (FXR, PXR, vitamin D) and different cell signalling pathways (ERK1/2, JNK1/2, AKT, PKC). The farnesoid X receptor (FXR) has emerged as a key regulator of multiple metabolic pathways in the liver. Its activation by bile acids allows for the regulation of bile acid synthesis and transport as well as lipid and glucose metabolism[4]. In this regard, FXR null mice develop fatty liver and have elevated serum levels of cholesterol, triglycerides, and glucose[4]. Bile acids, through their activation of FXR, have been reported to be involved in regulating glucose homeostasis in the liver by down-regulating genes encoding enzymes involved in gluconeogenesis[5,6].

Bile acids regulate their own synthesis as well as glucose and lipid metabolism in the liver by activating different cell signalling pathways.

Activation of the JNK1/2 pathway by either bile acids or specific cytokines down-regulates the genes encoding key enzymes in the bile acid biosynthetic pathway[7–10]. Bile acids also activate the ERK1/2 and AKT cell signalling pathways in hepatocytes[11]. Activation of the ERK1/2 and AKT pathways goes through the epidermal growth factor receptor (ERBB1) in primary rodent hepatocytes[12] (Figure 1). Bile acids have been reported to enhance the activity of the insulin receptor and activate glycogen synthase activity in primary hepatocytes[13]; however, the mechanisms of activation of these signalling pathways by bile acids have not been elucidated. Activation of the AKT pathway by conjugated bile acids has been reported to be via a pertussis toxin-sensitive mechanism in primary rodent and human hepatocytes[11]. These data strongly indicated that conjugated bile acids are activating the AKT signalling pathway through a Gαi protein-coupled receptor (GPCR) mechanism. In this chapter we report evidence for the activation of a conjugated bile acid Gi protein-coupled receptor in primary hepatocytes and in the chronic bile fistula rat. Activation of this receptor causes activation of the insulin signalling pathway (AKT) and glycogen synthase activity in each model system (Figure 1).

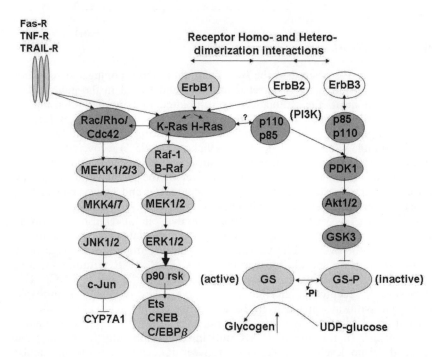

Figure 1 Cell signalling pathways in hepatocytes activated by bile acids. Pathways include the JNK1/2, ERK1/2 and AKT. Glycogen synthase (GS) activity is regulated by glycogen synthase kinase 3β (GSK3)

MATERIALS AND METHODS

Primary hepatocyte cultures

Primary adult rat hepatocyte monolayer cultures were prepared using the collagenase-perfusion technique described by Bissel and Guzelian[14]. Primary hepatocytes were plated on collagen-coated plates in serum-free Williams E medium containing insulin, L-thyroxine, and dexamethasone as described[13]. In some experiments the cells were plated in the absence of insulin. In other experiments the cells were pretreated with either vehicle or pertussis toxin (PTX) (300 ng/ml) 16 h before bile acid exposure. In other experiments the hepatocytes were treated with either PP2 (Src kinase inhibitor) (10 μM) or AG1478 (EGFR inhibitor) (1 μM) 30 min prior to bile acid exposure.

Western blot analysis of AKT

The phosphorylation state of AKT, following the addition of bile acids to primary hepatocytes, was determined as previously described[11]. In brief, hepatocytes were lysed in whole cell lysis buffer (0.5 M Tris-HCl, pH 6.8, 2% SDS, 10% glycerol, 1% 2-mercaptoethanol, 0.02% bromophenol blue) and samples boiled for 30 min. The denatured samples were loaded onto 10% SDS-polyacrylamide gels and electrophoresis was run overnight. Size-separated proteins were electrophoretically transferred onto nitrocellulose paper and immunoblotted with primary antibodies against ATK. All immunoblots were visualized by way of enhanced chemiluminescence. Immunoblots were quantitated by digital scanning as described previously[11].

Glycogen synthase (GS) activity assays in primary hepatocytes and chronic bile fistula rats

Male Sprague-Dawley rats weighing 280–350 g were housed under controlled lighting conditions on a natural light–dark cycle (0600–1800 light phase). Groups of age- and weight-matched animals were used in all experiments. Under brief methoxyflurane anaesthesia, biliary fistulas and intraduodenal cannulas were inserted as previously described[15]. To inhibit the putative conjugated bile acid-activated G protein-coupled receptor, Gαi dominant negative plasmid (100 μg), in 0.1 ml water, was injected directly into the rat liver at three or four lobes using a 26-gauge needle. Negative control rats were injected with 100 μg PCDNA3.1 plasmid. All animals received continuous intraduodenal infusion of glucose-salts solution throughout the experiment. Forty-eight hours after Gαi dominant negative plasmid injections, taurocholate (TCA) was added to the intraduodenal infusate at a rate of 36 μmol per 100 g of rat per hour for 1.5 h. Rats were anaesthetized and killed humanely by exsanguination. Livers were removed from treated and control rats and frozen immediately. For analysis, livers were homogenized with lysis buffer (50 mM Tris-HCl pH 7.8, 10 mM EDTA, 100 mM NaCl, 50 mM NaF, 1 μM Microcystin-LR, 1% (v/v) NP40, 1 mM PMSF, 40 μg/ml TPCK, 40 μg/ml TLCK) and centrifuged at 10 000 rpm. Fifty microlitres of the supernatant fluid

(100–200 µg of protein) were added to an equal volume of GS assay buffer (50 mM Tris/HCl pH 7.8, 10 mM EDTA, 50 mM NaF, 1 µM Microcystin-LR containing UDP-[^{14}C] glucose (0.5 µCi/mmol) and 15 mg/ml glycogen and 10 mM G-6-P. After 15 min incubation at 37°C, tubes were then chilled for 15 min on ice, after which the entire tube contents were spotted onto Whatman GF/A 2.4-cm filter papers (Maidstone, Kent, UK). Spotted filter papers were immediately immersed in 25 ml of 70% (v/v) ethanol (4°C), and washed twice for 30 min each time. Filter papers were air-dried; radioactivity incorporated into glycogen was determined by liquid scintillation spectrometry.

Primary hepatocytes were transfected with either control adenovirus protein or adenovirus protein to express dominant negative Gi plasmid for 24 h. After TCA treatment cells were washed with cold phosphate buffered saline (PBS) and scraped into lysis buffer. Glycogen synthase activity was assayed as described above.

RESULTS AND DISCUSSION

Both conjugated and free bile acids are capable of activating ERK1/2 and AKT pathways in primary rat hepatocytes in a concentration-dependent manner (Figure 2). At a concentration of 10 µM, taurocholate and deoxycholate were the best activators of the AKT pathway. The activation of AKT by conjugated bile acids in these cells appears to saturate around 50 µM. In contrast, the activation of AKT by deoxycholate shows a linear increase in AKT activation (Figure 2). Different activation kinetics may indicate differences in the mechanism of activation of these pathways by conjugated and unconjugated bile acids.

Experiments were next carried out to determine the possible mechanisms of activation of the ERK1/2 and AKT pathways by conjugated and unconjugated bile acids. Primary rat hepatocytes were pretreated with pertussis toxin 16 h prior to bile acid addition. Once pertussis toxin enters mammalian cells it specifically catalyses an ADP-ribosylation of the Gαi subunit of G proteins which then inhibits cell signalling from Gi protein-coupled receptors. Both conjugated bile acids and deoxycholate (all at 50 µM) activated the ERK1/2 and AKT pathways (Figure 3); however, only conjugated bile acid activation of these pathways was sensitive to PTX. These results suggest that conjugated bile acids may activate these pathways via a Gαi protein-coupled receptor[11]. In other experiments the hepatocytes were treated with either PP2 or AG1478 at 30 min before bile acid addition. The results show that the activation of both ERK1/2 and AKT by either conjugated bile acids or deoxycholate was inhibited by these compounds (Figure 3). These results indicate a possible role for Src kinase and the epidermal growth factor receptor (ErbB1) in activating these signalling pathways by bile acids.

Next, experiments were performed to determine if activation of the AKT pathway by different bile acids resulted in the activation of glycogen synthase activity in primary hepatocytes and if expression of a gene encoding a dominant negative Gαi protein would inhibit this activation. Hepatocytes were infected with poly-L-lysine conjugated adenoviruses to express either a

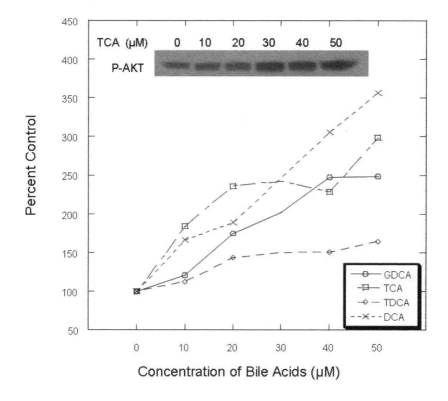

Figure 2 Effect of bile acid concentration on the activation of AKT in primary rat hepatocytes. Individual bile acids were added to primary hepatocytes, cells harvested 30 min after treatment, cell extracts prepared, proteins separated by SDS-PAGE, and immunoblotted. Abbreviations: TCA, taurocholate; GDCA, glycodeoxycholate; TDCA, taurodeoxycholate: DCA, deoxycholate

control plasmid or a plasmid encoding a dominant negative Gαi. The results indicate that either deoxycholate or taurocholate increased glycogen synthase activity. However, only TCA activation of glycogen synthase activity was sensitive to inhibition to by the dominant negative Gαi (Figure 4).

In additional experiments using the chronic bile fistula rat model, it was observed that the intraduodenal infusion of taurocholate (36 μmol/100 g rat per hour) resulted in a marked activation of AKT, glycogen synthase kinase 3 (GSK3) and glycogen synthase activity within 1 h. This activation was strongly inhibited by the expression of a dominant negative Gαi protein (data not shown).

The current data add another piece to the puzzle of how bile acids may function as regulatory molecules in the liver. It appears that bile acids help regulate lipid, glucose and cholesterol metabolism in the liver by their ability to activate specific nuclear receptors (i.e. FXR) and cell signalling pathways (i.e. JNK1/2 and AKT) (Figure 5). Bile acids regulate their own synthesis by

15

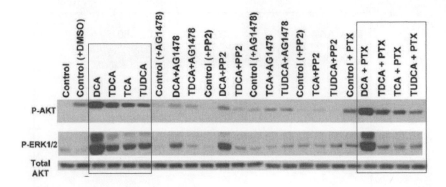

Figure 3 Conjugated bile acids activate the ERK1/2 and AKT signalling pathways via a pertussis toxin (PTX)-sensitive mechanism that also requires Src and the epidermal growth factor receptor (EGFR). Primary hepatocytes were pretreated 16 h with PTX or vehicle control before bile acid addition. In other experiments, cells were pretreated 30 min with PP2 (Src inhibitor) or AG1478 (EGFR) inhibitor as described in Methods. Cells were isolated 20 min after bile acid treatment, lysed, proteins separated on SDS-PAGE and immunoblotted for phosphorylation of ERK and AKT

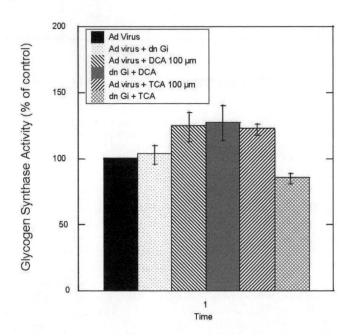

Figure 4 Effect of dominant negative Gαi expression on glycogen synthase (GS) activity by bile acids. Primary rat hepatocytes were isolated as described in Methods and cultured in the absence of insulin. Cells were treated (24 h) with a recombinant plasmid encoding the gene for dominant negative Gαi. Hepatocytes were then treated for 30 min with either deoxycholate (DCA) or taurocholate (TCA), cell extracts prepared and the activity of GS determined as described in Methods

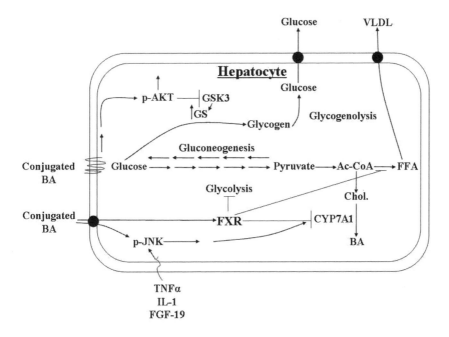

Figure 5 Regulation of hepatic glucose, lipid and bile acid metabolism by bile acids. Bile acids (BA) appear to function as regulatory molecules in the liver by activation of specific nuclear receptors (FXR) and cell signalling pathways (JNK and AKT). Activation of JNK and FXR by either conjugated or free bile acids results in the down-regulation of cholesterol 7α-hydroxylase (CYP7A1), the rate-limiting enzyme in bile acid synthesis. Activation of FXR also down-regulates glycolysis, and decreases the synthesis of free fatty acids (FFA) and triglycerides. Conjugated bile acids can activate glycogen synthase (GS) activity via Gαi protein-coupled receptor

inhibiting the gene encoding cholesterol 7α-hydroxylase (CYP7A1). In this regard, bile acids, via activation of FXR, induce the gene encoding the small heterodimeric partner (SHP) which can interact with positive-acting transcription factors (i.e. LRH-1) down-regulating the gene encoding CYP7A1[16,17]. In addition, bile acids can directly activate the JNK1/2 signalling pathway by stimulating ceramide synthesis in hepatocytes[8]. Alternatively, bile acids can induce intestinal cells and macrophages to produce specific cytokines (i.e. TNF-α, IL-1, FGF-19)[7,9,10]. These cytokines activate the JNK1/2 pathway in hepatocytes via specific membrane receptors, resulting in the down-regulation of the gene encoding CYP7A1.

Bile acids have also been reported to regulate glucose and lipid metabolism in the liver. The gene encoding FXR has been reported to be induced by glucose and repressed by insulin[18]. Moreover, FXR[−/−] mice have increased serum levels of free fatty acids (FFA), and glucose and display insulin resistance[4]. Moreover, it has been reported that the genes encoding PEP carboxykinase (PEPCK) and glucose-6-phosphatase (G-6-Pase) are down-regulated in a FXR-

SHP-dependent manner in HepG2 cells[5]. However, others have reported induction of the genes encoding these key enzymes in gluconeogenesis in primary hepatocytes[19]. The current study shows that conjugated bile acids can regulate glycogen synthesis activity via a $G\alpha i$ linked G protein-coupled receptor. Bile acids also appear to down-regulate the rates of fatty acid and VLDL biosynthesis in the liver. This may be through their ability to decrease SREBP-1 expression, which is a major transcription factor up-regulating genes involved in fatty acid synthesis[2]. In conclusion, bile acids appear to use multiple molecular mechanisms to control major pathways of metabolism in the liver.

Acknowledgements

This work was supported by National Institutes of Health Grants P01-DK38030 and DK-52825.

References

1. Dawson PA, Shneider BL, Hofmann AF. Bile formation and the enterohepatic circulation. In: Johnson, LR, Barrett, KE, Ghishan FK, Merchant JL, Said HM, Wood JD, editors. Physiology of the Gastroenterology Tract, Vol. 2, 4th edn, London: Academic Press, 2006: 1437–62.
2. Duran-Sandoval D, Cariou B, Fruchart J-C, Stael B. Potential regulatory role of the farnesoid X receptor in the metabolic syndrome. Biochimie. 2005;87:93–8.
3. Claudel T, Staels B, Kuipers F. The farnesoid X receptor – a molecular link between bile acid and lipid and glucose metabolism. Arterioscler Thromb Vasc Biol. 2005;25:2020–30.
4. Ma K, Saha PK, Chan L, Moore DD. Farnesoid X receptor is essential for normal glucose homeostasis. J Clin Invest. 2006;116:1102–9.
5. Fabian ED, Mitro N, Gilardi F, Caruso D, Galli G, Crestani M. Coordinated control of cholesterol catabolism to bile acids and of gluconeogenesis via a novel mechanism of transcription regulation linked to the fasted-to-fed cycle. J Biol Chem. 2003;278:39124–32.
6. Yamagata K, Daitoku H, Shimamoto Y et al. Bile acids regulate gluconeogenic gene expression via small heterodimeric partner-mediated repression of hepatocyte nuclear factor 4 and Foxo1. J Biol Chem. 2004;279:23158–65.
7. Gupta S, Stravitz RT, Dent P, Hylemon PB. Down-regulation of cholesterol 7α-hydroxylase (CYP7A1) gene expression by bile acids in primary rat hepatocytes is mediated by the c-Jun-N-terminal kinase pathway. J Biol Chem. 2001;276:15816–22.
8. Gupta S, Natarajan R, Payne SG et al. Deoxycholic acid activates the c-jun-N-terminal kinase (JNK) pathway via FAS receptor activation in primary hepatocytes: role of acidic sphingomyelinase-mediated ceramide generation in FAS receptor activation J Biol Chem. 2004;279:5821–8.
9. Holt JA, Luo G, Billin AN et al. Definition of a novel growth factor-dependent signal cascade for the suppression of bile acid biosynthesis. Genes Dev. 2003;17:1581–91.
10. Inagaki T, Choi M, Moschetta A et al. Fibroblast growth factory 15 functions as an enterohepatic signal to regulate bile acid homeostasis. Cell Metab. 2005;2:217–25.
11. Dent P, Fang Y, Gupta S et al. Conjugated bile acids promote ERK1/2 and AKT activation via a pertussis toxin-sensitive mechanism in murine and human hepatocytes. Hepatology. 2005;42:1291–9.
12. Rao YP, Studer EJ, Stravitz RT et al. Activation of the Raf-1/MEK/ERK cascade by bile acids occurs via the epidermal growth factor receptor in primary rat hepatocytes. Hepatology. 2002;35:307–14.
13. Han SI, Studer E, Gupta S et al. Bile acids enhance the activity of the insulin receptor and glycogen synthase in primary rodent hepatocytes. Hepatology. 2004;39:456–63.
14. Bissell DM, Guzelian PS. Phenotypic stability of adult rat hepatocytes in primary monolayer culture. Ann NY Acad Sci. 1980;349:85–98

15. Pandak WM, Li YC, Chiang JY et al. Regulation of cholesterol 7α-hydroxylase mRNA and transcriptional activity by taurocholate and cholesterol in the chronic biliary diverted rat. J Biol Chem. 1991;266:3416–21.
16. Goodwin B, Jones SA, Price RR et al. A regulatory cascade of the nuclear receptors FXR, SHP-1, and LRH-1 represses bile acid biosynthesis. Mol Cell. 2000;6:517–26.
17. Lee YK, Dell H, Dowhan DH, Hadzopoulou-Cladaras M, Moore DD. The orphan nuclear receptor SHP inhibits hepatocyte nuclear factor 4 and retinoid X receptor transactivation: two mechanisms for repression. Mol Cell Biol. 2000;20:187–95.
18. Duran-Sandoval D, Mautino G, Martin G et al. Glucose regulates the expression of the farnesoid X receptor in liver. Diabetes. 2004;53:890–8.
19. Stayrook KR, Bramlett KS, Savkur RS et al. Regulation of carbohydrate metabolism by the farnesoid X receptor. Endocrinology. 2005:146:984–91.

4
Discovery of a novel oxysterol, 5-cholesten-3β, 25-diol 3-sulphate, in nuclei and mitochondria following over-expression of the gene encoding StarD1

S. REN, P. B. HYLEMON, X. LI, D. RODRIGUEZ-AGUDO, H. ZHOU, S. ERICKSON, G. GIL and W. M. PANDAK

INTRODUCTION

The metabolism of cholesterol to primary bile acids occurs via two main pathways in hepatocytes[1]. The 'neutral' pathway is considered to be the major pathway in most species[2]. The highly regulated microsomal enzyme, cholesterol 7α-hydroxylase (CYP7A1), is the first and rate-limiting step of this pathway[3]. A possibly equally important alternative pathway, the 'acidic' pathway, is initiated by the mitochondrial enzyme, sterol 27-hydroxylase (CYP27A1). Oxysterol intermediates of the 'acidic' pathway such as 27-hydroxycholesterol have been implicated as regulators of cholesterol homeostasis[4], including expression of many genes encoding enzymes involved in cholesterol biosynthesis and transport[5]. Increased CYP27A1 activity in peripheral tissues may both down-regulate cholesterol synthesis through the SREBP pathway, and enhance the efflux of cholesterol and its elimination via LXR[6]; however, the *in-vivo* ligand is currently unknown[7]. Thus, characterizing endogenous oxysterols and their mechanism of action is critical for a better understanding of sterol homeostasis.

Overexpression of CYP27A1 in hepatocyte culture results in minimal increases (~50%) in the rates of bile acid biosynthesis, as compared to the 7-fold increases seen following overexpression of CYP7A1[8]. A mitochondrial cholesterol delivery protein, steroidogenic acute regulatory protein (StarD1), is present in liver and hepatocytes and its expression is highly regulated[9]. Recently, we found that overexpression of StarD1 dramatically increases cholesterol catabolism to bile acids both in cultured primary hepatocytes and *in vivo*[10,11]. Overexpression of StarD1 *in vivo* increases the rates of bile acid synthesis to the same level as overexpression of CYP7A1, and produced a similar composition of bile acids *in vivo*[11]. Based on these findings, we hypothesized that oxysterols generated in the mitochondria play an important role in the maintenance of intracellular cholesterol homeostasis. In this chapter we present evidence for increased formation of a sulphated oxysterol in primary rat hepatocytes following overexpression of the gene encoding StarD1. The identity of this sterol was confirmed and its mode of synthesis identified. In addition, some of its properties were investigated.

MATERIALS AND METHODS

Cell culture reagents and supplies were purchased from Gibco BRL (Grand Island, NY); [14C]cholesterol and [3H]25-hydroxy cholesterol from New England Nuclear (Boston, MA). [14C]27-hydroxy cholesterol was prepared as previously described[8]. Cyclodextrin was purchased from Cyclodextrin Technologies Development Inc. (Gainsville, FL); normal human liver samples were obtained from Liver Tissue Procurement Distribution System, University of Minnesota. All other reagents were from Sigma Chemical Co (St Louis, MO), unless otherwise indicated.

Adenovirus preparation and propagation

The adenovirus construct used in this study was obtained through the Massey Cancer Center Shared Resource Facility of the Virginia Commonwealth University as previously described[10].

Cyp27A1⁻ knockout mice

Cyp27A1 gene knockout heterozygote breeding pairs from the VAMC, San Francisco colony[4] were used to found the colony at Richmond VAMC. At 3 months of age the male mice were sacrificed in the morning, and livers were immediately collected for preparation of mitochondria as described below.

Culture and subcellular fractionation of primary rat hepatocytes and lipid fractionation

Primary rat hepatocyte cultures, prepared as previously described[10], were plated on 150 mm tissue culture dishes ($\sim 2.5 \times 10^7$ cells) in Williams' E medium containing dexamethasone (0.1 μM). Cells were maintained in the absence of thyroid hormone. Twenty-four hours after plating the culture medium was removed, and 4 ml of fresh medium was added. Cells were then infected with recombinant adenovirus encoding either the StarD1 (Ad-CMV-StarD1) or CYP7A1, cDNA in front of the human cytomegalovirus promoter (CMV) or no cDNA, as a control virus. The viruses were allowed to incubate for 2 h in minimal culture medium with gentle shaking of the plates every 15 min. After 2 h incubation the unbound virus was removed, replaced with 20 ml of fresh media, and 2.5 μCi of [14C]cholesterol was added. After 48 h the cells were harvested and processed for nuclear isolation as described[12], with minor modification. Briefly, cells were disrupted by Dounce homogenization in buffer A (10 mM Hepes-KOH at pH 7.6, 1.5 mM $MgCl_2$, 10 mM KCl, 0.5 mM dithiothreitol, 1 mM sodium EDTA, 1 mM EGTA) and centrifuged at 1000g for 10 min. The nuclear pellet was further fractionated by resuspension in 2.5 ml of a 1:1 mixture of buffer A and buffer B (2.4 M sucrose, 15 mM KCl, 2 mM sodium EDTA, 0.15 mM spermine, 0.15 mM spermidine, 0.5 mM dithiothreitol) and centrifuged at 100 000g for 1 h at 4°C through a 1 ml cushion of 3:7 mixture of buffer A and B. The washed nuclear pellet was resuspended in buffer A containing 0.5% (v/v) Nonidet P-40 and centrifuged at 1000g for 10 min at 4°C. The pellets as purified nuclei were resuspended and digested by 2 mg/ml of DNase I in 50 mM of acetic buffer, pH 5.0, 10 mM $MgCl_2$ at 37°C for 2 h. After centrifugation at 10 000g for 20 min the pellets were further digested by 2 mg/ml of proteinase K in phosphate buffered saline solution (PBS) at 50°C for 16 h and the solution was designed as nuclear protease digests. Total lipids in the nuclear protease digests were extracted by adding 3.3 volumes of chloroform:methanol (1:1) and separated into two phases, methanol/water and chloroform phases as previously described[13]. The counts of [14C]cholesterol/cholesterol derivatives in the methanol/water and chloroform phases were measured by liquid scintillation counting.

Mitochondria were isolated from primary hepatocytes and human liver tissues as described previously[14]. NADP-linked isocitrate dehydrogenase activity was used as a mitochondrial marker. Glucose 6-phosphatase activity, an endoplasmic reticulum marker, was used to monitor the purity of the isolated mitochondrial fractions.

HPLC analysis of cholesterol derivatives

[14C]Cholesterol derivatives in the chloroform phase were analysed by HPLC on an Ultrasphere Silica column (5 μm × 4.6 mm × 25 cm; Backman, USA) using an HP Series 1100 solvent delivery system (Hewlett Packard) at 1.3 ml/min flow rate. The column was equilibrated and run in a solvent system of hexane:isopropanol:glacial acetic acid (965:25:10, v/v/v), as the mobile phase. The effluents were collected every 0.5 min (0.65 ml per fraction) except as indicated. The counts in [14C]cholesterol/cholesterol derivatives were determined by scintillation counting. The column was calibrated with [14C] cholesterol, [3H]25-hydroxycholesterol, and [14C]27-hydroxycholesterol.

Total [14C]cholesterol derivatives found in methanol/water phases were analysed on an Ultrasphere PTH C-18 column (5 μm × 4.6 mm × 25 cm; Backman, USA) at 0.8 ml/min flow rate. The column was equilibrated and run in 20 mM of KH_2PO_4, pH 4.2:acetonitrile:methanol (1:3:6, v/v/v) as the mobile phase. The effluents were monitored at 195 nm and collected every 0.5 min (0.4 ml per fraction) except as indicated. The column was calibrated with tauroursodeoxycholic acid, glycoursodeoxycholic acid, taurocholic acid, glycocholic acid, taurochenodeoxycholic acid, taurodeoxycholic acid, and progesterone as standards.

Sulphatase treatment of the purified nuclear [¹⁴C]cholesterol derivatives

The purified nuclear [14C]cholesterol derivatives were digested with 2 mg/ml of sulphatase (EC 3.1.6.1) (Sigma, St Louis, MO) in 50 mM of acetic buffer, pH 5.0 by incubation at 37°C for 4 h. The products were extracted into chloroform phase from methanol/water phase by adding 3.3 volumes of methanol: chloroform (1:1, v/v) to the reaction mixture. [14C]Cholesterol derivatives in both chloroform and methanol/water phases were then analysed by HPLC as described above.

Mass spectrometry/mass spectrometry (MS/MS) analysis of nuclear cholesterol derivatives

A purified sample in methanol/water (80:20, v/v) was introduced into a MDS Sciex ABI 4000 Triple Quadrapole Mass Spectrometer (MDS Sciex, Toronto, Canada) with a Turbo IonSpray ionization (ESI) source for the analyses. The mass spectrometer was operated in negative ion modes and data were acquired using a full-scan mode as well as the product ion mode for MS/MS. The optimized parameters for Q1 full scan under the negative mode were: CUR:10; GS1: 40; GS2: 40; TEM:400; IS: –4500; DP: –150; EP: –10. The optimized parameters for the product scan of 481 under the negative mode were: CUR:10; GS1:40; GS2: 40; TEM: 400; IS: –4500; CAD: 5; DP: –150; EP: –10; CE: 50; CXP: –15.

Chemical synthesis of 5-cholesten-3β, 25-diol 3-sulphonate

A mixture of 25-hydroxycholesterol (0.1 mmol) and triethylamine-sulphur trioxide complex (0.12 mmol) in a dry toluene was incubated at 60°C for 24 h under nitrogen. The reaction was stopped by cooling at 4°C for 5 min, and the solvent was evaporated under reduced pressure. The residue was purified by flash chromatography to afford the product as a white solid. The yield is 30%. The colourless solid was >90% pure as determined by ESI-MS and 1H-NMR analysis (the data will be published in another article).

Determination of the synthesis of 25-hydroxy- and 27-hydroxycholesterol in hepatocyte mitochondria

The synthesis of 25-hydroxy and 27-hydroxycholesterol was determined as previously described[15]. Briefly, in a total volume of 500 μl containing 40 nmol of cholesterol dissolved in 10 μl of β-CD (45% in water), 500 μg of mitochondria protein, 18 units of proteinase K, 100 mM of sodium phosphate, pH 7.5, 0.2 mM of EDTA, 1 mM of DTT, 5.0 mM of trisodium isocitrate, and 0.2 units of isocitrate dehydrogenase, the reaction was initiated by adding 60 μl of 10 mM β-NADPH, and incubated with shaking at 37°C for 60 min. The reactions were stopped by adding 40 μl of 40% sodium cholate. Blanks were prepared by adding sodium cholate before adding mitochondrial solution. After stopping the reaction, 1.5 μg of testosterone was added to the reaction mixture as an internal standard. The sterol products were incubated with two units of cholesterol oxidase at 37°C for 20 min. The oxidation reaction was terminated by adding 1.5 ml of methanol followed by 0.5 ml of saturated KCl. The sterols were extracted twice using 3 ml of hexane. The hexane phase was collected and evaporated under a stream of nitrogen. The residues were dissolved in mobile phase solvents for HPLC and TLC analysis as previously described[16].

HPLC and TLC analysis of the 25-hydroxy- and 27-hydroxycholesterol

The sterol products synthesized by CYP27A1 were analysed by HPLC on an Ultrasphere Silica column (5 μm × 4.6 mm × 25 cm; Backman, USA) using an HP Series 1100 solvent delivery system (Hewlett Packard) at 1.3 ml/min flow rate. The chromatograph was run in a solvent system of hexane:isopropanol: glacial acetic acid (965: 25: 10, v/v/v), as the mobile phase. The elution profiles were monitored at 240 nm. The column was calibrated with cholesterol, testosterone, 25-hydroxycholesterol, and 27-hydroxycholesterol as previously described[16]. The individual ^{14}C-oxysterols were identified by TLC in a solvent system of ethyl acetate/toluene (2:3, v/v) and visualized with a PhosphorImager.

Detection of the synthesis of the 25-hydroxycholesterol 3β-sulphate in hepatocytes

Cell lysates were prepared from human liver tissues or primary rat hepatocytes. Following incubation of the lysates (250 μg protein) with [3H]25-hydroxycholesterol (12 μM)-cyclodextrin, 5 mM MgCl$_2$, 4% (v/v) ethanol, and 100 μM of 3'-phosphoadenosyl 5'-phosphosulphate (PAPS) in 100 μM tris buffer at 37°C for 1 h. The total lipids were extracted with 10 volumes of ethanol. The extracts were dried under the stream of nitrogen and the pellets were dissolved in the mobile phase (water:acetyl nitrile:methanol; 45:5:50, v/v/v). The products of [3H]25-hydroxycholesterol derivatives were analysed by HPLC using a silica gel column with a gradient elution system. An initial double-solvent system of A (45%, methanol with 5% (v:v) of acetonitrile) and B (55%, water with 5% (v:v) of acetonitrile) was used, with an initial flow rate of 0.5 ml/min. During a 25 min period the flow rate and the ratio of A:B changed linearly to 1.5 ml/min and 0:100, respectively, followed by an additional isocratic period of 15 min, for a total duration of 40 min. Five hundred microlitres/fraction were collected. The eluted fractions were analysed for radioactivity by liquid scintillation counting.

RT-PCR and real-time RT-PCR analysis

Total RNA was purified from human liver, primary human hepatocytes, HepG2 cells, rat liver, primary rat hepatocytes and rat testis tissue using a SV Total RNA Isolation Kit (Promega). Two micrograms of total RNA was used for first-strand cDNA synthesis as the manufacturer recommended (Invitrogen). The sequences of primers were used for determination of SULT expression as previously described[17]. The target genes were amplified by PCR. The PCR fragments were visualized on a 1.5% agarose gel containing 5 μg/ml ethidium bromide.

Real-time PCR was performed using SYBER Green on an ABI 7500 Fast Real-Time PCR System (Applied Biosystems). The final reaction mixture contained 10 ng of cDNA, 100 nM of each primer, 10 μl of $2 \times$ SYBR$^®$ Green PCR Master Mix (Applied Biosystems), and RNase-free water to complete the reaction mixture volume to 20 μl. All reactions were performed in triplicate. The PCR was performed with a hot-start denaturation step at 95°C for 10 min, and then was carried out for 40 cycles at 95°C for 15 s and 60°C for 1 min. The fluorescence was read during the reaction, allowing a continuous monitoring of the amount of PCR product. The data were normalized to internal control-β-actin mRNA. The sequences of primers used in real-time PCR are shown in Table 1.

Table 1   Primers for real-time RT-PCR analysis

Primer	Forward	Reverse
ABCA1	GCACTGAGGAAGATGCTGAAA	AGTTCCTGGAAGGTCTTGTTCAC
ABCG5	TCTCTTGGCCCCCACTTA	CTATATTTGGATTTTGGACGATACCA
ABCG8	TCGTACCCTCTCTACGCCATCT	GGACACGTAGTACAGGACCATGAA
ABCG1	CCGACCGACGACACAGAGA	GCACGAGACACCCACAAACC
LDLR	GCTTGTCTGTCACCTGCAAA	AACTGCCGAGAGATGCACTT
HMGCOA-R	ACCTTTCCAGAGCAAGCACATT	AGGACCTAAAATTGCCATTCCA
CYP7A1	CTTTACCCACAGTTAATGCACTTAGATC	GGTAGTCTTTGTCTTCCCGTTTTC

Statistics

Data are reported as mean ± standard deviation (SD). Where indicated, data were subjected to t-test analysis and determined to be significantly different if $p < 0.05$.

RESULTS

A novel nuclear oxysterol is synthesized in primary rat hepatocytes following StarD1 overexpression

Primary rat hepatocytes infected with recombinant adenovirus encoding either StarD1 or CYP7A1, as described in Materials and Methods, showed increased bile acid synthesis as previously reported[10,11]. Approximately 50% of the total cellular counts from [^{14}C]cholesterol metabolites were found in the nuclear fraction; the other 50% were recovered in other organelles including cytosol, plasma membranes, lysosomes, and mitochondria. Only a small number of counts were detected in the DNase digested fractions. The total extractable [^{14}C]cholesterol metabolite counts in nuclear fractions from StarD1-infected cells were slightly higher than those of CYP7A1-infected or control nuclear extracts.

After Folch partitioning, [^{14}C]cholesterol metabolites in the methanol/water phase extracted from the nuclear fractions were dramatically increased in the StarD1-overexpressing cells compared to control ($p < 0.001$, n = 5) or CYP7A1-overexpressing cells ($p < 0.001$, n = 5) (Figure 1). The [^{14}C] cholesterol metabolites could be extracted only after DNase and proteinase K treatments, suggesting that [^{14}C]cholesterol metabolites present inside the nuclei may be protein-bound. We characterized the composition of the cholesterol metabolites in the different subcellular fractions of StarD1-overexpressing hepatocytes by reverse-phase HPLC analysis of [^{14}C] cholesterol metabolites in the methanol/water phase from the nuclear and non-nuclear fractions. The data in Figure 2 show the elution profiles of these lipid extracts. The elution profiles were relatively similar in the nuclear fraction (fraction D) from cells infected either with the StarD1 or null recombinant viruses, except for a peak with retention time of 11.51 min (Figures 2A, 2C) that was detectable only in StarD1-overexpressing cells (Figures 2C and 2D).

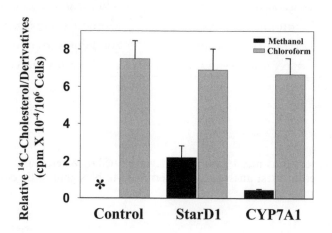

Figure 1 Phase distribution of [^{14}C]cholesterol derivatives in nuclei of primary rat hepatocytes following overexpression of StarD1 and CYP7A1. Rat primary hepatocytes were infected with the indicated viruses. Forty-eight hours later cells were harvested and subcellular fractions prepared. Fractions of nuclear digests were processed for lipid analysis as explained under 'Materials and Methods'. *[^{14}C]Cholesterol derivatives were not detected. The values represent means $\pm$ SD (n =5)

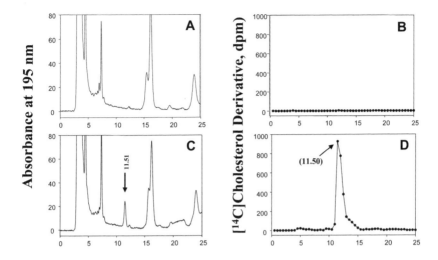

Figure 2 HPLC analysis of [¹⁴C]cholesterol derivatives in the nuclear digests. Twenty-four hours following the indicated recombinant adenovirus infection the cells were harvested, nuclear fractions were isolated, total lipids were extracted by the Folch method and the methanol/water phase analysed. **A**: (control) and **C** (StarD1), nuclear extract profiles at 195 nm. **B**: (control) and **D** (StarD1), nuclear extracts ¹⁴C-sterols profiles. **C**: Non-nuclear extracts (fraction A) [¹⁴C]-sterols profiles. In each case nuclear methanol/water extracts of the equivalent of 5×10^6 cells were loaded. The elution profiles represent one of the five sets of experiments (the profiles are highly repeatable)

Further analysis of extracts of mitochondria from StarD1-overexpressing cells indicated the presence of two [¹⁴C]cholesterol metabolites with retention times at 5.00 min and 11.5 min (Figure 3A). The metabolite eluting at the 11.5 min peak was present only in mitochondria and nuclei, and was not in the culture media (Figures 3A and 3B), suggesting that this [¹⁴C]cholesterol metabolite might be synthesized in mitochondria and translocated to the nuclei. In contrast, the peak with retention time at 5.00 min was found in the culture medium; within the cell it was found only in mitochondria, and not in the nuclear fractions (Figures 3A and 3C), suggesting that this molecule was secreted from the cells.

To characterize its chemical structure, the purified nuclear metabolite was further analyzed by MS/MS mass spectrometry. The Q1 full-scan spectrum of the purified nuclear metabolite showed two major molecule ions, m/z 480.1 and 481.2 (Figure 4A). The product scans showed that the characteristic fragment ions of these two molecules were very similar. Fragment ions were observed at m/z = 80(a), 97(b), 107, 123(c), 288, 465, and 59(d) in the product scan spectrum of m/z 481 (Figure 4B). These observed fragment ions indicate that the nuclear meabolite is a sulphated oxysterol with a sulphate group on the 3-hydroxy position[18] and a hydroxyl group on side-chain, m/z 59 (molecular mass 482 = 80 (sulphate) + 16 (O) + 386 (cholesterol). Combined with data

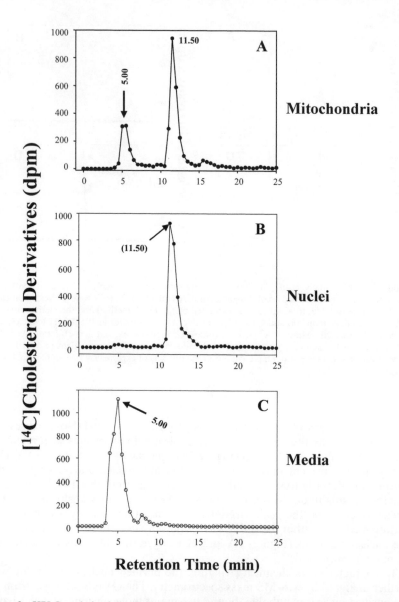

Figure 3 HPLC analysis of the cholesterol derivatives extracted from the nuclei, mitochondria, and culture media. Rat primary hepatocytes were infected with the StarD1 adenovirus and 2 h later [^{14}C]cholesterol was added to the media. Twenty-four hours following infections the cells and culture media were harvested. Nuclei and mitochondria were isolated as described under 'Experimental Procedures'. Total lipids were extracted from the nuclei, mitochondria, and culture media by Folch partitioning into methanol phase, and analysed by HPLC, and the radioactitivity in each elution fraction was counted by liquid scintillation counter as described in 'Experimental Procedures'. The elution profiles represent one of the five sets of experiments. **A–C**: radioactivity profiles

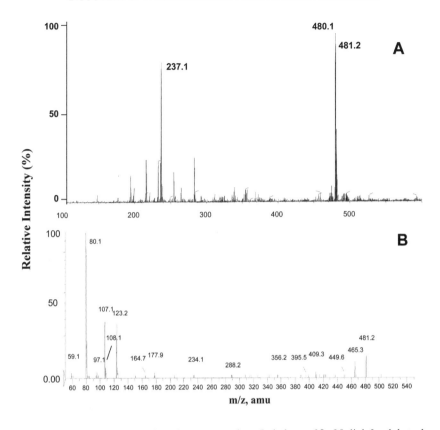

Figure 4 Characterization of nuclear oxysterol as 5-cholesten-3β, 25-diol 3-sulphate by negative ion-triple quadruple mass spectrometry. The mass spectrometer was operated in negative ion modes and data were acquired using full-scan mode as well as the product ion mode for MS/MS. The Q1 full-scan spectrum of the purified nuclear oxysterol (**A**); the product scan spectrum of m/z 481 (**B**) amu = atomic mass units

from enzymatic digestion and HPLC analysis (data not shown), the nuclear oxysterol derivative was identified as 5-cholesten-3β, 25-diol 3-sulphate (25-hydroxycholesterol 3-sulphate). The spectra are consistent with previously characterized sulphated cholesterol metabolites[18]. This structure is supported by high-resolution MS analysis showing its mass as 481.3118 with molecular formula $C_{27}H_{45}O_5S$ (calculated mass is 481.2988, PPM = 5.5).

CYP27A1 is responsible for the synthesis of 25-hydroxycholesterol in hepatocyte mitochondria

To determine whether 25-hydroxycholesterol was synthesized in hepatocyte mitochondria, the mitochondria were isolated from rat, mouse, or human liver tissues, and from HepG2 cells. After incubation of mitochondria with cholesterol/[^{14}C]cholesterol and treatment with proteinase K at 37°C for 90 min, the total cholesterol derivatives were extracted and analysed by TLC and HPLC as previously described[15]. The major products of the total [^{14}C]-cholesterol derivatives after incubation were 25-hydroxy- and 27-hydroxycholesterol and the amounts were time-dependent. HPLC analysis of sterol products after incubation of mitochondria with cholesterol showed that 28% of total cholesterol can be recovered as 27-hydroxy- and 3% to be 25-hydroxycholesterols, as shown in Figure 5B. A similar result was obtained when using liver tissues and HepG2 cells (data not shown). To determine whether CYP27A1 was responsible for the synthesis of 25-hydroxycholesterol, mitochondria isolated from cyp27A1 gene knockout mouse liver were assessed. As shown in Figure 5C, these mitochondria failed to synthesize both 25-hydroxy- and 27-hydroxycholesterol, supporting the notion that CYP27A1 is responsible for the synthesis of both oxysterols.

Hydroxysteoid sulphotransferase, SULT2B1b, is responsible for the synthesis of 5-cholesten-3β, 25-diol 3-sulphate

RT-PCR analysis showed that only two mRNA encoding hydroxysteroid sulphotransferases SULT2B1b and SULT2A2, are present in rat liver, lacking SULT2B1a and SULT2A1, and that levels of these mRNA are much higher in females than in males (Figure 6). Interestingly, after culture for 24 h, primary rat hepatocytes highly express SULT2B1b; in contrast SULT2A2 mRNA is barely detected (Figure 6). Incubation of rat hepatocyte mitochondria and cytosol fractions isolated from rat hepatocytes with [^{14}C]25-hydroxycholesterol or [^{14}C]cholesterol, resulted in a product with the same retention time as chemically synthesized 25HC3S (Figure 7), suggesting that SULT2B1b is responsible for the synthesis of 25HC3S.

5-Cholesten-3β, 25-diol 3-sulphate regulates expression of genes involved in cholesterol homeostasis

At 25 µM, cultured for 6 h, addition of 25HC3S inhibited the expression of HMG CoA reductase mRNA by 80% and LDLR by 70%; however, it increased CYP27A1, CYP7A1, StarD1, and ABCG5 about 50%, and ABCA1, ABCG8 by ~2-fold (Figure 8). The results suggest that the nuclear oxysterol, 25HC3S, serves as a potent regulatory molecule in the maintenance of cholesterol homeostasis.

DISCUSSION

In this chapter we report identification of the novel nuclear oxysterol, 5-cholesten-3β, 25-diol 3-sulphate, in nuclei of primary rat hepatocytes and normal human liver. The levels of this oxysterol were dramatically increased in mitochondria and nuclei following overexpression of the mitochondrial cholesterol delivery protein, StarD1, in primary rat hepatocytes. These results suggest that StarD1 may serve as a sensor of intracellular cholesterol levels in

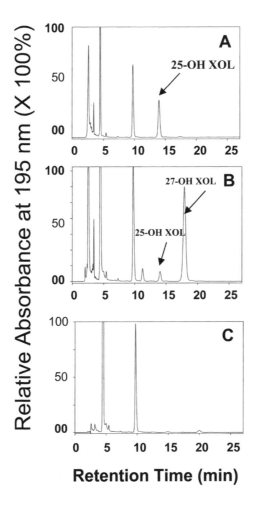

Figure 5 Synthesis of 25-hydroxy- and 27-hydroxycholesterol by Cyp27A1 in mouse hepatocyte mitochondria. After incubation of the isolated mitochondria from wild-type mouse (panel **B**) and Cyp27A1⁻ knockout mouse livers (panel **C**) with β-CD cholesterol, total sterol metabolites were extracted and analysed by HPLC using an ultrasphere silica column as described in detail in Materials and Methods. The indicated peaks are the ketones derived form 25-hydroxycholesterol (25-OH Xol) and 27-hydroxycholesterol (27-OH Xol); testosterone propionate was used as an internal standard to monitor sterol extraction. The data represent typical results from one of five experiments. Panel **A** shows standard retention time of 25-hydroxycholesterol

the liver. When cholesterol levels increase, StarD1 protein delivers cholesterol into mitochondria where it may be metabolized to 25-hydroxy-, 27-hydroxycholesterol, and 5-cholesten-3β, 25-diol 3-sulphate. These cholesterol metabolites were all found in the nuclei and may be involved in the regulation of gene expression.

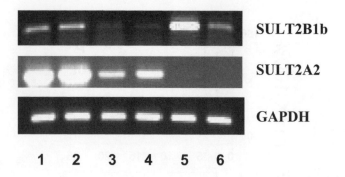

Figure 6 RT-PCR analysis of hydroxysteroid sulphate transferase expression in rat liver tissues and primary rat hepatocytes. Total RNA were purified from two individual primary rat hepatocyte preparations and rat liver tissues, respectively, using SV Total RNA Isolation Kit (Promega). RT-PCR was performed as the manufacturer recommended (Invitrogen). Lanes 1 and 2 represent two different samples (female rat liver); lanes 3 and 4, male rat liver; lane 5, primary rat hepatocytes (after culture for 48 h); lane 6, rat testis as positive control for SULT2B1a. The results were from 29 cycles. Each cycle consists of 94°C for 40 s, 60°C for 1 min, and 72°C for 1 min

25-Hydroxycholesterol has been reported to be a ligand of LXR and is believed to play an important role in the regulation of cholesterol degradation and secretion[19–23]. Known genes regulated by LXR include CYP7A1, ABCA1, ABCG5, and ABCG8. 25-Hydroxycholesterol has also been reported to inhibit HMGR and cholesterol biosynthesis by inhibiting activation of SREBP[19]. However, 25-hydroxycholesterol is not water-soluble and its metabolism and physiological significance is not clear[24,25]. In contrast, the sulphated derivative of 25-hydroxycholesterol is water-soluble. It has been reported that sulphated steroid hormones exhibit strong steroid hormone-like activity[26]. It is possible that the 5-cholesten-3β, 25-diol 3-sulphate could be a potent regulator of genes involved in cholesterol homeostasis. Our observations that this oxysterol sulphate is located in nuclei and its addition to HepG2 cells in culture inhibits the expression of HMG CoA reductase and LDL receptor, and increases expression of CYP7A1, CYP27A1, ABCA1, ABCG5/G8, and StarD1 strongly suggest that 25HC3S serves as a potent regulator of genes involved in cholesterol homeostasis. Since all of the increased mRNA are encoded by LXR targeting genes, 25HC3S could be an *in-vivo* ligand.

Several sulphated sterols have been reported to be widely distributed in steroidogenic tissues[27] and to circulate in plasma[28]. Sulphated sterols have been implicated in a wide variety of biological processes, e.g. regulation of cholesterol synthesis, sperm capacitation, thrombin and plasmin activities, and activation of protein kinase C isoenzymes[29]. Sulphated sterols can also serve as a substrate for adrenal and ovarian steroidogenesis[30,31]. They play an important, but unclear, role in the normal development and physiology of the skin, where an epidermal sterol sulphate cycle has been described[29].

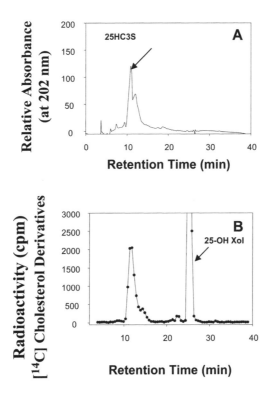

Figure 7 Synthesis of 25-hydroxycholesterol 3-sulphate by isolated mitochondrial and cytosol fractions from rat liver. After incubation of the isolated mitochondrial and cytosol fractions with β-CD [^{14}C]25-hydroxycholesterol (**B**) or [^{14}C]cholesterol (**C**), total sterol metabolites were extracted and the [^{14}C]sterol derivatives were analysed by HPLC using a C18 reverse-phase column as described in detail in Materials and Methods. Panel **A**, elution profile of the chemical synthesized 25-hydroxycholesterol 3β-sulphate (25HC3S) used as a standard. The data represent typical results from one of three experiments

This chapter demonstrates the presence of 25-hydroxycholesterol 3-sulphate in both the mitochondria and the nuclei of primary rat hepatocytes, but not in culture media. Two reactions must be involved in the generation of this oxysterol sulphate. In the present study we found that cyp27A1 is responsible for the biosynthesis of mitochondrial 25-hydroxycholesterol. We think that this is followed by sulphation at the 3β position via a sulphotransferase.

To date, hydroxycholesterol sulphotransferases have not been systematically investigated in liver. Four isoenzymes, SULT2B1a, SULT2b1b, SULT2A1, and SULT2A2 in rat[17,32], and three isoenzymes, SULT2B1a, SULT2B1b, and SULT2A1 in human have been reported[29,33]. Their physiological significance is still unclear[34]. In this chapter we have shown that only two isoenzymes, SULT2B1b and SULT2A2, are expressed in the rat liver and that the cultured

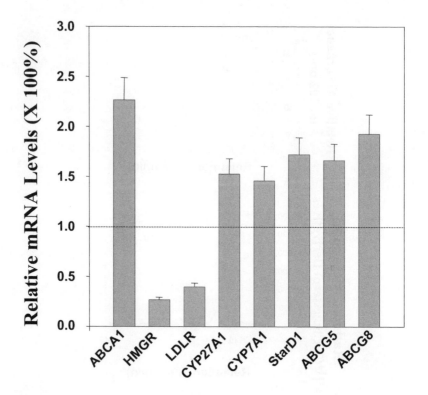

Figure 8 Real-time RT-PCR analysis of expression of genes involved in maintenance of intracellular cholesterol homeostasis. At 6 h following addition of 25HC3S to HepG2 cell culture the cells were harvested, the total RNA was extracted, and each mRNA level was analysed as described in Materials and Method. Two micrograms of total RNA were used for cDNA preparation (RT) and 10 ng of cDNA were used for PCR. The expression levels were normalized to β-actin. The values represent means ± SD (n =3)

primary rat hepatocytes express only SULT2B1b mRNA. Thus, our observation that the mitochondrial plus cytosol fractions were able to synthesize 25HC3S suggests that the SULT2B1b is responsible for the synthesis of the oxysterol sulphate, 25HC3S.

Acknowledgements

We acknowledge excellent technical help from Dalila Marques, Kaye Redford, and Pat Bohdan. This work was supported by grants from the National Institutes of Health (R01 HL078898 and P01 DK38030), and the Veterans Administration. D.R-A. is the Recipient of an American Liver Foundation Research Fellowship.

References

1. Pandak WM, Heuman DM, Hylemon PB, Vlahcevic ZR. Regulation of bile acid synthesis. IV. Interrelationship between cholesterol and bile acid biosynthesis pathways. J Lipid Res. 1990;31:79–90.
2. Hylemon PB, Stravitz RT, Vlahcevic ZR. Molecular genetics and regulation of bile acid biosynthesis. Prog Liver Dis. 1994;12:99–120.
3. Chiang JY. Regulation of bile acid synthesis. Front Biosci. 1998;3:d176–93.
4. Dubrac S, Lear SR, Ananthanarayanan M et al. Role of CYP27A in cholesterol and bile acid metabolism. J Lipid Res. 2005;46:76–85.
5. Bjorkhem I, Andersson O, Diczfalusy U et al. Atherosclerosis and sterol 27-hydroxylase: evidence for a role of this enzyme in elimination of cholesterol from human macrophages. Proc Natl Acad Sci USA. 1994;91:8592–6.
6. Fu X, Menke JG, Chen Y et al. 27-Hydroxycholesterol is an endogenous ligand for liver X receptor in cholesterol-loaded cells. J Biol Chem. 2001;276:38378–87.
7. Bjorkhem I, Diczfalusy U. Oxysterols: friends, foes, or just fellow passengers? Arterioscler Thromb Vasc Biol. 2002;22:734–42.
8. Hall E, Hylemon P, Vlahcevic Z et al. Overexpression of CYP27 in hepatic and extrahepatic cells: role in the regulation of cholesterol homeostasis. Am J Physiol Gastrointest Liver Physiol. 2001;281:G293–301.
9. Hall EA, Ren S, Hylemon PB et al. Detection of the steroidogenic acute regulatory protein, StAR, in human liver cells. Biochim Biophys Acta. 2005;1733:111–19.
10. Pandak WM, Ren S, Marques D et al. Transport of cholesterol into mitochondria is rate-limiting for bile acid synthesis via the alternative pathway in primary rat hepatocytes. J Biol Chem. 2002;277:48158–64.
11. Ren S, Hylemon PB, Marques D et al. Overexpression of cholesterol transporter StAR increases *in vivo* rates of bile acid synthesis in the rat and mouse. Hepatology. 2004;40:910–17.
12. Dignam JD, Lebovitz RM, Roeder RG. Accurate transcription initiation by RNA polymerase II in a soluble extract from isolated mammalian nuclei. Nucleic Acids Res. 1983;11:1475–89.
13. Ren S, Hylemon P, Marques D et al. Effect of increasing the expression of cholesterol transporters (StAR, MLN64, and SCP-2) on bile acid synthesis. J Lipid Res. 2004;45:2123–31.
14. Stravitz RT, Vlahcevic ZR, Russell TL, Heizer ML, Avadhani NG, Hylemon PB. Regulation of sterol 27-hydroxylase and an alternative pathway of bile acid biosynthesis in primary cultures of rat hepatocytes. J Steroid Biochem Mol Biol. 1996;57:337–47.
15. Li X, Hylemon P, Pandak WM, Ren S. Enzyme activity assay for cholesterol 27-hydroxylase in mitochondria. J Lipid Res. 2006;47:1507–12.
16. Ren S, Hylemon P, Zhang ZP et al. Identification of a novel sulfonated oxysterol, 5-cholesten-3beta,25-diol 3-sulfonate, in hepatocyte nuclei and mitochondria. J Lipid Res. 2006;47:1081–90.
17. Kohjitani A, Fuda H, Hanyu O, Strott CA. Cloning, characterization and tissue expression of rat SULT2B1a and SULT2B1b steroid/sterol sulfotransferase isoforms: divergence of the rat SULT2B1 gene structure from orthologous human and mouse genes. Gene. 2006;367:66–73.
18. Lemonde HA, Johnson AW, Clayton PT. The identification of unusual bile acid metabolites by tandem mass spectrometry: use of low-energy collision-induced dissociation to produce informative spectra. Rapid Commun Mass Spectrom. 1999;13:1159–64.
19. Adams CM, Reitz J, De Brabander JK et al. Cholesterol and 25-hydroxycholesterol inhibit activation of SREBPs by different mechanisms, both involving SCAP and Insigs. J Biol Chem. 2004;279:52772–80.
20. Corsini A, Verri D, Raiteri M, Quarato P, Paoletti R, Fumagalli R. Effects of 26-aminocholesterol, 27-hydroxycholesterol, and 25-hydroxycholesterol on proliferation and cholesterol homeostasis in arterial myocytes. Arterioscler Thromb Vasc Biol. 1995;15:420–8.
21. Javitt NB. 25R,26-Hydroxycholesterol revisited: synthesis, metabolism, and biologic roles. J Lipid Res. 2002;43:665–70.

22. Saucier SE, Kandutsch AA, Taylor FR, Spencer TA, Phirwa S, Gayen AK. Identification of regulatory oxysterols, 24(S),25-epoxycholesterol and 25-hydroxycholesterol, in cultured fibroblasts. J Biol Chem. 1985;260:14571–9.
23. Zhang Y, Repa JJ, Gauthier K, Mangelsdorf DJ. Regulation of lipoprotein lipase by the oxysterol receptors, LXRalpha and LXRbeta. J Biol Chem. 2001;276:43018–24.
24. Bjorkhem I. Do oxysterols control cholesterol homeostasis? J Clin Invest. 2002;110:725–30.
25. Mellon SH,.Bair SR. 25-Hydroxycholesterol is not a ligand for the orphan nuclear receptor steroidogenic factor-1 (SF-1). Endocrinology. 1998;139:3026–9.
26. Kumar R, Londowski JM, Murari MP, Nagubandi S. Synthesis and biological activity of vitamin D2 3 beta-glucosiduronate and vitamin D2 3 beta-sulfate: role of vitamin D2 conjugates in calcium homeostasis. J Steroid Biochem. 1982;17:495–502.
27. Meng LJ, Griffiths WJ, Nazer H, Yang Y, Sjovall J. High levels of (24S)-24-hydroxycholesterol 3-sulfate, 24-glucuronide in the serum and urine of children with severe cholestatic liver disease. J Lipid Res. 1997;38:926–34.
28. Gurpide E, Roberts KD, Welch MT, Bandy L, Lieberman S. Studies on the metabolism of blood-borne cholesterol sulfate. Biochemistry. 1966;5:3352–62.
29. Javitt NB, Lee YC, Shimizu C, Fuda H, Strott CA. Cholesterol and hydroxycholesterol sulfotransferases: identification, distinction from dehydroepiandrosterone sulfotransferase, and differential tissue expression. Endocrinology. 2001;142:2978–84.
30. Korte K, Hemsell PG, Mason JI. Sterol sulfate metabolism in the adrenals of the human fetus, anencephalic newborn, and adult. J Clin Endocrinol Metab. 1982;55:671–5.
31. Tuckey RC. Side-chain cleavage of cholesterol sulfate by ovarian mitochondria. J Steroid Biochem Mol Biol. 1990;37:121–7.
32. Liu L, LeCluyse EL, Liu J, Klaassen CD. Sulfotransferase gene expression in primary cultures of rat hepatocytes. Biochem Pharmacol. 1996;52:1621–30.
33. Lee KA, Fuda H, Lee YC, Negishi M, Strott CA, Pedersen LC. Crystal structure of human cholesterol sulfotransferase (SULT2B1b) in the presence of pregnenolone and 3'-phosphoadenosine 5'-phosphate. Rationale for specificity differences between prototypical SULT2A1 and the SULT2BG1 isoforms. J Biol Chem. 2003;278:44593–9.
34. Strott CA, Higashi Y. Cholesterol sulfate in human physiology: what's it all about? J Lipid Res. 2003;44:1268–78.

Section II
Hepatobiliary transport of bile acids

Chair: W KRAMER and FJ SUCHY

5
Role of Ntcp phosphorylation in cAMP-mediated stimulation of hepatic bile acid uptake

M. S. ANWER, M. ANANTHANARAYANAN and F. J. SUCHY

INTRODUCTION

It is becoming more evident that the activities of biomolecules are regulated by phosphorylation and dephosphorylation[1]. For example, enzymes and signalling molecules can be activated by phosphorylation and deactivated by dephosphorylation or vice versa, with phosphorylation and dephosphorylation being carried out by specific kinases and phosphatases, respectively. Recent studies suggest that transporters can also be regulated by the phosphorylation and dephosphorylation process. In the case of a transporter, phosphorylation may affect the transporter activity (function) and/or its location; a transporter has to be at the right location to carry out its function. The regulation of transporters has lagged behind other biomolecules and we are beginning to unravel the regulation of hepatocyte transporters by phosphorylation.

A number of transporters are involved in solute transport across hepatocellular membranes[2]. Many of these transporters play an important function in biliary secretion of solutes and hence bile formation. One of the major determinants of bile formation is bile acids which are transported from blood to bile by specific transporters located in the sinusoidal and canalicular membranes[2-4]. Bile acid uptake by Na^+/taurocholate cotransporting polypeptide (NTCP, SLC10A1) at the sinusoidal membrane, and bile acid excretion by bile salt export pump (BSEP, ABCB11) at the canalicular membrane represent the major mechanisms of transhepatic transport of bile acids. In addition, multidrug resistance associated protein 2 (MRP2, ABCC2) is involved in canalicular transport of bile acids conjugated with sulphate and glucuronide, and organic anion transporting proteins (Oatp) and microsomal epoxide hydroxylase may also be involved in hepatic uptake of bile acids[4,5].

It is now apparent that malfunction of these transporters, due to mutations and/or defective post-transcriptional regulation, is associated with various cholestatic liver diseases[2,3]. A transporter has to be inserted into the membrane for it to transport solutes across that membrane. This is a complex regulated process requiring participation of various signalling molecules. A breakdown in this regulated process can lead to a decreased amount or an absence of a transport protein at its intended site, resulting in decreased or no transport function and hence cholestasis. In addition, the transporter activity may be decreased directly, leading to cholestasis. Recent studies indicate that phosphorylation may play an important role in regulating activity and localization of hepatic bile acid transporters. The following is a summary of what is currently known about regulation of hepatic bile acid transporters, more specifically Ntcp, by phosphorylation.

Cyclic AMP stimulates Na^+/taurocholate cotransport by translocating Ntcp to the plasma membrane. Further studies showed that the effect of cAMP is dependent on phosphoinositide-3-kinase and $Ca2^+$-mediated signalling pathways[2]. It is also known that NTCP is a serine/threonine phosphoprotein and is dephosphorylated by cAMP[6]. This finding raised two questions: (i) what is the mechanism of cAMP-mediated Ntcp dephosphorylation and (ii) what is the role of phosphorylation in cAMP-mediated NTCP translocation?

MECHANISM OF cAMP-MEDIATED Ntcp DEPHOSPHORYLATION

Many effects of cAMP are mediated via cAMP-dependent protein kinase (PKA). The cAMP/PKA pathway has been suggested in cAMP-mediated increases in cytosolic Ca^{2+}, stimulation of Na^+/taurocholate cotransport[7] and vesicle movement[8]. The increase in cytosolic Ca^{2+} by cAMP involves both release of stored Ca^{2+} and influx of extracellular Ca^{2+} (see ref. 9); the release of stored Ca^{2+} is due to phosphorylation of the inositol trisphosphate (IP3) receptor with consequent increase in IP3 sensitivity[10,11]. Since cAMP dephosphorylates Ntcp, this effect is likely to be mediated via activation of a protein phosphatase and/or inhibition of a kinase involved in Ntcp phosphorylation. However, the identity of the kinase involved in Ntcp phosphorylation has not been established, although a role for extracellular signal-regulated kinase (ERK1/2) is indicated by preliminary data from the author's laboratory. Other studies suggest that protein phosphatase 2B may be involved in cAMP-mediated Ntcp dephosphorylation.

Typical amino acids phosphorylated in a protein are tyrosine, serine and threonine, and protein phosphatases (PP) are broadly divided into protein tyrosine phosphatases (PTP) and protein serine/threonine phosphatases (PSP). Since Ntcp is a serine/threonine phosphoprotein, a PSP is likely to dephosphorylate Ntcp. There are four major types of cytosolic PSP[1,12]: (i) PP1 and PP2A are inhibited by okadaic acid and do not require divalent cation for activation, (ii) PP2B (calcineurin) is inhibited by pyrethroids and is activated by Ca^{2+}, and (iii) PP2C is activated by Mg^{2+} with no known inhibitor. If any of these PSP are involved in cAMP-mediated Ntcp dephosphorylation, cAMP should activate the PP, and inhibition of the PP should result in increased Ntcp phosphorylation.

Studies with okadaic acid to define the role of PP1/2A showed that okadaic acid inhibited cAMP-mediated stimulation of taurocholate uptake, Ntcp translocation and reversed cAMP-mediated Ntcp dephosphorylation[13].

However, cAMP failed to activate either PP1 or PP2A. Thus, it is unlikely that cAMP-mediated Ntcp dephosphorylation involves PP1/2A. Interestingly, okadaic acid inhibited cAMP-induced increases in cytosolic Ca^{2+} in hepatocytes, suggesting that PP1/2A may facilitate cAMP-mediated intracellular Ca^{2+} release. This result raised the possibility that okadaic acid may affect cAMP-induced Ntcp dephosphorylation by inhibiting Ca^{2+}-dependent protein phosphatase, PP2B. The activation of PP2B involves Ca^{2+}-dependent binding of calmodulin to PP2B, resulting in a displacement of an auto-inhibitory domain[12].

The role of Ca^{2+} was studied with a Ca^{2+} chelator, bis-(2-amino-5-methylphenoxy)-ethane-tetraacetic acid (MAPTA). In MAPTA loaded hepatocytes, cAMP failed to induce translocation and dephosphorylation of Ntcp[6]. The role of PP2B was studied using known PP2B inhibitors, cypermethrin and FK506[14]. These inhibitors inhibited cAMP-mediated stimulation of taurocholate uptake in hepatocytes. Cypermethrin also reversed cAMP-mediated Ntcp translocation and phosphorylation without affecting cAMP-mediated increases in cytosolic Ca^{2+}. Thus, the effect of PP2B inhibitor is subsequent to cAMP-mediated increases in cytosolic Ca^{2+}. In addition, PP2B directly dephosphorylated Ntcp immunoprecipitated from control, but not from cAMP-treated hepatocytes. Cyclic AMP stimulated PP2B activity in hepatocytes and this effect was completely inhibited by cypermethrin.

Taken together, these results suggest that both PP1/2A and 2B are involved in cAMP-induced translocation of Ntcp. A likely mechanism may be as follows: cAMP, in a PP2A-dependent manner, increases $[Ca^{2+}]_i$, which activates PP2B and PP2B in turn dephosphorylates Ntcp (Figure 1).

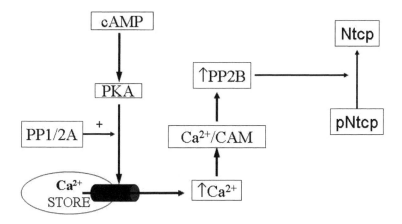

Figure 1 Proposed mechanism of cAMP-mediated Ntcp dephosphorylation. Cyclic AMP increases cytosolic Ca^{2+} by inducing IP3-mediated release of stored Ca^{2+} and this process is facilitated by PP1/2A. The increase in cytosolic Ca^{2+} activates PP2B by facilitating binding of calmodulin to PP2B. The activation of PP2B results in dephosphorylation of Ntcp

ROLE OF PHOSPHORYLATION IN Ntcp TRANSLOCATION

Experimental manipulations that inhibit cAMP-mediated Ntcp dephosphorylation also inhibit cAMP-mediated Ntcp translocation[6,13,15]. Thus, cAMP-mediated Ntcp translocation may involve Ntcp dephosphorylation by PP2B. However, the identity of Ntcp phosphorylation site(s) is needed to design experiments to determine whether dephosphorylation of a specific site facilitates cAMP-mediated Ntcp translocation. Thus, studies were conducted to determine whether a specific site is dephosphorylated by cAMP and whether dephosphorylation of such a site facilitates Ntcp translocation.

We approached these questions by conducting phosphopeptide analysis on proteolytic digestion products of phosphorylated Ntcp isolated from hepatocytes treated with or without cAMP[16]. Ntcp is a $\cong 51$ kDa glycoprotein protein with seven transmembrane domains and three cytoplasmic loops with intracellular localization of the C-terminal end[17]. An analysis of the potential protease cleavage site showed that clostripain (cleavage site RX) could cleave Ntcp at five different sites resulting in five peptides ranging in estimated molecular sizes from 2.1 to 15.7 kDa (Figure 2). Analysis of clostripain-treated phospho-Ntcp revealed that 7.8 and 15.7 kDa peptides were phosphorylated.

Pretreatment with cAMP decreased the phosphorylation of 7.8 kDa peptide containing the third cytoplasmic loop, suggesting the possibility that the phosphorylation site(s) on this peptide may be involved in Ntcp translocation. The 7.8 kDa peptide fragment contains 12 serine and threonine residues with three serine and two threonine residues contained in the cytoplasmic loop. Since the phosphorylation is likely to occur on the cytoplasmic site of a transmembrane protein, any of these three serine and two threonine residues may be involved in cAMP-mediated Ntcp dephosphorylation.

Studies were first conducted to determine whether any of these serine (S213, -226 and -227) and threonine (T-219 and -225) residues in the cytoplasmic loop was phosphorylated. The rationale was that, if any of these residues was phosphorylated, then replacement by alanine should decrease Ntcp phosphorylation. Thus, these residues in Ntcp were each mutated to alanine and the mutated Ntcp was expressed in HuH-7 cells followed by determination of Ntcp phosphorylation. Results showed that the phosphorylation of only S226A-Ntcp was significantly decreased by 35% compared to wild-type Ntcp (WT-Ntcp). Thus, Ntcp is phosphorylated at S226. However, phosphorylation was not abolished, indicating other phosphorylation sites. We speculate that these other phosphorylation sites are located in the cytoplasmic loops of the 15.7 kDa fragment containing seven serine and threonine residues (Figure 2).

Further studies showed that plasma membrane expression of S226A-Ntcp was significantly higher (3-fold) than that of WT-Ntcp. Taurocholate uptake in HuH-7 cells expressing S-226A-Ntcp was also significantly higher compared to WT-Ntcp expressing cells. These results suggested that dephosphorylation at S226 may facilitate plasma membrane retention of Ntcp.

We next studied whether cAMP stimulates taurocholate uptake and Ntcp translocation by dephosphorylating Ntcp at S226. If this is the case, cAMP

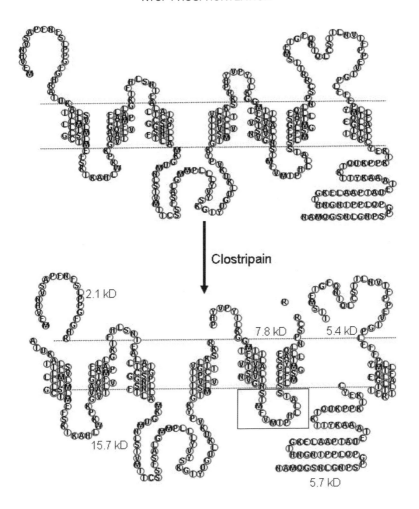

Figure 2 Predicted peptide products of Ntcp cleaved by clostripain with cleavage site at RX. The third cytoplasmic loop in the 7.8 kDa fragment is shown in the box

should not further decrease and increase phosphorylation and plasma membrane retention, respectively, of S226A-Ntcp. In addition, cAMP should not further increase taurocholate uptake induced by S226A-Ntcp. Studies in HuH-7 cells transfected with either WT-Ntcp or S226A-Ntcp showed that the increases in taurocholate uptake and Ntcp translocation and the decrease in Ntcp phosphorylation in S226A-Ntcp transfected cells were not further affected by cAMP (Figure 3). These results suggest that cAMP dephosphorylates Ntcp at S226, and this leads to increased Ntcp translocation

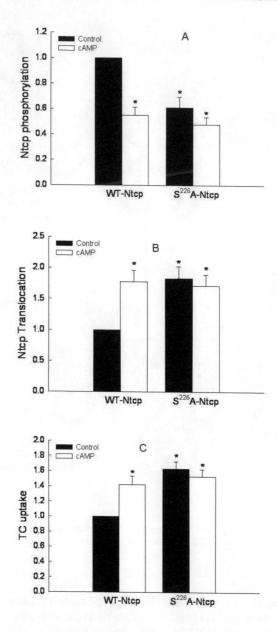

Figure 3 Effect of cAMP on Ntcp phosphorylation (**A**), Ntcp translocation (**B**) and taurocholate (TC) uptake (**C**) in HuH-7 cells transfected with either WT-Ntcp or S^{226}A-Ntcp. *Significantly ($p < 0.05$) different from WT-Ntcp control values

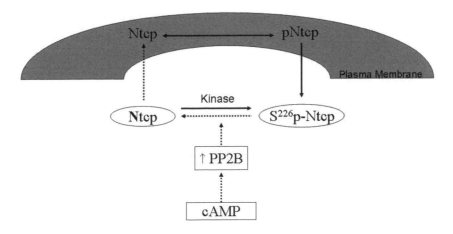

Figure 4 Proposed role of phosphorylation in cAMP-mediated Ntcp translocation. Ntcp is present in phosphorylated (pNtcp) and dephosphorylated (Ntcp) forms, and undergoes recycling between plasma membrane and cytoplasmic storage vesicles (endosomes). The cycling is regulated by phosphorylation in that dephosphorylation favours retention in the plasma membrane and phosphorylation favours internalization. When stimulated by cAMP this equilibrium shifts from pNtcp to Ntcp because of S^{226} dephosphorylation of pNtcp by PP2B. This allows for more Ntcp to be translocated and retained in the plasma membrane. Since PP2b is a cytoplasmic protein, PP2B-mediated Ntcp dephosphorylation is considered to take place in the cytoplasm

and taurocholate uptake. Based on these results we propose that S226 in the third cytoplasmic loop is one of the sites phosphorylated in Ntcp and cAMP facilitates Ntcp translocation to the plasma membrane by dephosphorylating Ntcp at this site (Figure 4).

PHOSPHORYLATION OF OTHER HEPATIC BILE ACID TRANSPORTERS

Other hepatic bile transporters that are also phosphorylated include Bsep, Mrp2 and Oatp1a1. Studies conducted with mouse Bsep expressed in SF9 cells showed that Bsep is a phosphoprotein and one of the protein kinase C (PKC), PKCα, increases Bsep phosphorylation[18]. Like Ntcp, Bsep also undergoes translocation to the plasma membrane[2]. However, it is not known whether phosphorylation affects the activity or translocation of Bsep. It is of interest that bile acids can activate PKC[19]. Thus, this study raises the possibility that bile acids, acting via PKC, may regulate bile acid efflux by phosphorylating Bsep.

Mrp2, like Bsep, is a member of the ATP-binding cassette transporter family and a number of studies suggest that Mrp2 is regulated by various kinases[2]. For example, PKC may be involved in the translocation of Mrp2[20,21]. A recent study showed that Mrp2 is a phosphoprotein and the co-expression of PKCα and Mrp2 in SF9 cells increases Mrp2 phosphorylation and its transport activity without changing Mrp2 expression[22]. However, this study was unable to separate the effect of phosphorylation on Mrp2 transport activity and translocation. Thus, it remains to be established whether PKCα-mediated phosphorylation of Mrp2 also affects its translocation in addition to its transport activity.

Some Oatp are able to transport bile acids, and Oatp1a1, located at the sinusoidal membrane, may be involved in Na$^+$-independent bile acid uptake by hepatocytes[4,5]. Extracellular ATP inhibits Oatp1a1 transport activity and this is associated with serine phosphorylation[23]. ATP-induced phosphorylation was not associated with a redistribution of Oatp1a1. In addition, okadaic acid decreases Oatp1a1 activity, suggesting a role for PP2A in the regulation of Oatp1[23]. In a recent study the phosphorylation sites of Oatp1a1 were found to be S634 and S635 located in the C-terminus with phosphorylation of S634 preceding that of S635[24]. Whether phosphorylation near the C-terminus inhibits oligomerization of Oatp1a1 and thereby inhibits transport functions remains to be established.

In summary, phosphorylation is involved in post-transcriptional regulation of bile acid transporters in hepatocytes. Phosphorylation may affect the transport activity, as in the case of Oatp1a1 and Mrp2, or transporter translocation, as in the case of Ntcp. To what extent regulation by phosphorylation is adversely affected in cholestatic liver diseases remains to be determined. Based on our current understanding of the role of various kinases in hepatic bile acid transport and bile formation, it is likely that altered phosphorylation of bile acid transporters may play an important role in cholestatic liver diseases.

ACKNOWLEDGEMENTS

This study was supported in part by National Institutes of Health (USA) grants DK-33436 (to M.S.A.) and HD-20632 (to F.J.S.). We thank Holly Jameson, Henry Gillin and Natarajan Balasubramaniyan for providing excellent technical assistance and helpful comments.

References

1. Hunter T. Protein kinases and phosphatases: the yin and yang of protein phosphorylation and signaling. Cell. 1995;80:225–36.
2. Anwer MS. Cellular regulation of hepatic bile acid transport in health and cholestasis. Hepatology. 2004;39:581–9.
3. Trauner M, Boyer JL. Bile salt transporters: molecular characterization, function, and regulation. Physiol Rev. 2003;83:633–71.
4. Wolkoff AW, Cohen DE. Bile acid regulation of hepatic physiology: I. Hepatocyte transport of bile acids. Am J Physiol Gastrointest Liver Physiol. 2003;284:G175–9.
5. Hagenbuch B, Meier PJ. The superfamily of organic anion transporting polypeptides. Biochim Biophys Acta. 2003;1609:1–18.

6. Mukhopadhayay S, Ananthanarayanan M, Stieger B, Meier PJ, Suchy FJ, Anwer MS. Sodium taurocholate cotransporting polypeptide is a serine, threonine phosphoprotein and is dephosphorylated by cyclic AMP. Hepatology. 1998;28:1629–36.

7. Grüne S, Engelking LR, Anwer MS. Role of intracellular calcium and protein kinases in the activation of hepatic Na+/taurocholate cotransport by cyclic AMP. J Biol Chem. 1993;268: 17734–41.

8. Davidson HW, McGowan CH, Balch WE. Evidence for the regulation of exocytic transport by protein phosphorylation. J Cell Biol. 1992;116:1343–55.

9. Exton JH. Role of phosphoinositides in the regulation of liver-function. Hepatology. 1988; 8:152–66.

10. Joseph SK, Ryan SV. Phosphorylation of the inositol trisphosphate receptor in isolated rat hepatocytes. J Biol Chem. 1993;268:23059–65.

11. Burgess GM, Bird GS, Obie JF, Putney Jr JW. The mechanism for synergism between phospholipase C- and adenylylcyclase-linked hormones in liver. Cyclic AMP-dependent kinase augments inositol trisphosphate-mediated Ca^{2+} mobilization without increasing the cellular levels of inositol polyphosphates. J Biol Chem. 1991;266:4772–81.

12. Cohen P. Classification of proten serine/threonine phosphatases: identification and quantification in cell extracts. Methods Enzymol. 1991;201:389–98.

13. Mukhopadhayay S, Webster CRL, Anwer MS. Role of protein phosphatase in cyclic AMP-mediated stimulation of hepatic Na^+/taurocholate cotransport. J Biol Chem. 1998;273: 30039–45.

14. Webster CRL, Blanch C, Anwer MS. Role of PP2B in cAMP-induced dephosphorylation and translocation of NTCP. Am J Physiol Gastrointest Liver Physiol. 2002;283:G44–50.

15. Lavoie L, Band CJ, Kong M, Bergeron JJ, Posner BI. Regulation of glycogen synthase in rat hepatocytes. Evidence for multiple signaling pathways. J Biol Chem. 1999;274:28279–85.

16. Anwer MS, Gillin H, Mukhopadhyay S, Balasubramaniyam N, Suchy FJ, Ananthanarayanan M. Dephosphorylation of Ser-226 facilitates plasma membrane retention of Ntcp. J Biol Chem. 2005;280:33687–92.

17. Hagenbuch B, Stieger B, Foguet M, Lubbert H, Meier PJ. Functional expression cloning and characterization of the hepatocyte Na^+/bile acid cotransport system. Proc Natl Acad Sci USA. 1991;88:10629–33.

18. Noe J, Hagenbuch B, Meier PJ, St Pierre MV. Characterization of the mouse bile salt export pump overexpressed in the baculovirus system. Hepatology. 2001;33:1223–31.

19. Stravitz RT, Rao YP, Vlahcevic ZR, Gurley EC, Jarvis WD, Hylemon PB. Hepatocellular protein kinase C activation by bile acids: implications for regulation of cholesterol 7 alpha-hydroxylase. Am J Physiol. 1996;271:G293–303.

20. Beuers U, Bilzer M, Chittattu A et al. Tauroursodeoxycholic acid inserts the apical conjugate export pump, Mrp2, into canalicular membranes and stimulates organic anion secretion by protein kinase C-dependent mechanisms in cholestatic rat liver. Hepatology. 2001;33:1206–16.

21. Kubitz R, Huth C, Schmitt M, Horbach A, Kullak-Ublick G, Haussinger D. Protein kinase C-dependent distribution of the multidrug resistance protein 2 from the canalicular to the basolateral membrane in human HepG2 cells. Hepatology. 2001;34:340–50.

22. Ito K, Wakabayashi T, Horie T. Mrp2/Abcc2 transport activity is stimulated by protein kinase C alpha in a baculo virus co-expression system. Life Sci. 2005;77:539–50.

23. Glavy JS, Wu SM, Wang PJ, Orr GA, Wolkoff AW. Down-regulation by extracellular ATP of rat hepatocyte organic anion transport is mediated by serine phosphorylation of Oatp1. J Biol Chem. 2000;275:1479–84.

24. Xiao YS, Nieves E, Angeletti RH, Orr GA, Wolkoff AW. Rat organic anion transporting protein 1A1 (Oatp1a1): purification and phosphopeptide assignment. Biochemistry. 2006; 45:3357–69.

6

The concept of basolateral efflux pumps of the hepatocyte

D. KEPPLER and M. RIUS

INTRODUCTION

The molecular basis of the efflux of bile acids and other organic anions from hepatocytes into blood under conditions of cholestasis was poorly understood until recently. We have localized three members of the multidrug resistance protein subfamily, MRP3 (ABCC3)[1], MRP4 (ABCC4)[2], and MRP6 (ABCC6) to the basolateral membrane of human hepatocytes[3]. These transport proteins are ATP-driven efflux pumps mediating the unidirectional release of organic anions from cells[4]. The broad substrate specificity of human MRP3 includes bile acids[5] and, importantly, monoglucuronosyl and bisglucuronosyl bilirubin[6]. MRP3 seems to be the best glucuronoside efflux transporter in the basolateral membrane of hepatocytes. The substrate specificity of human MRP4 is also broad[2,7–10] and includes the cotransport of bile acids with reduced glutathione[2,10]. MRP6 accepts glutathione S-conjugates as substrates[11]; however, its physiologically most important substrates have not yet been elucidated. It should be mentioned that we have not obtained evidence for the localization of MRP1 to the basolateral membrane of human hepatocytes[3].

Basolateral efflux systems for bile acids and other organic anions include, in addition to the members of the MRP subfamily mentioned above, the recently discovered heterodimer OSTα-OSTβ[12]. We have not obtained evidence to support a role of the organic anion transporters of the OATP family[13] in the efflux of bile acids. In spite of the observation that the hepatic Oatp transporters catalyse the exchange of substrates *in vitro*[14], studies with positron-emitting organic anions *in vivo* indicate an apparently unidirectional uptake into hepatocytes[3].

A compensatory function of members of the MRP family in the basolateral hepatocyte membrane, particularly when the activity of canalicular efflux pumps is impaired, was first proposed on the basis of immunodetection of MRP isoforms using antibodies with broad specificity[15,16]. This concept has been supported by the observed up-regulation of rodent Mrp3 protein in Mrp2-deficient and cholestatic livers[17–19], and by the specific detection of basolateral MRP3[1] and MRP4[2] in human hepatocytes. Most recently the up-regulation of

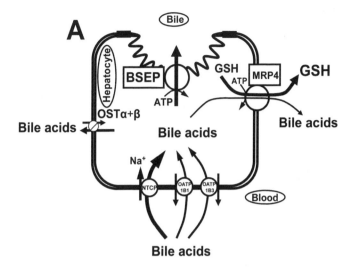

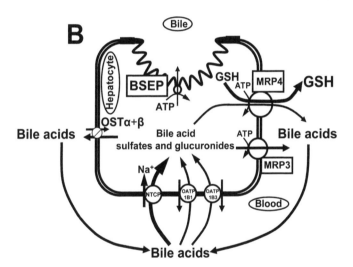

Figure 1 Scheme of bile acid transport processes of the human hepatocyte. **A**: Under normal conditions bile acids enter hepatocytes predominantly via the sodium-dependent cotransporter NTCP, in addition to the sodium-independent uptake transporters OATP1B1 and OATP1B3. ATP-dependent efflux of glycine and taurine conjugates of bile acids into bile is mediated by the bile salt export pump BSEP (ABCB11). Basolateral efflux is mediated by MRP4 (ABCC4) in a co-transport process with reduced glutathione[2,10]. Efflux into sinusoidal blood is also possible via OSTα+OSTβ[12]. **B**: Under conditions of impaired BSEP activity[20] or in obstructive cholestasis, MRP4 is up-regulated[19–21] and serves as a pathway for bile acid efflux from hepatocytes into sinusoidal blood. Cycling of bile acids enhances the time for bile acid conjugation in hepatocytes. Bile acid sulphates and glucuronosides are substrates for MRP3, in addition to the excretion of sulphoconjugates via MRP4, via canalicular MRP2, and via BCRP (not indicated in the scheme)

human MRP4 was demonstrated in patients with hereditary deficiency of BSEP (ABCB11)[20]; this is in line with the function of MRP4 as a bile acid efflux pump[2,10]. Moreover, knockout mice lacking Mrp4 were more susceptible to liver damage associated with bile duct ligation[21].

THE CONCEPT OF HEPATOCELLULAR BILE ACID CYCLING

The discovery and localization of basolateral efflux pumps in the hepatocyte[1–3,15,16] raised the question of the cycling of bile acids and their conjugates (Figure 1). Efflux into sinusoidal blood via MRP4 and possibly OSTα+OSTβ is required when the rate of sinusoidal bile acid uptake into hepatocytes via NTCP, OATP1B1, and OATP1B3 exceeds the capacity of the bile acid efflux pump (BSEP) in the canalicular membrane. Re-entry from the sinusoidal blood into (neighbouring) hepatocytes provides for a higher probability for the formation of bile acid conjugates that are substrates for MRP3 and MRP2, in addition to MRP4. It is of interest in this context that cholate is not a substrate for human BSEP[22] and must undergo conjugation prior to efflux into bile. It has been known for a long time that obstructive cholestasis is associated with hepatic formation of bile acid glucuronosides and sulphates that are ultimately excreted into urine[23–26]. Thus, bile acid cycling, particularly under conditions of cholestasis, extends the time of exposure of bile acids to conjugating enzymes and the possibility of efflux of the conjugates via MRP3 and MRP4, ultimately resulting in renal excretion (Figure 1). In case of a selectively impaired function of BSEP in the canalicular membrane, glucuronosyl and sulphoconjugates can be effluxed into bile via MRP2 (ABCC2) or BCRP (ABCG2).

CONCLUSION

Basolateral efflux pumps serve to maintain the balance when the rate of uptake of bile acids exceeds canalicular secretion. The major efflux pumps involved in this process are MRP4 and MRP3. OSTα+OSTβ may contribute to basolateral bile acid efflux. Cycling of bile acids via basolateral efflux and re-entry into hepatocytes increases the time for hydroxylation and conjugation, leading to metabolites that are substrates for additional efflux pathways including MRP2. In cholestasis, basolateral efflux pumps serve as overflow pathways releasing sulphoconjugates (MRP4) and glucuronosides (MRP3) into sinusoidal blood, leading to the renal elimination of these metabolites.

References

1. König J, Rost D, Cui Y, Keppler D. Characterization of the human multidrug resistance protein isoform MRP3 localized to the basolateral hepatocyte membrane. Hepatology. 1999;29:1156–63.
2. Rius M, Nies AT, Hummel-Eisenbeiss J, Jedlitschky G, Keppler D. Cotransport of reduced glutathione with bile salts by MRP4 (ABCC4) localized to the basolateral hepatocyte membrane. Hepatology. 2003;38:374–84.

3. Keppler D, König J, Nies AT. Conjugate export pumps of the multidrug resistance protein (MRP) family in liver. In: Arias IM, Boyer JL, Chisari FV, Fausto N, Schachter D, Shafritz DA, editors. The Liver: Biology and Pathobiology. New York: Lippincott Williams & Wilkins, 2001:373–82.
4. Deeley RG, Westlake C, Cole SP. Transmembrane transport of endo- and xenobiotics by mammalian ATP-binding cassette multidrug resistance proteins. Physiol Rev. 2006;86:849–99.
5. Akita H, Suzuki H, Hirohashi T, Takikawa H, Sugiyama Y. Transport activity of human MRP3 expressed in Sf9 cells: comparative studies with rat MRP3. Pharm Res. 2002;19:34–41.
6. Lee YM, Cui Y, König J et al. Identification and functional characterization of the natural variant MRP3-Arg1297His of human multidrug resistance protein 3 (MRP3/ABCC3). Pharmacogenetics. 2004;14:213–23.
7. Kruh GD, Belinsky MG. The MRP family of drug efflux pumps. Oncogene. 2003;22:7537–52.
8. Zelcer N, Reid G, Wielinga P et al. Steroid and bile acid conjugates are substrates of human multidrug-resistance protein (MRP) 4 (ATP-binding cassette C4). Biochem J. 2003;371:361–7.
9. van Aubel RA, Smeets PH, Peters JG, Bindels RJ, Russel FG. The MRP4/ABCC4 gene encodes a novel apical organic anion transporter in human kidney proximal tubules: putative efflux pump for urinary cAMP and cGMP. J Am Soc Nephrol. 2002;13:595–603.
10. Rius M, Hummel-Eisenbeiss J, Hofmann AF, Keppler D. Substrate specificity of human ABCC4 (MRP4)-mediated cotransport of bile acids and reduced glutathione. Am J Physiol Gastrointest Liver Physiol. 2006;290:G640–9.
11. Ilias A, Urban Z, Seidl TL et al. Loss of ATP-dependent transport activity in pseudoxanthoma elasticum-associated mutants of human ABCC6 (MRP6). J Biol Chem. 2002;277:16860–7.
12. Ballatori N, Christian WV, Lee JY et al. OSTalpha-OSTbeta: a major basolateral bile acid and steroid transporter in human intestinal, renal, and biliary epithelia. Hepatology. 2005;42:1270–9.
13. Hagenbuch B, Meier PJ. Organic anion transporting polypeptides of the OATP/ SLC21 family: phylogenetic classification as OATP/SLCO superfamily, new nomenclature and molecular/functional properties. Pflugers Arch. 2004;447:653–65.
14. Li L, Meier PJ, Ballatori N. Oatp2 mediates bidirectional organic solute transport: a role for intracellular glutathione. Mol Pharmacol. 2000;58:335–40.
15. Mayer R, Kartenbeck J, Büchler M, Jedlitschky G, Leier I, Keppler D. Expression of the *MRP* gene-encoded conjugate export pump in liver and its selective absence from the canalicular membrane in transport-deficient mutant hepatocytes. J Cell Biol. 1995;131:137–50.
16. Keppler D, Kartenbeck J. The canalicular conjugate export pump encoded by the *cmrp/ cmoat* gene. In: Boyer JL, Ockner RK, editors. Progress in Liver Diseases. Philadelphia: Saunders, 1996:55–67.
17. Donner MG, Keppler D. Up-regulation of basolateral multidrug resistance protein 3 (Mrp3) in cholestatic rat liver. Hepatology. 2001;34:351–9.
18. Soroka CJ, Lee JM, Azzaroli F, Boyer JL. Cellular localization and up-regulation of multidrug resistance-associated protein 3 in hepatocytes and cholangiocytes during obstructive cholestasis in rat liver. Hepatology. 2001;33:783–91.
19. Wagner M, Fickert P, Zollner G et al. Role of farnesoid X receptor in determining hepatic ABC transporter expression and liver injury in bile duct-ligated mice. Gastroenterology. 2003;125:825–38.
20. Keitel V, Burdelski M, Warskulat U et al. Expression and localization of hepatobiliary transport proteins in progressive familial intrahepatic cholestasis. Hepatology. 2005;41:1160–72.
21. Mennone A, Soroka CJ, Cai SY et al. Mrp4$^{-/-}$ mice have an impaired cytoprotective response in obstructive cholestasis. Hepatology. 2006;43:1013–21.
22. Noe J, Stieger B, Meier PJ. Functional expression of the canalicular bile salt export pump of human liver. Gastroenterology. 2002;123:1659–66.
23. Frohling W, Stiehl A. Bile salt glucuronides: identification and quantitative analysis in the urine of patients with cholestasis. Eur J Clin Invest. 1976;6:67–74.

24. Stiehl A, Raedsch R, Rudolph G, Gundert-Remy U, Senn M. Biliary and urinary excretion of sulfated, glucuronidated and tetrahydroxylated bile acids in cirrhotic patients. Hepatology. 1985;5:492–5.
25. Takikawa H, Beppu T, Seyama Y. Urinary concentrations of bile acid glucuronides and sulfates in hepatobiliary diseases. Gastroenterol Jpn. 1984;19:104–9.
26. Back P. Bile acid glucuronides. Isolation and identification of a chenodeoxycholic acid glucuronide from human plasma in intrahepatic cholestasis. Hoppe Seylers Z Physiol Chem. 1976;357:213–17.

7
Insights into the regulation of expression of human OSTα-OSTβ

C. J. SOROKA, S. XU, S.-Y. CAI, N. BALLATORI and J. L. BOYER

INTRODUCTION

The organic solute transporter (OSTα-OSTβ) is a heteromeric transporter of bile acids and other organic solutes and steroids. In humans, OSTα-OSTβ is found predominantly in epithelial cells of liver, intestine, kidney, adrenal gland, and testis[1]. It is expressed on the basolateral membrane of these cells and has been shown[1,2] to transport oestrone 3-sulphate, taurocholate, digoxin, dehydroepiandrosterone 3-sulphate and prostaglandin E_2.

This transporter was originally cloned from the liver of the small skate, *Leucoraja erinacea*, and was subsequently found to have orthologues in mammals, including humans, rats and mice[2]. In the process of cloning the transporter it was noted that transport activity required the coexpression of two distinct gene products. The first was a predicted 340-amino acid protein with seven membrane-spanning domains that was given the name Ostα. The second gene product was a 128-amino acid, single membrane-spanning protein named Ostβ. Transport with these two gene products was found to be sodium-independent and saturable[2]. Furthermore, transport did not require ATP and was not affected by changes in transmembrane Na^+, K^+, Cl^-, or H^+ gradients[3]. Transport is bidirectional across the plasma membrane, and most likely occurs by facilitated diffusion of substrates down their electrochemical gradients[3].

REGULATION OF EXPRESSION

In rodents, Ostα-Ostβ is expressed predominantly in the ileum and kidney[3,4]. This led Dawson and colleagues[4] to investigate its role in the basolateral efflux of bile acids from the terminal ileum into the mesenteric circulation. Using the Slc10a2 (Asbt) null mouse they demonstrated that Ostα-Ostβ is most likely the elusive intestinal basolateral bile acid efflux transporter[4]. Thus, in the absence of Slc10a2, ileal bile acid uptake was decreased, resulting in decreased Ostα-Ostβ expression. On the other hand, the increased flux of bile acids into the caecum and colon of these animals resulted in an increase in Ostα-Ostβ expression in these segments, suggesting that bile acids can regulate the expression of these proteins. Bile acid regulation of Ostα and Ostβ expression has now been confirmed in a number of studies[5-9].

Cholestasis is a condition in which bile acids cannot be properly excreted from the hepatocyte into the bile. In this situation the hepatocyte regulates expression of both bile acid uptake and efflux mechanisms in order to prevent further liver injury due to the accumulation of toxic bile acids. When livers from patients with primary biliary cirrhosis were examined, OSTα-OSTβ was significantly up-regulated at both the mRNA and protein levels[5]. This effect of cholestasis was confirmed in rodents subjected to common bile duct ligation (CBDL), although there appeared to be significant species variability primarily due to the low level of liver expression of Ostα-Ostβ in rodents. The significant increase in rat Ostβ mRNA was found primarily in the hepatocytes rather than cholangiocytes. Also, treatment of a human hepatoma cell line, HepG2 cells, with chenodeoxycholic acid (CDCA) significantly induced the expression of OSTα-OSTβ[5].

The ability of bile acids to regulate the expression of OSTα-OSTβ was subsequently determined to be through the action of the bile acid-activated nuclear receptor, the farnesoid X receptor (FXR). FXR null mice demonstrated no up-regulation of Ostβ mRNA after CBDL, unlike their wild-type controls[5]. This regulation of Ostα-Ostβ by FXR has been confirmed for liver, adrenal gland and intestine[6-9]. FXR response elements also have been identified in human OSTα-OSTβ[7].

REGULATION OF CELLULAR LOCALIZATION AND FUNCTION

As noted above, functional transport activity requires the expression of both subunits. Early experiments using the oocyte expression system determined that there was complete functional complementation between the alpha and beta subunits from different species. Thus, human OSTα was activated not only by human OSTβ, but by the beta subunits of mouse or skate, and likewise, human OSTβ was activated not only by human OSTα, but by the alpha subunits of mouse or skate[1]. Although expression of single subunits in the oocyte system could result in membrane expression of at least some of the proteins, transport activity required the expression of both subunits[1]. In a mammalian expression system, Dawson and colleagues[4] demonstrated that plasma membrane expression and functional transport required expression of both subunits. Furthermore, they demonstrated that glycosylation of Ostα occurred only in the presence of Ostβ, thus suggesting that expression of both subunits was necessary for trafficking of the transporter out of the Golgi to the plasma membrane. However, it is still unclear how the two subunits are interacting, the relative contribution of the individual subunits to the functional activity, and the stoichiometry of their interaction.

Recent studies in HepG2 cells indicate that the stimulated expression and functional activity of OSTα-OSTβ by CDCA require both transcription and translation[10]. This suggests that a significant pool of transporters is not waiting within the cell to be trafficked to the plasma membrane. Furthermore, plasma membrane localization of human OSTα and functional activity of the intact transporter was not affected when N-glycosylation was inhibited with tunicamycin[10]. However, the presence of OSTβ is essential for the movement of OSTα to the plasma membrane. This again suggests that OSTβ is acting as a chaperone to move the transporter out of the Golgi and to the plasma membrane.

Preliminary studies by Sun and co-workers[11] show that trafficking of OSTα-OSTβ to the apical membrane in stably transfected MDCK cells is not affected by treatment with nocodazole or colchicine. However, the apical localization was effected by treatment with cytochalasin D and bafilomycin A1, suggesting a role for actin microfilaments and vacuolar H^+-ATPase in the plasma membrane sorting. Brefeldin A treatment resulted in the accumulation of OSTα-OSTβ in the ER region of the cell.

SUMMARY

The organic solute transporter, OSTα-OSTβ, is a heteromeric transporter on the basolateral membrane of epithelial cells in the liver, intestine, testis, kidney, and adrenal gland. Its expression is regulated by bile acids in an FXR-dependent manner. Thus, it is up-regulated in cholestatic liver injury and is down-regulated in the ileum if bile acids cannot be taken up into the ileocyte. Both the alpha and beta subunits are required for the functional activity of the transporter, although it is still unclear whether this requirement is solely for the trafficking of the transporter or is also necessary for solute transport. Additional studies are needed to understand the mechanism by which the subunits interact.

Acknowledgements

This study was supported by National Institutes of Health grants DK25636 and DK P30-34989.

References

1. Seward DJ, Koh AS, Boyer JL, Ballatori N. Functional complementation between a novel mammalian polygenic transport complex and an evolutionarily ancient organic solute transporter, OSTα-OSTβ. J Biol Chem. 2003;278:27473–82.
2. Wang W, Seward DJ, Li L, Boyer JL, Ballatori N. Expression cloning of two genes that together mediate organic solute and steroid transport in the liver of a marine vertebrate. Proc Natl Acad Sci USA. 2001;98:9431–6.
3. Ballatori N, Christian WV, Lee JY et al. OSTα-OSTβ: a major basolateral bile acid and steroid transporter in human intestinal, renal, and biliary epithelia. Hepatology. 2005;42:1270–9.
4. Dawson PA, Hubbert M, Haywood J et al. The heteromeric organic solute transporter alpha-beta, Ostα-Ostβ, is an ileal basolateral bile acid transporter. J Biol Chem. 2005;280: 6960–8.
5. Boyer JL, Trauner M, Mennone A et al. Up-regulation of a basolateral FXR-dependent bile acid efflux transporter, OSTalpha-OSTbeta, in cholestasis in humans and rodents. Am J Physiol Gastrointest Liver Physiol. 2006;290:G1124–30.

6. Frankenberg T, Rao A, Chen F, Haywood J, Shneider BL, Dawson PA. Regulation of the mouse organic solute transporter alpha-beta, Ostalpha-Ostbeta, by bile acids. Am J Physiol Gastrointest Liver Physiol. 2005;290:G912–22.
7. Landrier JF, Eloranta JJ, Vavricka SR, Kullak-Ublick GA. The nuclear receptor for bile acids, FXR, transactivates the human organic solute transporter-alpha and -beta genes. Am J Physiol Gastrointest Liver Physiol. 2005;290:G476–85.
8. Lee H, Zhang Y, Lee FY, Nelson SF, Gonzalez FJ, Edwards PA. FXR regulates organic solute transporters alpha and beta in the adrenal gland, kidney, and intestine. J Lipid Res. 2006;47:201–14.
9. Zollner G, Wagner M, Moustafa T et al. Coordinated induction of bile acid detoxification and alternative elimination in mice: role of FXR-regulated organic solute transporter-alpha/beta in the adaptive response to bile acids. Am J Physiol Gastrointest Liver Physiol. 2006;290:G923–32.
10. Soroka, CJ, Xu S, Cai S-Y, Ballatori N, and Boyer JL. Mechanism of OSTαlpha-OSTβeta subunit expression and function in HepG2 cells. Hepatology. 2006;44(Suppl. 1):93A.
11. Sun A-Q, Balasubramaniyan N, Ponamgi V, Suchy F. Mechanisms of plasma membrane trafficking of human organic solute transporter (HOST). Hepatology. 2006;44(Suppl. 1): 380A.

8
Regulation of hepatobiliary transport proteins in chronic cholestasis

R. KUBITZ, V. KEITEL, M. BURDELSKI and D. HÄUSSINGER

Bile salts are essential for cholesterol excretion and lipid absorption. Nonetheless, increased bile salt concentrations have numerous injurious effects. These effects result from intrahepatic or extrahepatic accumulation of bile salts. Intrahepatic rise of bile salt concentration disturbs cholesterol biosynthesis[1], may cause cell damage and hepatocellular apoptosis[2] and can influence the responsiveness of hepatocytes towards antiviral interferon signalling[3]. An extrahepatocytic increase in bile salt levels may alter general metabolism[4], and influences cytokine secretion by immune cells[5]. Furthermore, elevated bile salt levels are responsible for pruritus and adverse effects for the fetus in intrahepatic cholestasis of pregnancy[6] and may increase the susceptibility to gallstone formation.

Under healthy conditions intracellular and extracellular bile salt homeostasis is controlled by phase I and II metabolizing enzymes as well as a number of uptake and efflux transporters, distributed over the sinusoidal and canalicular membrane of hepatocytes[7-10]. These enzymes and transporters are regulated by a complex signalling network, including bile salt sensors (nuclear receptors, kinases, membrane receptors) and downstream signalling pathways (MAP kinases, PKC, Src kinases, etc.). This network protects the liver and the body from toxic effects of bile salts. In cholestasis bile salt levels are increased, which may indicate active as well as impaired protective mechanisms.

The pathogenesis of cholestasis has mostly been studied in animal models[11-13]; however, significant species differences prohibit a direct transposition of the results to humans. We have studied livers of 10 children with progressive familial intrahepatic cholestasis type 2 and 3 (PFIC-2 and -3), who carried genetic mutations within the genes of the bile salt export pump *BSEP* (*ABCB11*) or the multidrug resistance protein 3 (*MDR3; ABCB4*)[14]. These genetic defects resulted in bile salt concentrations ranging between 47 and 616 µmol/L (normal <8 µmol/L). All children received a liver transplant between $2\frac{1}{2}$ and $10\frac{1}{2}$ years of age. Transporters were studied in explanted livers in terms of mRNA, protein expression and localization, comprising three of five major levels of transporter regulation.

Bilirubin levels were increased to 9.3 ± 8.9 mg/dl (normal < 1.1 mg/dl) and ranged from 0.5 to 22.7 mg/dl. In PFIC livers multidrug resistance associated protein 2 (MRP2; ABCC2)-mRNA and MRP2-protein were diminished to 60% and 53%, respectively, as compared to controls. There was no correlation between bilirubin concentrations and MRP2-mRNA, MRP2-protein or bile salt concentrations. However, jaundice roughly paralleled to the severity of liver cirrhosis.

Expressions of the sinusoidal bile salt uptake transporter OATP2 (OATP1B1) and OATP8 (OATP1B3) was reduced at the mRNA (to 83% and 44%) and protein (to 30% and 24%) level, whereas NTCP (SCL10A1) was only reduced at the protein level (46% compared to controls). NTCP-mRNA in PFIC livers was similar to mRNA levels in control livers (115%), pointing to a post-transcriptional mechanism of NTCP down-regulation. On immunofluorescence staining, OATP2, OATP8 and NTCP were all significantly reduced.

MRP3 (ABCC3)[15,16] and MRP4 (ABCC4)[17], two potential sinusoidal bile salt efflux pumps, were regulated differently: MRP3-mRNA and protein were not significantly changed in PFIC livers compared to controls. MRP4-mRNA was increased by 2.8- and 6.1-fold in PFIC-2 and PFIC-3 livers, respectively. MRP4 protein was even more increased, by 7.6-fold (PFIC-2) and 14.1-fold (PFIC-3) as compared to controls, which was confirmed by immunofluorescence. MRP4 has recently been shown to transport bile salts

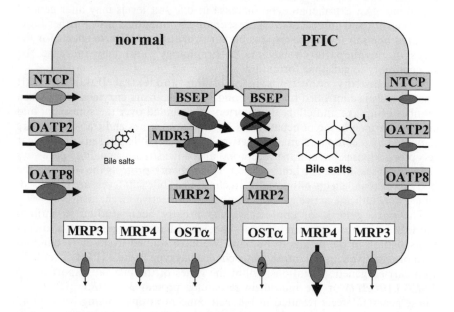

Figure 1 Simplified scheme of changes in hepatic transporter proteins under normal and cholestatic conditions as observed in progressive familial intrahepatic cholestasis (PFIC). The sizes of the ovals and arrows represent the level of protein expression and assumed activity of the respective transporter.

with similar K_m values as reported for BSEP[18], thus up-regulation of MRP4 may represent a mechanism for hepatocytes to eliminate intracellular bile salts across the sinusoidal membrane at the expense of the extracellular space. In line with our findings, MRP4 knockout mice were more susceptible to liver damage after common bile duct ligation than wild-type mice, and had lower serum bile salt levels[19]. MRP3 and OSTα/OSTβ were up-regulated in these animals but were unable to compensate for the loss of MRP4[19]. Mice lacking MRP3 showed a reduced sinusoidal excretion of glucuronidated compounds and decreased serum bilirubin levels as compared to wild-type[20]. Changes in bile salt homeostasis were not observed in these animals[20]. OSTα-OSTβ is a heterodimeric bile salt transporter, which is localized in the sinusoidal membrane of hepatocytes[21,22]. A recent study in patients with primary biliary cirrhosis, and mice with common bile duct ligation, found a significant up-regulation of both OSTα- and OSTβ-mRNA and protein, indicating that OSTα-OSTβ may represent yet another protective mechanism by which bile salts are transported out of the hepatocyte into the sinusoidal blood under cholestatic conditions[22].

CONCLUSION

Our results suggest that down-regulation of all sinusoidal uptake transporters involved in bile acid uptake represents an important adaptive response when canalicular bile salt secretion is compromised. Up-regulation of MRP4 but not of MRP3 seems to be a major escape mechanism, which shifts bile salts from hepatocytes into the blood in order to protect liver parenchymal cells. Thus, regulation of transporter proteins in severe cholestasis includes protective and compensative mechanisms.

Acknowledgement

The work of the authors was supported by grants from the Deutsche Forschungsgemeinschaft through Sonderforschungsbereich 575 Düsseldorf.

References

1. Oude Elferink RP, Groen AK. Genetic defects in hepatobiliary transport. Biochim Biophys Acta. 2002;1586:129–45.
2. Reinehr R, Becker S, Wettstein M, Haussinger D. Involvement of the Src family kinase yes in bile salt-induced apoptosis. Gastroenterology. 2004;127:1540–57.
3. Podevin P, Rosmorduc O, Conti F, Calmus Y, Meier PJ, Poupon R. Bile acids modulate the interferon signalling pathway. Hepatology. 1999;29:1840–7.
4. Watanabe M, Houten SM, Mataki C et al. Bile acids induce energy expenditure by promoting intracellular thyroid hormone activation. Nature. 2006;439:484–9.
5. Kawamata Y, Fujii R, Hosoya M et al. A G protein-coupled receptor responsive to bile acids. J Biol Chem. 2003;278:9435–40.
6. Glantz A, Marschall HU, Mattsson LA. Intrahepatic cholestasis of pregnancy: relationships between bile acid levels and fetal complication rates. Hepatology. 2004;40: 467–74.
7. Kullak-Ublick GA, Stieger B, Meier PJ. Enterohepatic bile salt transporters in normal physiology and liver disease. Gastroenterology. 2004;126:322–42.

8.   Chiang JY. Bile acid regulation of gene expression: roles of nuclear hormone receptors. Endocrinol Rev. 2002;23:443–63.
9.   Eloranta JJ, Kullak-Ublick GA. Coordinate transcriptional regulation of bile acid homeostasis and drug metabolism. Arch Biochem Biophys. 2005;433:397–412.
10. Zollner G, Marschall HU, Wagner M, Trauner M. Role of nuclear receptors in the adaptive response to bile acids and cholestasis: pathogenetic and therapeutic considerations. Mol Pharm. 2006;3:231–51.
11. Pawlikowska L, Groen A, Eppens EF et al. A mouse genetic model for familial cholestasis caused by ATP8B1 mutations reveals perturbed bile salt homeostasis but no impairment in bile secretion. Hum Mol Genet. 2004;13:881–92.
12. Wang R, Salem M, Yousef IM et al. Targeted inactivation of sister of P-glycoprotein gene (spgp) in mice results in nonprogressive but persistent intrahepatic cholestasis. Proc Natl Acad Sci USA. 2001;98:2011–16.
13. Smit JJ, Schinkel AH, Oude Elferink RP et al. Homozygous disruption of the murine mdr2 P-glycoprotein gene leads to a complete absence of phospholipid from bile and to liver disease. Cell. 1993;75:451–62.
14. Keitel V, Burdelski M, Warskulat U et al. Expression and localization of hepatobiliary transport proteins in progressive familial intrahepatic cholestasis. Hepatology. 2005;41: 1160–72.
15. Kiuchi Y, Suzuki H, Hirohashi T, Tyson CA, Sugiyama Y. cDNA cloning and inducible expression of human multidrug resistance associated protein 3 (MRP3). FEBS Lett. 1998; 433:149–52.
16. König J, Rost D, Cui Y, Keppler D. Characterization of the human multidrug resistance protein isoform MRP3 localized to the basolateral hepatocyte membrane. Hepatology. 1999;29:1156–63.
17. Rius M, Nies AT, Hummel-Eisenbeiss J, Jedlitschky G, Keppler D. Cotransport of reduced glutathione with bile salts by MRP4 (ABCC4) localized to the basolateral hepatocyte membrane. Hepatology. 2003;38:374–84.
18. Rius M, Hummel-Eisenbeiss J, Hofmann AF, Keppler D. Substrate specificity of human ABCC4 (MRP4)-mediated cotransport of bile acids and reduced glutathione. Am J Physiol Gastrointest Liver Physiol. 2006;290:G640–9.
19. Mennone A, Soroka CJ, Cai SY et al. Mrp4$^{-/-}$ mice have an impaired cytoprotective response in obstructive cholestasis. Hepatology. 2006;43:1013–21.
20. Zelcer N, van de Wetering K, de Waart R et al. Mice lacking Mrp3 (Abcc3) have normal bile salt transport, but altered hepatic transport of endogenous glucuronides. J Hepatol. 2006;44:768–75.
21. Ballatori N, Christian WV, Lee JY et al. OSTalpha-OSTbeta: a major basolateral bile acid and steroid transporter in human intestinal, renal, and biliary epithelia. Hepatology. 2005; 42:1270–9.
22. Boyer JL, Trauner M, Mennone A et al. Upregulation of a basolateral FXR-dependent bile acid efflux transporter OSTalpha-OSTbeta in cholestasis in humans and rodents. Am J Physiol Gastrointest Liver Physiol. 2006;290:G1124–30.

9
Assessment of inhibitory effect of many therapeutically important drugs on bile acid transport by NTCP, BSEP and other transporters

K. MAEDA, Y. TIAN, S. MITA, H. SUZUKI, H. AKITA, H. HAYASHI, R. ONUKI, A. F. HOFMANN and Y. SUGIYAMA

INTRODUCTION

The vectorial transport of bile acids from blood into bile is one of the major driving forces of bile flow, and active transporters are involved in this process. In general, bile acids are taken up into liver, mainly by NTCP (Na^+-taurocholate cotransporting polypeptide) and excreted into bile mainly by BSEP (bile salt export pump), which results in their effective enterohepatic circulation. Many reports have shown that biliary excretion of bile acids can be interrupted by several factors such as pathophysiological conditions, mutations in transporters and some compounds. Especially some drugs such as cyclosporin A, bosentan, rifampicin and ritonavir unfavourably caused drug-induced intrahepatic cholestasis, and these drugs are reported to inhibit BSEP function potently[1–3]. The thiazolidinediones (TZD) (troglitazone, pioglitazone and rosiglitazone) are a new class of drugs targeting to PPARγ nuclear receptor for the treatment of diabetes mellitus. Troglitazone, the first TZD, launched in 1997, appeared to be harmless during pre-marketing clinical trials. However, because some people have been killed by serious liver damage induced by troglitazone, it was withdrawn from the market in 2000. The mechanisms underlying troglitazone-associated hepatotoxicity have not yet been clarified. Though the severe hepatotoxicity caused by troglitazone seems to be idiosyncratic, one of the possible mechanisms of hepatotoxicity is that troglitazone sulphate, which is the main metabolite of troglitazone and highly concentrated into liver, potently inhibits the BSEP-mediated transport of bile acids[4,5]. Recently case reports concerning the pioglitazone-induced liver damage have also been published[6], but it is unknown whether these drugs can also inhibit the transport of bile acids.

Certain type of drugs also inhibited the transporters involving hepatic uptake (OATP1B1 and OATP1B3) and efflux (MRP2 and BCRP) of organic anions. This sometimes caused transporter-mediated drug–drug interactions. For example, drug interaction between cerivastatin and gemfibrozil, a novel PPARα agonist for the treatment of hyperdyslipidaemia, is caused by the inhibition of CYP2C8-mediated metabolism as well as OATP1B1-mediated uptake of cerivastatin by gemfibrozil glucuronide, which is extensively formed in liver[7]. Now several PPARα/γ dual agonists are being developed for the treatment of diabetes with avoidance of obesity, a well-known side-effect of PPARα agonists. Because PPAR is a novel important target of drugs for the treatment of lifestyle-related diseases, we checked the inhibitory effects of PPARα, γ and α/γ dual agonists on the transporter-mediated uptake and efflux of bile acids and organic anions, and especially for PPARγ agonists. We also investigated the relationship between the hepatic concentration of PPARγ agonists and increase in plasma bile acid level.

To avoid drug-induced cholestasis in the early phase of drug development, it is desirable to predict the inhibitory effects of drugs on bile acid transport easily and rapidly. Therefore, we have constructed a novel *in-vitro* assay system, NTCP/BSEP double transfectant[8] and characterized the inhibitory effects of some cholestatic drugs on bile acid transport (Figure 1).

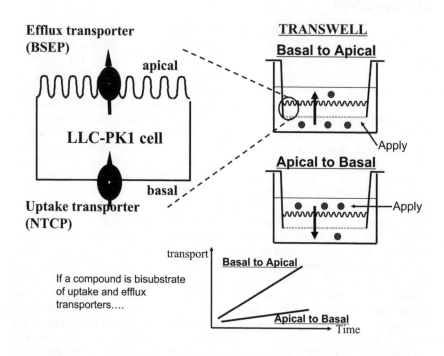

Figure 1   Schematic diagram of the experiments using double transfectants

METHODS

In-vitro experiments to clarify the inhibitory effects of drugs on uptake and efflux transporters

For uptake transporters (OATP1B1, OATP1B3, NTCP), we have constructed stable transfectants expressing each transporter as described previously[8,9]. Cells were seeded on 12-well plates (OATP) or transwell membrane inserts (NTCP) and cultured for 2 days. Then the expression of each transporter was induced by replacing the medium with fresh medium containing 10 mM sodium butyrate. After induction for 24 h an uptake assay was performed as described previously[8,9]. Oestradiol-17β-glucuronide ($O_2$17βG) (for OATP1B1), cholecystokinin octapeptide (for OATP1B3) and taurocholate (for NTCP) were selected as typical substrates.

For efflux transporters (BSEP, MRP2, BCRP), the vesicle transport study was performed using the rapid filtration technique described previously[10]. HEK293 cells were infected with the recombinant adenovirus for each transporter, and transporter-expressing membrane vesicles were prepared in the normal procedure. Then ATP-dependent uptake of substrate into membrane vesicles was evaluated in the presence of several concentrations of inhibitors. Sulphobromophthalein (for MRP2), taurocholate (for BSEP) and oestrone-3-sulphate (for BCRP) were selected as typical substrates.

In-vivo analysis of the cholestatic potentials of PPARγ agonists

Following anaesthesia using an intraperitoneal injection of urethane (1.5 g/kg), male SD rats (200–250 g) were given a single intravenous dose of PPARγ agonists (troglitazone (10 mg/kg), pioglitazone (2.5 or 10 mg/kg) and rosiglitazone (0.5 or 2 mg/kg)), dissolved in glycofurol. Control rats were treated with the same volume of glycofurol. After drug application, the blood samples were collected at designated times. Rats were sacrificed at the end of the experiment and the liver was excised. The concentration of troglitazone, troglitazone sulphate, pioglitazone and rosiglitazone in plasma and liver was determined by LC/MS and the plasma level of total bile acids was measured colorimetrically using a commercially available test kit (TBA Wako test kit).

Transcellular transport study using NTCP/BSEP double-transfected cells

We have constructed double-transfected LLC-PK1 cells expressing human NTCP and BSEP as described previously[8] (Figure 1). Cells were seeded on transwell culture inserts and cultured for 2 days. Then the expression of transporters was induced by replacing the medium with fresh medium containing 10 mM sodium butyrate. After induction for 24 h, the transcellular transport study was performed. After wash and preincubation with transport buffer, this experiment was initiated by the addition of substrate into the apical or basal compartment. At a designated time an aliquot of medium in the opposite compartment was sampled and the amount of ligand was measured. If a compound is a bisubstrate of uptake and efflux transporters, the basal-to-apical transcellular transport is significantly larger than that in the opposite direction. Basal-to-apical trancellular transport clearance (PS_{b-a}) was calculated by dividing the increasing velocity of compound in the apical compartment (V_{apical}) by the initial concentration in the basal compartment. The efflux clearance across the apical membrane (PS_{apical}) was calculated by dividing V_{apical} by intracellular concentration. In the inhibition assay, [^{3}H] taurocholate was used as a typical substrate of NTCP/BSEP.

RESULTS AND DISCUSSION

Inhibitory effects of PPAR agonists on transporter-mediated transport

We checked the inhibitory effects of several kinds of PPARα agonists (gemfibrozil, clofibrate, bezafibrate and fenofibrate), PPARγ agonists (troglitazone, pioglitazone, rosiglitazone) and PPARα/γ dual agonists (tesaglitazar, muraglitazar and LM4156) on the transport activity of uptake (NTCP, OATP1B1, OATP1B3) and efflux (BSEP, BCRP, MRP2) transporters. We also compared the inhibition potency of the conjugated metabolites of troglitazone, troglitazone sulphate and troglitazone glucuronide, with that of troglitazone itself. Among these compounds PPARγ agonists and metabolites of troglitazone potently inhibited the NTCP-mediated uptake of taurocholate. Dual PPARα/γ agonists moderately inhibited the uptake of taurocholate, while PPARα agonists showed relatively weak inhibitory effects on its uptake (> 58% of control (100 μM)). K_i values of troglitazone and troglitazone sulphate were 0.886 ± 0.132 and 0.739 ± 0.246 μM, respectively. Regarding OATP1B1 and OATP1B3, PPARα agonists had slight inhibitory effects on OATP1B1- and OATP1B3-mediated uptake. Among PPARα agonists, gemfibrozil showed the strongest inhibitory effect on OATP1B1-mediated $O_2 17βG$ uptake with a K_i value of 51.4 ± 17.8 μM. For PPARγ agonists, troglitazone and its metabolites showed the potent inhibitory effects on OATP1B1 and OATP1B3. Especially K_i values of troglitazone, its sulphate and glucuronide for OATP1B1 were 0.278 ± 0.033, 0.0374 ± 0.0072 and 0.113 ± 0.031 μM, respectively. Dual PPARα/γ agonists also inhibited the uptake mediated by OATP1B1 and OATP1B3 to some extent. Among them, K_i values of muraglitazar and LM4156 were relatively low (0.733 ± 0.180 and 1.45 ± 0.13 μM, respectively). After oral administration of 600 mg troglitazone, the clinical maximum unbound concentration of troglitazone and its sulphate in plasma is about 12 nM and 0.4 μM, respectively. The K_i value of troglitazone sulphate for OATP1B1 was lower than its clinical concentration, suggesting that the troglitazone sulphate may inhibit the OATP1B1-mediated uptake in the clinical situation. Though the other PPARγ agonists potently inhibited some uptake transporters, the clinical maximum unbound concentration of pioglitazone and rosiglitazone in plasma was less than 30 and 2.5 nM, respectively, which is much smaller than their K_i values, indicating that inhibition of uptake transporters by pioglitazone and rosiglitazone in the clinical situation unlikely occurred.

Regarding the efflux transporters, PPARγ agonists relatively showed strong inhibition potency for each transporter compared with other categories of drugs. Among PPARγ agonists, troglitazone and its conjugates showed the potent inhibitory effects on the transport by all efflux transporters we tested; 100 μM of PPARα/γ dual agonists almost inhibited the BCRP-mediated uptake of oestrone-3-sulphate. On the other hand, except for bezafibrate for BCRP, PPARα agonists did not affect the transport mediated by BSEP, BCRP and MRP2 even at a concentration of 100 μM. For BSEP, other than troglitazone and its metabolites as previously reported[4], pioglitazone, rosiglitazone and muraglitazar showed a relatively high affinity for human BSEP with K_i values of 0.183 ± 0.044, 2.36 ± 0.27 and 4.53 ± 1.04 μM, respectively.

Species difference in the inhibitory effects of PPARγ agonists on the BSEP-mediated transport of taurocholate

Interestingly, species differences in the inhibitory effects of PPARγ agonists on the BSEP-mediated taurocholate transport between rats and humans were observed. The K_i values of troglitazone sulphate for human BSEP and rat Bsep were almost the same (5.44 ± 1.07 and 2.47 ± 0.48 μM, respectively). However, in the case of pioglitazone and rosiglitazone, human BSEP-mediated transport drastically decreased even at 10 μM, whereas rat Bsep-mediated transport was not significantly inhibited by 100 μM ligands (Figure 2). This result suggested that information on the cholestatic potencies of drugs in animal experiments is sometimes not adequate for the prediction of cholestatic effects in humans due to the great species difference in K_i values between human BSEP and rat Bsep.

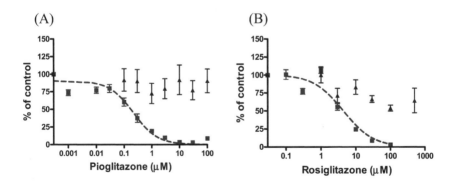

Figure 2 Inhibitory effects of pioglitazone (**A**) and rosiglitazone (**B**) on the transport of taurocholate in membrane vesicles expressing rat Bsep and human BSEP. Squares and triangles represent the data for human BSEP and rat Bsep, respectively

Rat *in-vivo* experiments to observe the PPARγ agonist-induced increase in the total bile acids in plasma and its relation with plasma and hepatic concentration of compounds

We observed an apparent increase in the average values of plasma total bile acid level after administration of troglitazone and pioglitazone, but not rosiglitazone; but looking into the data for individual rats, the total bile acid levels of all rats treated with troglitazone were increased, but in the case of pioglitazone the total bile acid levels of most of the rats we tested were not changed so much (Figure 3). Therefore, the *in-vivo* cholestatic effect of troglitazone may be more potent than that of pioglitazone. We also measured the plasma and hepatic concentration of PPARγ agonists. After administration of 10 mg/kg troglitazone the hepatic concentration of troglitazone sulphate exceeded 100 μM and was much higher than its plasma concentration and that of troglitazone itself. In the case of pioglitazone its plasma concentration is almost the same as the intrahepatic concentration (101 μM). Considering the results of *in-vitro* experiments, pioglitazone did not inhibit rat Bsep-mediated transport of taurocholate even at 100 μM, so we thought that the increase in total bile acid in plasma observed in some rats treated with pioglitazone was not caused by the inhibition of BSEP. On the other hand, the K_i value of troglitazone sulphate, but not troglitazone itself, for rat Bsep was more than 50-fold lower than the intrahepatic concentration of troglitazone sulphate,

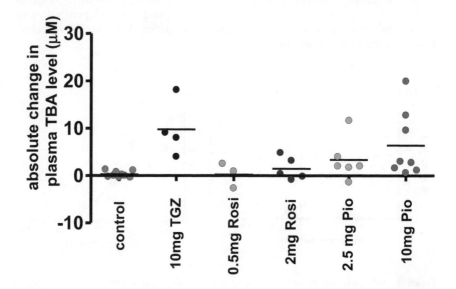

Figure 3 PPARγ agonist-induced increase in the concentration of total bile acids in plasma. The Y axis represents the increase in the total bile acid concentration in plasma after the treatment of each drug in rats. Each point represents the result obtained from individual rats and the bar indicates the median value in each group

suggesting that the increase in total bile acid in plasma after treatment with troglitazone can be explained by the inhibition of BSEP by troglitazone sulphate.

Inhibitory effects of cholestasis-inducing drugs on the transport of taurocholate across NTCP/BSEP double transfectants

We investigated the inhibitory effects of several cholestasis-inducing drugs on bile acid transport using NTCP/BSEP double-transfected cells. Transcellular transport of taurocholate was significantly inhibited by rifampicin, rifamycin SV and glibenclamide, but not by 100 μM captopril and cimetidine[11]. It is therefore suggested that the cholestatic effect induced by captopril and cimetidine was not caused by the inhibition of BSEP, but by other mechanisms. The efflux clearance on the apical membrane of taurocholate (PS_{apical}), which is calculated by its efflux rate divided by its intracellular concentration, was also inhibited by three drugs, suggesting that BSEP is inhibited by these drugs[11]. If the efflux process is solely inhibited, intracellular concentration should be increased; however, in the case of rifamycin SV and glibenclamide, it is not changed or decreased. These results suggested that at least rifamycin SV and glibenclamide can inhibit NTCP, as well as BSEP. We never exclude the possibility that rifampicin can inhibit NTCP-mediated uptake and a detailed kinetic analysis will be needed. For the high-throughput screening we searched for the fluorescent bile acids which can be used as a substrate of NTCP/BSEP. As a result, fluorescein-conjugated glycocholate and glycochenodeoxycholate are bisubstrates of NTCP/BSEP[11]. Therefore, these compounds enable us to check the inhibitory effects of many drugs on the transcellular transport of bile acids using a microplate fluorescence reader.

CONCLUSIONS

Some PPAR agonists can inhibit the hepatic uptake and efflux of bile acids and organic anions. We found the tendency with which PPARγ agonists potently inhibited the activities of hepatic uptake and efflux transporters: dual PPAR α/γ agonists showed a moderate inhibition, while PPARα agonists (except bezafibrate for BCRP) showed relatively weak inhibitory effects on several transporters. The inhibitory effects of PPARγ agonists on BSEP-mediated transport showed large species differences between rats and humans. *In-vivo* analysis revealed that the cholestatic effect induced by troglitazone can be caused by the inhibition of BSEP by troglitazone sulphate. For the high-throughput screening for the selection of cholestatic drugs which cause the inhibition of transport of bile acids in human liver, NTCP/BSEP double transfectant is very useful.

References

1. Kostrubsky VE, Strom SC, Hanson J et al. Evaluation of hepatotoxic potential of drugs by inhibition of bile-acid transport in cultured primary human hepatocytes and intact rats. Toxicol Sci. 2003;76:220–8.
2. Fattinger K, Funk C, Pantze M et al. The endothelin antagonist bosentan inhibits the canalicular bile salt export pump: a potential mechanism for hepatic adverse reactions. Clin Pharmacol Ther. 2001;69:223–31.
3. McRae MP, Lowe CM, Tian X et al. Ritonavir, saquinavir, and efavirenz, but not nevirapine, inhibit bile acid transport in human and rat hepatocytes. J Pharmacol Exp Ther. 2006;318:1068–75.
4. Funk C, Pantze M, Jehle L et al. Troglitazone-induced intrahepatic cholestasis by an interference with the hepatobiliary export of bile acids in male and female rats. Correlation with the gender difference in troglitazone sulfate formation and the inhibition of the canalicular bile salt export pump (Bsep) by troglitazone and troglitazone sulfate. Toxicology. 2001;167:83–98.
5. Funk C, Ponelle C, Scheuermann G, Pantze M. Cholestatic potential of troglitazone as a possible factor contributing to troglitazone-induced hepatotoxicity: *in vivo* and *in vitro* interaction at the canalicular bile salt export pump (Bsep) in the rat. Mol Pharmacol. 2001; 59:627–35.
6. May LD, Lefkowitch JH, Kram MT, Rubin DE. Mixed hepatocellular–cholestatic liver injury after pioglitazone therapy. Ann Intern Med. 2002;136:449–52.
7. Shitara Y, Hirano M, Sato H, Sugiyama Y. Gemfibrozil and its glucuronide inhibit the organic anion transporting polypeptide 2 (OATP2/OATP1B1:SLC21A6)-mediated hepatic uptake and CYP2C8-mediated metabolism of cerivastatin: analysis of the mechanism of the clinically relevant drug-drug interaction between cerivastatin and gemfibrozil. J Pharmacol Exp Ther. 2004;311:228–36.
8. Mita S, Suzuki H, Akita H et al. Vectorial transport of unconjugated and conjugated bile salts by monolayers of LLC-PK1 cells doubly transfected with human NTCP and BSEP or with rat Ntcp and Bsep. Am J Physiol Gastrointest Liver Physiol. 2006;290:G550–6.
9. Hirano M, Maeda K, Shitara Y, Sugiyama Y. Contribution of OATP2 (OATP1B1) and OATP8 (OATP1B3) to the hepatic uptake of pitavastatin in humans. J Pharmacol Exp Ther. 2004;311:139–46.
10. Hayashi H, Takada T, Suzuki H et al. Transport by vesicles of glycine- and taurine-conjugated bile salts and taurolithocholate 3-sulfate: a comparison of human BSEP with rat Bsep. Biochim Biophys Acta. 2005;1738:54–62.
11. Mita S, Suzuki H, Akita H et al. Inhibition of bile acid transport across Na^+/taurocholate cotransporting polypeptide (SLC10A1) and bile salt export pump (ABCB 11)-coexpressing LLC-PK1 cells by cholestasis-inducing drugs. Drug Metab Dispos. 2006;34:1575–81.

ASBT expression has not been shown[4]. The liver receptor homologue-1 (LRH-1) activates the mouse but not rat ASBT gene due to the coincident presence (mouse) or absence (rat) of both the LRH-1 transcription factor and its *cis* element[5]. Two fat-soluble vitamins, retinoic acid and 1α,25-dihydroxyvitamin D_3, activate human ASBT via the RAR and VDR receptors, respectively[6,7]. Glucocorticoids and cibrofibrate also increase human ASBT transcription via the GR and PPARα receptors[8,9].

In contrast to the large number of activators of ASBT, only two systems to date have been shown to repress ASBT, c-fos and the FXR-SHP cascade. Inflammatory cytokines, which are elaborated in the setting of intestinal inflammation, lead to phosphorylation and nuclear translocation of c-fos[10]. Binding of c-fos to the rat, mouse or human ASBT promoter leads to transcriptional repression[11]. The physiological relevance of this process is evident in c-fos null mice, where ileitis is associated with activation rather than repression of ASBT[11]. The bile acid responsiveness of the ASBT gene has been an area of ongoing controversy, with conflicting results reported from different laboratories using different assays, model systems and species. Strong evidence has been reported that suggests that in mice, rabbits and humans ASBT is under negative feedback regulation by bile acids[5,6,12]. The molecular mechanism of the repression involves the well-described cascade of bile acid-induced, FXR-mediated activation of the transcription of the short heterodimer partner (Figure 2). In the mouse and rabbit the repression works through inactivation of LRH-1, while in humans SHP deactivates RAR.

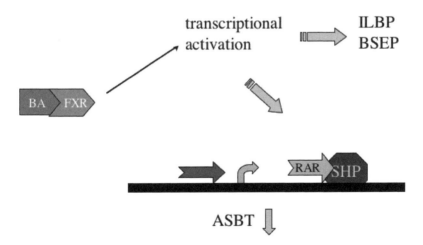

Figure 2 Bile acid-mediated negative feedback regulation of ASBT. Bile acids (BA) bind to the farnesoid X-receptor (FXR) and transcriptionally activate the ileal lipid-binding protein (ILBP), the bile salt excretory pump (BSEP) and the short heterodimer partner (SHP). SHP deactivates the retinoic acid receptor (RAR), which normally transactivates ASBT. Thus the overall effect of bile acids is to repress the transcription of ASBT

The physiological relevance of regulation of ASBT is clearly manifest in human disease, especially as it pertains to loss of function. The most striking example is in the setting of inherited defects in ASBT, which lead to intractable bile acid-induced diarrhoea[13]. These findings have been recapitulated after targeted deletion of ASBT in mice[14]. Loss of ASBT function and mRNA can be observed in patients with various forms of ileitis including Crohn's disease[8,15]. Bile acid-induced effects in the colon are likely to exacerbate the diarrhoea observed in inflammatory bowel disease and could predispose to an increased risk of carcinoma of the colon. Glucocorticoid therapy in inflammatory bowel disease may serve two distinct functions *vis-à-vis* ASBT: first by diminishing ileal inflammation and secondary effects of inflammatory cytokines, and second by activating ASBT via the glucocorticoid receptor[8].

The potential relevance of gain of function of ASBT in human disease is more controversial. Analysis of [75]SeHCAT retention in primary biliary cirrhosis indicated that bile acid retention was enhanced in this form of cholestasis, leading to the comment by Alan Hofmann that this represented 'homeostasis gone awry'[16,17]. If in fact ASBT is under negative feedback by luminal bile acids, then one might observe up-regulation of ASBT expression in cholestasis. This could lead to relatively inappropriate retention of bile acids in a circumstance where bile acid wasting might be more appropriate/beneficial. Fat-soluble vitamin malabsorption is common in cholestatic liver disease and supplementation is often required to avoid complications of nutritional deficiencies. The recent finding that retinoic acid and 1α,25-dihydroxyvitamin D_3 activate human ASBT suggests that there could be a detrimental effect of this supplementation. At present this is only theoretical, bears future investigation and should not lead to a reluctance to provide appropriate nutritional support to patients with chronic cholestasis.

One of the intriguing circumstances where ASBT gain of function may impact on human disease is in the setting of Byler's disease (also know as PFIC1 or FIC1 disease). Early investigations of a mouse model of Byler's disease suggested that intestinal handling of bile acids might be deranged[18]. Analysis of ASBT mRNA levels in a limited number of ileal samples suggested that there might be gain of function in FIC1 disease[19]. This was modelled in Caco-2 cells by siRNA-mediated knock-down of FIC1. Changes in the expression of ILBP suggested that there was a central problem in FXR activity. The effect of FIC1 knock-down could not be corrected by overexpression of FXR mRNA, suggesting a post-translational effect on FXR. Alterations in FXR expression were associated with changes in nuclear localization of FXR and thus downstream targets of FXR were affected. A unifying hypothesis for the pathophysiology of FIC1 disease is that FXR activity is reduced, leading to a direct reduction in BSEP (bile salt excretory pump) expression and an indirect activation in ASBT expression (Figure 3). This hypothesis is not completely supported by current human and mouse investigations, although much more work is required to assess this concept. Interestingly, and supportive of this hypothesis, interruption of the enterohepatic circulation of bile acids by either partial biliary diversion (Figure 4) or ileal exclusion is very successful in treating both low-γGTP cholestasis and Alagille syndrome[20–22]. It remains to be seen whether these

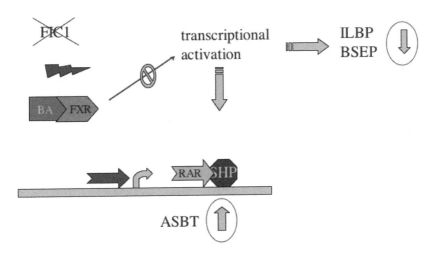

Figure 3 Potential role of FIC1 on bile acid homeostasis. FIC1 normally activates FXR, whereas in FIC1 disease (Byler's disease) this process is absent. As such BSEP expression is reduced, although not absent. In addition, SHP expression is reduced so there is a relative induction of ASBT due to diminished deactivation of RAR

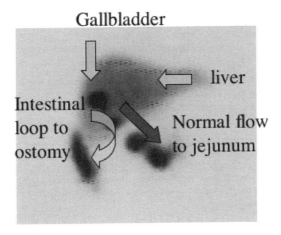

Figure 4 Hepatobiliary scintigraphy after partial biliary diversion. Radioisotope is shown in the liver with flow going to the gallbladder with subsequent normal progression to the jejunum and partial diversion through an intestinal loop to an external ostomy

surgical techniques and potential pharmacological equivalents may be of use in chronic cholestasis in a general sense. Certainly, in the setting of hypercholesterolaemia, partial ileal exclusion has been shown to be of clinical benefit[23].

In summary, loss of ASBT function is clearly associated with human disease, and methods to increase ASBT function in those settings may ameliorate the problems associated with bile acid malabsorption. It is less clear whether ASBT gain of function is associated with human disease, but it seems likely that surgical and/or pharmacological interruption of the enterohepatic circulation of bile acids will be useful in the treatment of cholestatic liver disease.

Acknowledgements

This work was supported by grants from the National Institutes of Health to Benjamin Shneider (NIDDK DK 54165 and DK 69942).

References

1. Wong MH, Oelkers P, Craddock AL, Dawson PA. Expression cloning and characterization of the hamster ileal sodium-dependent bile acid transporter. J Biol Chem. 1994;269:1340–7.
2. Dawson PA, Hubbert M, Haywood J et al. The heteromeric organic solute transporter alpha-beta, Ostalpha-Ostbeta, is an ileal basolateral bile acid transporter. J Biol Chem. 2005;280:6960–8.
3. Shih D, Bussen M, Sehayek E et al. Hepatocyte nuclear factor-1alpha is an essential regulator of bile acid and plasma cholesterol metabolism. Nature Genet. 2001;27:375–82.
4. Chen F, Ma L, Al-Ansari N, Shneider B. The role of AP-1 in the transcriptional regulation of the rat apical sodium-dependent bile acid transporter. J Biol Chem. 2001;276:38703–14.
5. Chen F, Ma L, Dawson P et al. Liver receptor homologue-1 mediated species- and cell line-specific bile acid dependent negative feedback regulation of the apical sodium-dependent bile acid transporter. J Biol Chem. 2003;278:19909–16.
6. Neimark E, Chen F, Li X, Shneider BL. Bile acid-induced negative feedback regulation of the human ileal bile acid transporter. Hepatology. 2004;40:149–56.
7. Chen X, Chen F, Liu S et al. Transactivation of rat apical sodium-dependent bile acid transporter and increased bile acid transport by 1alpha,25-dihydroxyvitamin D3 via the vitamin D receptor. Mol Pharmacol. 2006;69:1913–23.
8. Jung D, Fantin AC, Scheurer U, Fried M, Kullak-Ublick GA. Human ileal bile acid transporter gene ASBT (SLC10A2) is transactivated by the glucocorticoid receptor. Gut. 2004;53:78–84.
9. Jung D, Fried M, Kullak-Ublick G. Human apical sodium-dependent bile salt transporter gene (SLC10A2) is regulated by the peroxisome proliferator-activated receptor *a*. J Biol Chem. 2002;277:30559–66.
10. Chen F, Ma L, Sartor B et al. Inflammatory-mediated repression of the rat ileal sodium-dependent bile acid transporter by c-fos nuclear translocation. Gastroenterology. 2002;123:2005–16.
11. Neimark E, Chen F, Li X et al. c-Fos is a critical mediator of inflammatory-mediated repression of the apical sodium-dependent bile acid transporter. Gastroenterology. 2006;131:554–67.
12. Li H, Chen F, Shang Q et al. FXR-activating ligands inhibit rabbit ASBT expression via FXR-SHP-FTF cascade. Am J Physiol Gastrointest Liver Physiol. 2005;288:G60–6.
13. Oelkers P, Kirby LC, Heubi JE, Dawson PA. Primary bile acid malabsorption caused by mutations in the ileal sodium-dependent bile acid transporter gene (SLC10A2). J Clin Invest. 1997;99:1880–7.
14. Dawson PA, Haywood J, Craddock AL et al. Targeted deletion of the ileal bile acid transporter eliminates enterohepatic cycling of bile acids in mice. J Biol Chem. 2003;278:33920–7.

15. Suchy FS, Balistreri WF. Ileal dysfunction in Crohn's disease assessed by the postprandial serum bile acid response. Gut. 1981;22:948–52.
16. Lanzini A, De Tavonatti MG, Panarotto B et al. Intestinal absorption of the bile acid analogue 75Se-homocholic acid-taurine is increased in primary biliary cirrhosis, and reverts to normal during ursodeoxycholic acid administration. Gut. 2003;52:1371–5.
17. Hofmann AF. Inappropriate ileal conservation of bile acids in cholestatic liver disease: homeostasis gone awry. Gut. 2003;52:1239–41.
18. Pawlikowska L, Groen A, Eppens EF et al. A mouse genetic model for familial cholestasis caused by ATP8B1 mutations reveals perturbed bile salt homeostasis but no impairment in bile secretion. Hum Mol Genet. 2004;13:881–92.
19. Chen F, Ananthanarayanan M, Emre S et al. Progressive familial intrahepatic cholestasis, type 1, is associated with decreased farnesoid X receptor activity. Gastroenterology. 2004;126:756–64.
20. Whitington PF, Whitington GL. Partial external diversion of bile for the treatment of intractable pruritus associated with intrahepatic cholestasis. Gastroenterology. 1988;95:130–6.
21. Hollands CM, Rivera-Pedrogo J, Gonzalez-Vallina R, Loret-de-Mola O, Nahmad M, Burnweit CA. Ileal exclusion for Byler's disease: an alternative surgical approach with promising early results for pruritus. J Pediatr Surg. 1998;33:220–4.
22. Emerick K, Whitington P. Partial external biliary diversion for intractable pruritus and xanthomas in Alagille syndrome. Hepatology. 2002;35:1501–6.
23. Buchwald H, Varco RL, Matts JP et al. Effect of partial ileal bypass surgery on mortality and morbidity from coronary heart disease in patients with hypercholesterolemia. Report of the program on the surgical control of the hyperlipidemias (POSCH). N Engl J Med. 1990;323:946–55.
24. Chen F, Ma L, Al-Ansari N, Shneider B. The role of AP-1 in the transcriptional regulation of the rat apical sodium-dependent bile acid transporter. J Biol Chem. 2001;276:38703–14.
25. Jung D, Fried M, Kullak-Ublick GA. Human apical sodium-dependent bile salt transporter gene (SLC10A2) is regulated by the peroxisome proliferator-activated receptor alpha. J Biol Chem. 2002;277:30559–66.

13

Evidence for a role of the FXR-driven intestinal regulatory factor FGF-19 upon cholestyramine and chenodeoxycholic acid treatment and during the diurnal regulation of bile acid synthesis in humans

M. RUDLING, T. LUNDÅSEN, B. ANGELIN and C. GÄLMAN

INTRODUCTION

Bile acid metabolism is central in metabolic homeostasis and disturbances in this system are associated with several clinically important disease entities. Regulation of the potentially toxic bile acids is thus a delicate matter in order to maintain an adequate pool of circulating bile acids in the body. In the classic pathway for bile acid synthesis hepatic cholesterol 7α-hydroxylase, Cyp7a1, is the rate-limiting enzyme.

The liver contains most components in the regulatory machinery for Cyp7a1, and it has been generally assumed that the major events in the regulation of bile acid synthesis occur in this organ. There are however animal experimental data that indicate that the gut may suppress hepatic bile acid synthesis since the suppressive effects exerted by bile acids themselves on their synthesis are present only following oral administration, and not when given by a parenteral route[1]. However, there are several major species differences between humans and rodents as regards bile acid metabolism precluding direct conclusions obtained from rodent models for the human situation. For instance, the important feedforward response of Cyp7a1 following cholesterol feeding present in mice and rats does not occur in humans. We recently demonstrated that bile acid synthesis has a unique diurnal rhythm in humans with two major peaks during the day[2], which is opposite to that seen in rodents, where bile acid synthesis shows one single peak in the middle of the night.

We could not identify the reason for this unique rhythm in humans. However, the temporal changes in bile acid synthesis observed indicated that the postprandial return of bile acids to the liver might explain the suppression of bile acid synthesis and may thus be driving the suppressive phases of this diurnal rhythm[2].

Recent experiments have shown that, in mice, intestinal fibroblast growth factor 15 (FGF15) appears to function as a secretory signal from the gut to the liver where Cyp7a1 expression is repressed[3]. These conclusions have been drawn by use of genetically altered mice, although the direct demonstration of FGF15 in plasma has yet not been shown. The human homologue for FGF15 is FGF19. However, there is no information available in the literature on serum levels of FGF19 in humans.

In the present study we therefore tested the hypothesis that FGF19 may be an important suppressive regulator on hepatic bile acid synthesis in humans. The study is now published[4].

MATERIALS AND METHODS

Subjects and study design

Overnight fasting serum was obtained from 15 healthy volunteers (eight men, seven women). Studies on the effects of perturbation of bile acid enterohepatic circulation were made using serum samples from gallstone patients previously reported on[5]. They had been treated for >2 weeks with cholestyramine (Questran[®], Bristol-Myers), 16 g/day ($n = 4$), or with chenodeoxycholic acid (Chenofalk, Dr Falk Pharma GmbH, Freiburg, Germany), 15 mg/kg per day ($n = 6$) as described[5]. For the studies on diurnal variation, previously obtained samples from five healthy volunteers[2] were used. All subjects gave informed consent to participation in the studies, which had been approved by the Ethics Committee of the Karolinska Institute.

Serum analyses

A sandwich ELISA kit (FGF19 Quantikine, R&D Systems, Minneapolis, MN) was used for assay of serum FGF19 in duplicate. Serum levels of 7α-hydroxy-4-cholesten-3-one (C4), corrected for total serum cholesterol, were measured[6] to monitor CYP7A1 enzymatic activity (bile acid synthesis). Total bile acids in serum were assayed by GC/MS[2]. Total serum cholesterol and triglyceride levels were determined enzymatically. For further details please see ref 4 .

RESULTS AND DISCUSSION

We first assayed the basal levels of FGF19 in serum samples from 15 normal volunteers (eight males, seven females). There was a wide interindividual variation (range 49–590 pg/ml) and no apparent gender difference.

We next evaluated whether pharmacologically induced changes in bile acid circulation, known to affect bile acid synthesis, would alter serum levels of FGF19. Treatment with the resin cholestyramine reduced serum FGF19 levels as much as 87% ($p < 0.02$) while serum C4 levels were increased by 18-fold ($p < 0.001$). On the other hand, administration of chenodeoxycholic acid (CDCA) increased FGF19 levels by 3-fold ($p < 0.004$) whereas serum C4 levels were reduced by 26% ($p < 0.003$). Thus, pharmacological interruption of bile acid circulation with a resin (cholestyramine) reduced serum FGF19 levels, whereas an increased circulation of bile acids induced by CDCA treatment resulted in increased serum levels of FGF19.

Thus FGF19 serum levels were increased in a situation when bile acid synthesis was suppressed (CDCA treatment) whereas there were strongly reduced FGF19 serum levels when bile acid circulation was disrupted by cholestyramine treatment in line with our hypothesis. This suggests that the hepatic synthesis of bile acids may be controlled from the intestine via FGF19.

We then wanted to evaluate whether FGF19 levels in serum may show any diurnal changes. We were particularly interested to know how FGF19 levels in serum would relate to the diurnal changes in bile acid synthesis we had previously shown in humans[2]. Serum samples previously collected over 25.5 h and assayed for C4 and bile acids[2] were analysed for this purpose. There were marked temporal changes of serum FGF19 in synchronicity with the temporal changes in C4. FGF19 displayed two major peaks around 3 and 9 pm. Analysis of serum bile acid levels, mirroring portal venous flow of bile acids from the intestine[7], showed that FGF19 in serum peaked about 1.5–3 h after serum bile acids. These results are in line with the thinking that FGF19 is released from the intestine following the postprandial flow of bile acids over the intestinal wall. The relationship between FGF19 and C4 levels in time where the suppression of bile acid synthesis was about 2 h after the peaking of FGF19 is in agreement with the thinking that circulating FGF19 reduces bile acid synthesis.

We have previously shown that the induction of bile acid synthesis in the morning to noon period occur independent of food intake[2]. If FGF19 is secreted from the intestine in response to bile acid flux over the intestinal wall the diurnal rhythm would be expected to be abolished during fasting. We therefore determined serum FGF19 levels in four of the five subjects sampled on a second session where food was omitted[2]. As expected, serum bile acids and triglycerides declined with time, whereas bile acid synthesis increased in the morning to noon period as shown previously[2]. In line with our hypothesis, serum FGF19 levels were unchanged when subjects were fasting. As discussed previously[2], the reduction of bile acid synthesis in the afternoon after 1:30 pm, when food was provided regularly, was less evident when fasting. This result is in line with the concept that the levels of circulating FGF19 are important for suppression of bile acid synthesis also at normal physiological conditions during regular feeding–fasting cycles.

Interestingly, circulating FGF19 may serve as a mediator of metabolic effects attributed to bile acids. Thus, animals treated with FGF19 also respond with a reduction in body weight and with reduced plasma levels of triglycerides and glucose and increased energy expenditure[8,9]. It has been shown that the hepatic synthesis of triglycerides is reduced by CDCA feeding of humans and increased upon resin treatment[10]; therefore altered FGF19 levels may be important for the changes in plasma lipids observed following treatment with cholestyramine and bile acids in humans. Considering the recently reported effects of FGF19 on glucose and energy metabolism in animals[8,9] it should be noted that treatment of mice with bile acids has been reported to induce similar effects (reduced plasma glucose and triglycerides, reduced body weight and increased energy expenditure[11]). These effects have been ascribed to the interaction of bile acids with TGR5[11]. The possible contribution of the FGF19–FGFR4 pathway here needs to be addressed in human studies. Our finding of a diurnal regulation of circulating FGF19 that relates to intestinal bile acid uptake also raises questions on how differences in endogenous FGF19 secretion in relation to bile acid metabolism may influence not only lipid but also carbohydrate and intermediary metabolism.

In conclusion, our results indicate that the transintestinal flux of bile acids in humans regulates the release of FGF19 from the intestine, and that circulating FGF19 in turn suppresses the synthesis of bile acids in the liver. This mechanism seems to operate not only during pharmacological interference with bile acid circulation but also during the physiological diurnal changes of bile acid synthesis in humans. The magnitude of the contribution of intestinal FGF19 in the regulation of hepatic bile acid synthesis, and the role of FGF19 as mediator of bile acid-induced effects on triglyceride and carbohydrate metabolism, are important questions to address in future studies.

Acknowledgements

We thank Ingela Arvidsson for technical assistance, and Ingemar Björkhem for advice. This work was supported by grants from the Swedish Research Council, the Swedish Foundation for Strategic Research, the Grönberg and the Swedish Heart–Lung Foundations, the Foundation of Old Female Servants, Novo Nordisk Fonden and the Karolinska Institute.

References

1.   Pandak WM, Li YC, Chiang JY et al. Regulation of cholesterol 7 alpha-hydroxylase mRNA and transcriptional activity by taurocholate and cholesterol in the chronic biliary diverted rat. J Biol Chem. 1991;266:3416–21.
2.   Galman C, Angelin B, Rudling M. Bile acid synthesis in humans has a rapid diurnal variation that is asynchronous with cholesterol synthesis. Gastroenterology. 2005; 129:1445–53.
3.   Inagaki T, Choi M, Moschetta A et al. Fibroblast growth factor 15 functions as an enterohepatic signal to regulate bile acid homeostasis. Cell Metab. 2005;2:217–25.
4.   Lundasen T, Galman C, Angelin B, Rudling M. Circulating intestinal fibroblast growth factor 19 has a pronounced diurnal variation and modulates hepatic bile acid synthesis in man. J Intern Med. 2006;260:530–6.
5.   Reihner E, Bjorkhem I, Angelin B, Ewerth S, Einarsson K. Bile acid synthesis in humans: regulation of hepatic microsomal cholesterol 7 alpha-hydroxylase activity. Gastroenterology. 1989;97:1498–505.
6.   Galman C, Arvidsson I, Angelin B, Rudling M. Monitoring hepatic cholesterol 7alpha-hydroxylase activity by assay of the stable bile acid intermediate 7alpha-hydroxy-4-cholesten-3-one in peripheral blood. J Lipid Res. 2003;44:859–66.
7.   Angelin B, Bjorkhem I, Einarsson K, Ewerth S. Hepatic uptake of bile acids in man. Fasting and postprandial concentrations of individual bile acids in portal venous and systemic blood serum. J Clin Invest. 1982;70:724–31.

8. Strack AM, Myers RW. Modulation of metabolic syndrome by fibroblast growth factor 19 (FGF19)? Endocrinology. 2004;145:2591–93.
9. Tomlinson E, Fu L, John L et al. Transgenic mice expressing human fibroblast growth factor-19 display increased metabolic rate and decreased adiposity. Endocrinology. 2002; 143:1741–7.
10. Angelin B, Einarsson K, Hellstrom K, Leijd B. Effects of cholestyramine and chenodeoxycholic acid on the metabolism of endogenous triglyceride in hyperlipo-proteinemia. J Lipid Res. 1978;19:1017–24.
11. Watanabe M, Houten SM, Mataki C et al. Bile acids induce energy expenditure by promoting intracellular thyroid hormone activation. Nature. 2006;439:484–9.

Section IV
Nuclear receptor regulation

Chair: DJ MANGELSDORF and DW RUSSELL

14

Bile acid-like hormones function as ligands for the nematode orphan nuclear receptor DAF-12 and govern dauer formation, reproduction and lifespan

Z. WANG, C. L. CUMMINS, D. L. MOTOLA and
D. J. MANGELSDORF

EVIDENCE FOR HORMONAL CONTROL OF *CAENORHABDITIS ELEGANS* DAUER FORMATION AND REPRODUCTIVE DEVELOPMENT

Nematodes, like other metazoans, coordinate their development, metabolism and homeostasis by responding to cues from their environment. A good example of this is seen in *C. elegans* larval development. Under favourable conditions L1 larvae develop directly into fertile adults through four larval stages (L1–L4); while in response to harsh environments – such as high temperature, overcrowding, and depletion of food sources – they will adopt the protective strategy of dauer diapause, in which they form the stress-resistant, L3-arrested dauer larvae. As dauer larvae, *C. elegans* can survive up to several months without feeding and can resume normal reproductive development to L4 adults when the environment again becomes favourable[1].

Molecular, cellular, and genetic studies have revealed that selection of either dauer diapause or reproductive growth is controlled by a neuroendocrine system that involves a collection of genes called the dauer formation genes (Daf). Mutations in DAF genes lead the animal to either constitutively enter dauer (Daf-c) or bypass dauer diapause (Daf-d, dauer defective) regardless of environmental cues[1]. Genetic epistasis studies have demonstrated that the most downstream genes involved in this decision are *daf-9* and *daf-12*. The product of the *daf-9* gene belongs to the superfamily of cytochrome P450 enzymes that in humans are critical for the formation and metabolism of bile acids and steroid hormones. *daf-12* encodes a protein in the nuclear hormone receptor superfamily[2–5]. These receptors are ligand-activated transcription factors whose mammalian homologues are regulated by a variety of lipid-soluble molecules such as retinoids, thyroid and steroid hormones to control important homeostatic functions including energy regulation and reproduction[6]. Analysis of Daf genes has revealed that favourable environments activate insulin/IGF-1 and TGF-β signalling pathways within the organism that converge upon DAF-12. Interestingly, mutations in *daf-9* and *daf-12* have been found to affect dauer formation, reproductive development, and lifespan[2–5]. From the genetic data placing the P450 enzyme upstream of the nuclear receptor we hypothesized that DAF-9 produces a hormone that prevents the initiation of dauer diapause through activation of DAF-12[2,4,7]. Indeed, the existence of such a pathway would be remarkably similar to the steroidogenic biosynthetic pathway that produces ligands for vertebrate nuclear receptors[6,8].

Several other lines of evidence suggest that DAF-12 ligands are derived from cholesterol. *C. elegans* requires cholesterol for normal reproductive development and must obtain it from its environment because it lacks the ability to synthesize it *de novo*[9,10]. Impairment of *C. elegans* cholesterol intake by either depleting the environmental cholesterol or mutating the intracellular cholesterol transporters (*ncr-1, ncr-2*) leads to constitutive dauer diapause[11,12]. In addition, only subtle traces of environmental cholesterol are required for normal development[10]. Furthermore, it has been shown that the structural enantiomer (mirror image) of cholesterol cannot sustain the normal development, growth, and reproduction of *C. elegans*, despite sharing the same biophysical and membrane properties of natural cholesterol[13]. Together, these data indicate that, in nematodes, cholesterol functions in a signalling pathway to prevent dauer diapause.

CONSERVATION OF THE NUCLEAR RECEPTOR PARADIGM

The superfamily of nuclear receptors consists of 48 members in humans, 20 members in fruit flies, and 284 members in *C. elegans*. About 30% of the *C. elegans* nuclear receptors exhibit similarity in their ligand-binding domain to nuclear receptors from other phyla[14]. The evolutionary conservation across species suggests that nematode nuclear receptors control very fundamental physiological events that are important for all animals, such as development, reproductive growth, and metabolic homeostasis. While several ligands have been identified for the human and *Drosophila* nuclear receptors, no ligand had yet been identified for any of the 284 *C. elegans* receptors prior to the initiation of this work.

Among the large family of worm nuclear receptors, DAF-12 is relatively well studied. As described previously, geneticists have placed this receptor at the end of the dauer formation pathway, controlling the critical decision between dauer formation and reproductive development. Previous studies have shown that DAF-12 preferentially binds to direct repeats with a five-nucleotide spacer (DR-5) DNA binding elements[15] and functionally interacts with a putative co-repressor, DIN-1S, a *C. elegans* gene that is homologous to the human co-repressor SHARP[16]. The bipotential action of DAF-12 on dauer formation and reproductive development is further substantiated by genetic evidence demonstrating that *daf-12* null mutants are dauer-defective (probably from the loss of co-repressor interaction) and that ligand-binding domain mutants of *daf-12* are dauer-constitutive (indicating the receptor is unable to interact with the putative hormone to prevent the animal from entering dauer)[2,3].

In this chapter we summarize the discovery of the dafachronic acids, bile acid-like molecules that bind to DAF-12 *in vivo* and represent the first nuclear receptor ligands discovered in *C. elegans*. This discovery, from the synthesis of dafachronic acids to their function *in vivo*, demonstrates the conservation of hormonal regulation of reproduction from worms to humans[17].

IDENTIFYING BILE ACID-LIKE MOLECULES AS PHYSIOLOGICAL LIGANDS FOR DAF-12

C. elegans metabolizes cholesterol in distinct ways compared to mammals. The major metabolites include two desmethyl sterols, 7-dehydrocholesterol and lathosterol, and two 4α-methyl sterols unique to nematodes, lophenol and its $\Delta^{8(14)}$ derivative[9]. When supplied as the sole dietary sterol, only the desmethyl sterols can substitute for cholesterol with respect to reproductive development, suggesting they might be intermediates in the synthesis of the steroidal ligand of DAF-12[18]. Because the ligands for nuclear receptors are usually in very low concentration, and are difficult to identify from their structurally similar relatives *in vivo*, we began by screening sterol-containing compound libraries for the DAF-12 ligand. The closest homologues of DAF-12 in vertebrates are PXR (pregnane X receptor), a xenobiotic receptor that can bind to bile acids; VDR (vitamin D receptor), which binds to 1,25 $(OH)_2$-vitamin D_3 as well as several bile acids; and LXR (liver X receptor), which binds to oxysterols[19–21]. This knowledge helped us to narrow the initial candidates to the cholesterol-derived molecules that are known ligands for the DAF-12 vertebrate orthologues. To perform the candidate screen we used a co-transfection assay in HEK293 cells in which GAL4-DAF-12 (containing the DAF-12 ligand-binding domain fused to the GAL4 DNA-binding domain) and a GAL4-responsive luciferase construct were transfected with or without the DAF-9 enzyme. We found that the bile acid, 3-ketolithocholic acid (3K-LCA), could activate DAF-12 independent of DAF-9. In contrast, lithocholic acid (LCA), which differs from 3K-LCA only by a 3α-hydroxyl group, failed to do so, implying the structural importance of a 3-keto group to activate DAF-12. Using this structural clue, we then tested the 3-keto derivatives of the worm's endogenous sterols, lathosterol and lophenol, as well as 4-cholesten-3-one, a natural 3-keto oxidation product of cholesterol. Incredibly, all these 3-keto steroids strongly activated DAF-12 in a DAF-9-dependent manner. More importantly, the metabolites of lathosterone and 4-cholesten-3-one produced by DAF-9 fully rescued the daf-c phenotypes of *daf-9* null mutants, indicating they functioned as DAF-12 ligands *in vivo*.

DAF-9 IS A 3-KETO-STEROL-26-MONOOXYGENASE

Using microsomes expressing DAF-9 from baculovirus infected *Sf*-9 cells we found that DAF-9 was metabolizing the side chain of the 3-keto worm sterols to a hydroxylated and carboxylated metabolite through successive oxidations[17]. To identify the location of the hydroxylation reaction we prepared synthetic standards of the side-chain hydroxylated 4-cholesten-3-one molecules (including 20(S)-OH, 22(R)-OH, 22(S)-OH, 24(S)-OH, 25-OH, 25R, 26-OH and 25S, 26-OH derivatives) to test in a co-transfection assay. From these compounds we determined that only 25R, 26-OH and 25S, 26-OH could activate DAF-12 and could be further metabolized by DAF-9 microsomes to the 25R, 26-COOH and 25S, 26-COOH metabolites, respectively (also known as C27 metabolites)[17]. Furthermore, we found that the 25S, 26-COOH derivative of 4-cholesten-3-one was more potent than the 25R diastereomer. Using the DAF-9 expressing microsomes, we also demonstrated that DAF-9 could successively oxidize lathosterone or 4-cholesten-3-one to generate their carboxylic acid derivatives, 3-keto-7,5α-cholestenoic acid or 3-keto-4-cholestenoic acid. These molecules were termed Δ^7-dafachronic or Δ^4-dafachronic acid, respectively. Preparation of the synthetic standard of Δ^4-dafachronic acid (the 25S, C26-carboxylated derivative of 4-cholesten-3-one) demonstrated that nanomolar concentrations of this acid could bind and activate DAF-12 independent of DAF-9, and fully rescue the daf-c and heterochronic phenotypes of daf mutants at physiological concentrations[17]. Moreover, both dafachronic acids were found to be present in the wild-type worms (but not *daf-9* null) at physiologically relevant (~ 200 nM) concentrations. Therefore, dafachronic acids are physiological bile acid-like hormones that control the developmental fate of the organism.

DAF-9 IS A FUNCTIONAL ORTHOLOGUE OF MAMMALIAN CYP27A1

The formation of mammalian bile acids shares many similarities with the dafachronic acids. Both are derived from cholesterol and require successive oxidations at the C26 position on the side-chain. In contrast to the *C. elegans* microsomal DAF-9 enzyme, mammals perform this C26-oxidation function using the mitochondrial P450, CYP27A1. *In vitro* studies have shown that CYP27A1 utilizes 4-cholesten-3-one more efficiently than cholesterol[22]. Indeed, CYP27A1 can functionally replace DAF-9 in a co-transfection assay testing for DAF-12 activation using 4-cholesten-3-one as a substrate[17]. However, co-transfection of CYP27A1 with lathosterone had no effect on DAF-12 activity, suggesting that, while DAF-9 and CYP27A1 have similar enzymatic activities, they have overlapping but distinct substrate specificities[17]. The finding that CYP27A1 can substitute for DAF-9 in generating a hormonal ligand for DAF-12 may have important pathophysiological implications for parasitic nematode diseases (see below).

CONSERVED PATHWAYS OF HORMONAL REGULATION IN WORMS AND HUMANS

Bile acids are known to function as signalling molecules to control bile acid homeostasis by physiologically activating the nuclear receptors FXR, PXR, and VDR[20,21,23]. Recently, circulating bile acids have also been shown to regulate energy expenditure in mice through activation of a GPCR, indicating a role for hormonal signalling by bile acids in mammals[24]. The work summarized herein provides the first direct evidence for the conservation of bile acid-like hormone signalling from worms to mammals. This conservation includes not only the nuclear receptors involved in regulating organism-wide homeostasis but also the enzymes required for generating the nuclear receptor ligands (Figure 1A). In this work we demonstrated that DAF-9 is a functional orthologue of mammalian CYP27A1 and lies at a critical juncture for the production of bile acid-like ligands (Δ^4 and Δ^7 dafachronic acids) for the nuclear receptor DAF-12 (Figure 1B). In humans, CYP27A1 is essential for the synthesis of all bile acids (including 3K-LCA) as well as the oxysterol 27-OH cholesterol, metabolites of cholesterol which are all involved in signalling through nuclear receptors (i.e. FXR, PXR, VDR and LXR) (Figure 1B)[20,21,23,25].

Similar to the many enzymatic steps important for mammalian bile acid synthesis, we propose that *C. elegans*, starting from cholesterol, must convert the unsaturation at C-5 in the steroid nucleus into a C-4 or C-7 unsaturation. To date we have identified DAF-36, a Rieske-like oxygenase that converts cholesterol into 7-dehydrocholesterol[7]. This reaction is the initial step in the transfer of the steroid unsaturation to C-7, providing a precursor to Δ^7-dafachronic acid. Next, there must also be oxidation of the 3β-alcohol into a 3-keto moiety for further conversion to the bile acid-like hormone by DAF-9. Mammals perform these reactions using 3β-hydroxysteroid dehydrogenases (3β-HSD), which are essential enzymes in the synthesis of all bile acids[26]. The *C. elegans* homologue to the mammalian 3β-HSD has not yet been identified; however, analysis of the *C elegans* genome revealed at least four potential candidates that are currently being explored.

DAFACHRONIC ACIDS IN THE CONTROL OF *C. ELEGANS* LIFESPAN

Ageing is a fundamental biological process in metazoans that is regulated by hormonal signalling. Much of our understanding of the pathways controlling ageing have come from numerous studies involving worms and flies, and involve the peptide hormone insulin/IGF-1[27]. Recently, a second signalling pathway known as the germline pathway, thought to involve a steroid hormone, was discovered. Mutant worms with ablated germline cells live 60% longer than their wild-type counterparts. This lifespan extension does not result from sterility of the animals since ablation of the whole gonad has no longevity phenotype[28]. Rather, it seems to depend on the absence of a steroid hormone made by the germline cells that shortens the lifespan of the worm, since ablation of the germline cells in *daf-9* or *daf-36* mutants, which are unable to

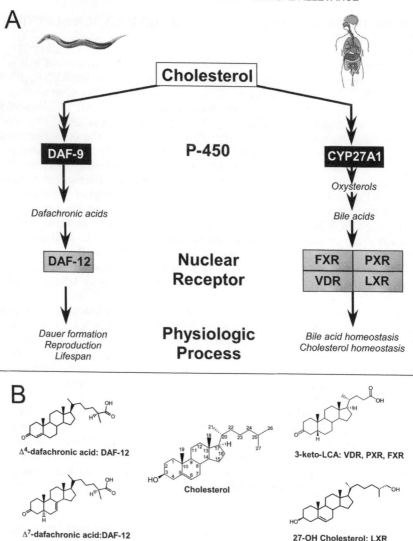

Figure 1 Conserved pathways of hormonal regulation in worms and humans. **A:** Sharing cholesterol as a common precursor, *C. elegans* and mammals carry out a series of enzymatic reactions to generate bile acid-like hormones that control critical physiological processes. The *C. elegans* P450 DAF-9 is a functional orthologue of mammalian CYP27A1 and lies at a critical juncture in the production of bile acid-like ligands (Δ^4 and Δ^7 dafachronic acids). Dafachronic acids bind and activate the nuclear receptor DAF-12 that controls the developmental fate of the organism. In humans, CYP27A1 is essential for the synthesis of all bile acids as well as the oxysterol 27-OH cholesterol. These cholesterol-derived metabolites are ligands for various nuclear receptors involved in maintaining basal bile acid and cholesterol homeostasis. **B:** Chemical structures of nuclear receptor ligands derived from cholesterol

synthesize dafachronic acids, has no effect on lifespan[4,7]. Since we already know that *daf-36* and *daf-9* are key enzymes in the synthesis of dafachronic acids, it is likely that this bile acid-like steroid hormone functions in the germline pathway to control worm lifespan. Experiments designed to address this hypothesis are currently ongoing.

TOWARDS THE TREATMENT OF PARASITIC NEMATODE INFECTIONS

Nematodes constitute one of the largest phyla in animals, with more than 40 000 species. Nematodes are divided into either free-living or parasitic species. Free-living nematodes such as *C. elegans* can live in soil or freshwater, whereas parasitic nematodes have to complete their life cycle in a suitable host[29]. Hookworms (e.g. *Ancylostoma*) are parasitic nematodes that attach to the small intestine of mammalian hosts such as dogs, cats or humans, where they thrive by feeding on the host's blood supply. As a direct consequence of their feeding behaviour hookworm infections are a major cause of iron-deficient anaemia, which can lead to irreversible effects on the growth and development of children. It is estimated that over 1 billion people worldwide suffer from hookworm infection, particularly in tropical and subtropical countries that have poor public health systems[29,30].

The process of hookworm transmission occurs through a series of steps that, depending on their local environment, can correlate with the stages of larval development. Sexually mature females lay eggs that leave the host body through the faeces. If the environment is favourable the eggs will hatch, moult twice in the soil and generate the infective L3 larva (iL3). The iL3 larvae are sheathed, stress-resistant, non-feeding and relatively long-lived. When the chance arises to contact and attach to the host, the L3 larvae can penetrate the host skin and migrate through the blood and lymphatic systems into the pulmonary microcirculation. After being extruded from the vasculature they begin a 'tracheal migration' and are coughed up and swallowed into the gut, where they enter the small intestine and resume reproductive development to L4 larvae and become fertile adults[29–31].

The developmentally arrested iL3 larvae of hookworm are strikingly similar to the dauer larvae of the free-living nematode *C. elegans* in function, morphology, anatomy, and behaviour[30,32]. In a pathway analogous to the re-entry of *C. elegans* into reproductive development, increased insulin signalling by either pharmacological activation of muscarinic receptors or addition of cGMP analogues can induce hookworm iL3 re-feeding[33,34]. Furthermore, blockage of insulin signalling with a PI3K inhibitor can prevent activation of iL3 *in vitro*[35]. Moreover, hookworms express a nuclear receptor that is homologous to the *C. elegans* DAF-12 (unpublished data). These data strongly suggest that a conserved hormone signalling pathway controls activation of the suspended reproductive development in both *C. elegans* and hookworm. When the infective L3 larvae successfully enter the host, the insulin-signalling pathway is activated in response to host-specific factors. We hypothesize that the hookworm would then either make a bile acid-like hormone from a host-derived sterol, or obtain a hormone that is functionally homologous to the dafachronic acids directly from the host. Activation of hookworm DAF-12 would then switch on the expression of genes that allows the parasite to resume reproductive development.

Using a co-transfection assay with the hookworm homologue of DAF-12, we found that cholestenoic acid, a bile acid-like compound made by alveolar macrophages in the lung[36,37], activates the hookworm DAF-12 of *Ancylostoma* spp. at a physiologically relevant concentration. CYP27A1 is responsible for the metabolism of cholesterol to cholestenoic acid in a manner almost identical to the reaction DAF-9 carries out to generate dafachronic acids. It is of interest to note that, to date, no DAF-9 homologues have been found in any hookworm species, leading to speculation that a host enzyme (i.e. CYP27A1) may fulfil this function. Although *in vivo* studies must still be performed, this finding provides compelling evidence that endogenous bile acid-like metabolites are the host-derived factors that permit parasitic nematodes to complete their life cycle and reproduce. Taken together, this work provides new avenues to explore the reproductive development of parasitic nematodes, and importantly provides a novel strategy for pharmacological intervention of parasitic nematode infections that affect plants, animals, and ~1 billion people worldwide.

Acknowledgements

We thank Veerle Rottiers and Adam Antebi (Baylor College of Medicine); Kamalesh Sharma, Tingting Li, and Richard Auchus (UT Southwestern); Yong Li, Kelly Suino-Powell and Eric Xu (Van Andel Research Institute) who co-authored the findings reviewed in this work[17]. C.L.C. is an associate and D.J.M is an investigator of the Howard Hughes Medical Institute. D.L.M. is supported by the Pharmacological Science training grant from the NIH. This work was funded by the Howard Hughes Medical Institute and the Robert A. Welch Foundation.

References

1. Riddle DL, Albert PS. Genetic and environmental regulation of dauer larva development. In: Riddle DL, Blumenthal T, Meyer BJ, R. PJ, editors. *C. Elegans* II. Cold Spring Harbor: Cold Spring Harbor Laboratory Press, 1997:739–68.
2. Antebi A, Culotti JG, Hedgecock EM. daf-12 regulates developmental age and the dauer alternative in *Caenorhabditis elegans*. Development. 1998;125:1191–205.
3. Antebi A, Yeh WH, Tait D, Hedgecock EM, Riddle DL. daf-12 encodes a nuclear receptor that regulates the dauer diapause and developmental age in *C. elegans*. Genes Dev. 2000;14: 1512–27.
4. Gerisch B, Weitzel C, Kober-Eisermann C, Rottiers V, Antebi A. A hormonal signaling pathway influencing *C. elegans* metabolism, reproductive development, and life span. Dev Cell. 2001;1:841–51.
5. Jia K, Albert PS, Riddle DL. DAF-9, a cytochrome P450 regulating *C. elegans* larval development and adult longevity. Development. 2002;129:221–31.
6. Mangelsdorf DJ, Thummel C, Beato M et al. The nuclear receptor superfamily: the second decade. Cell. 1995;83:835–9.
7. Rottiers V, Motola DL, Gerisch B et al. Hormonal control of *C. elegans* dauer formation and life span by a Rieske-like oxygenase. Dev Cell. 2006;10:473–82.

8. Payne AH, Hales DB. Overview of steroidogenic enzymes in the pathway from cholesterol to active steroid hormones. Endocrinol Rev. 2004;25:947–70.
9. Chitwood DJ. Biochemistry and function of nematode steroids. Crit Rev Biochem Mol Biol. 1999;34:273–84.
10. Kurzchalia TV, Ward S. Why do worms need cholesterol? Nat Cell Biol. 2003;5:684–8.
11. Li J, Brown G, Ailion M, Lee S, Thomas JH. NCR-1 and NCR-2, the *C. elegans* homologs of the human Niemann-Pick type C1 disease protein, function upstream of DAF-9 in the dauer formation pathways. Development. 2004;131:5741–52.
12. Matyash V, Entchev EV, Mende F et al. Sterol-derived hormone(s) controls entry into diapause in *Caenorhabditis elegans* by consecutive activation of DAF-12 and DAF-16. PLoS Biol. 2004;2:e280.
13. Crowder CM, Westover EJ, Kumar AS, Ostlund RE Jr, Covey DF. Enantiospecificity of cholesterol function *in vivo*. J Biol Chem. 2001;276:44369–72.
14. Sluder AE, Mathews SW, Hough D, Yin VP, Maina CV. The nuclear receptor superfamily has undergone extensive proliferation and diversification in nematodes. Genome Res. 1999;9:103–20.
15. Shostak Y, Van Gilst MR, Antebi A, Yamamoto KR. Identification of *C. elegans* DAF-12-binding sites, response elements, and target genes. Genes Dev. 2004;18:2529–44.
16. Ludewig AH, Kober-Eisermann C, Weitzel C et al. A novel nuclear receptor/coregulator complex controls *C. elegans* lipid metabolism, larval development, and aging. Genes Dev. 2004;18:2120–33.
17. Motola DL, Cummins CL, Rottiers V et al. Identification of ligands for DAF-12 that govern dauer formation and reproduction in *C. elegans*. Cell. 2006;124:1209–23.
18. Merris M, Kraeft J, Tint GS, Lenard J. Long-term effects of sterol depletion in *C. elegans*: sterol content of synchronized wild-type and mutant populations. J Lipid Res. 2004;45: 2044–51.
19. Janowski BA, Willy PJ, Devi TR, Falck JR, Mangelsdorf DJ. An oxysterol signalling pathway mediated by the nuclear receptor LXR alpha. Nature. 1996;383:728–31.
20. Makishima M, Lu TT, Xie W et al. Vitamin D receptor as an intestinal bile acid sensor. Science. 2002;296:1313–16.
21. Staudinger JL, Goodwin B, Jones SA et al. The nuclear receptor PXR is a lithocholic acid sensor that protects against liver toxicity. Proc Natl Acad Sci USA. 2001;98:3369–74.
22. Norlin M, von Bahr S, Bjorkhem I, Wikvall K. On the substrate specificity of human CYP27A1: implications for bile acid and cholestanol formation. J Lipid Res. 2003;44: 1515–22.
23. Makishima M, Okamoto AY, Repa JJ et al. Identification of a nuclear receptor for bile acids. Science. 1999;284:1362–5.
24. Watanabe M, Houten SM, Mataki C et al. Bile acids induce energy expenditure by promoting intracellular thyroid hormone activation. Nature. 2006;439:484–9.
25. Fu X, Menke JG, Chen Y et al. 27-Hydroxycholesterol is an endogenous ligand for liver X receptor in cholesterol-loaded cells. J Biol Chem. 2001;276:38378–87.
26. Russell DW. The enzymes, regulation, and genetics of bile acid synthesis. Annu Rev Biochem. 2003;72:137–74.
27. Tatar M, Bartke A, Antebi A. The endocrine regulation of aging by insulin-like signals. Science. 2003;299:1346–51.
28. Hsin H, Kenyon C. Signals from the reproductive system regulate the lifespan of *C. elegans*. Nature. 1999;399:362–6.
29. Anderson RC. The superfamily Ancylostomatoidea. In: Anderson RC, editor. Nematode Parasites of Vertebrates: Their Development and Transmission. New York: CABI Publishing, 2000:45–60.
30. Hawdon JM, Hotez PJ. Hookworm: developmental biology of the infectious process. Curr Opin Genet Dev. 1996;6:618–23.
31. Loukas A, Prociv P. Immune responses in hookworm infections. Clin Microbiol Rev. 2001; 14:689–703.
32. Hotez P, Hawdon J, Schad GA. Hookworm larval infectivity, arrest and amphiparatenesis: the *Caenorhabditis elegans* Daf-c paradigm. Parasitol Today. 1993;9:23–6.
33. Hawdon JM, Datu B. The second messenger cyclic GMP mediates activation in *Ancylostoma caninum* infective larvae. Int J Parasitol. 2003;33:787–93.

34. Tissenbaum HA, Hawdon J, Perregaux M, Hotez P, Guarente L, Ruvkun G. A common muscarinic pathway for diapause recovery in the distantly related nematode species *Caenorhabditis elegans* and *Ancylostoma caninum*. Proc Natl Acad Sci USA. 2000;97:460–5.
35. Brand A, Hawdon JM. Phosphoinositide-3-OH-kinase inhibitor LY294002 prevents activation of *Ancylostoma caninum* and *Ancylostoma ceylanicum* third-stage infective larvae. Int J Parasitol. 2004;34:909–14.
36. Babiker A, Andersson O, Lindblom D et al. Elimination of cholesterol as cholestenoic acid in human lung by sterol 27-hydroxylase: evidence that most of this steroid in the circulation is of pulmonary origin. J Lipid Res. 1999;40:1417–25.
37. Babiker A, Andersson O, Lund E et al. Elimination of cholesterol in macrophages and endothelial cells by the sterol 27-hydroxylase mechanism. Comparison with high density lipoprotein-mediated reverse cholesterol transport. J Biol Chem. 1997;272:26253–61.

15
Regulation of CYP7A1 by nuclear receptor signalling in human liver cells

J. Y. L. CHIANG, T. LI, K.-H. SONG, M. HAGHIAC and E. OWSLEY

INTRODUCTION

Transcription of the gene encoding cholesterol 7α-hydroxylase (CYP7A1), the first and rate-limiting enzyme in the bile acid biosynthetic pathway, is inhibited by bile acids, cytokines and insulin[1,2]. Several nuclear receptors have been implicated in regulating CYP7A1 gene transcription[1,2]. It is now well established that bile acid-activated FXR inhibits CYP7A1 gene transcription by an indirect mechanism. FXR induces a negative nuclear receptor SHP, which subsequently interacts with orphan nuclear receptors FTF (or LRH-1) and HNF4α and suppresses CYP7A1 gene transcription. FTF and HNF4α bind to an overlapping sequence in the bile acid response element (BARE), which is highly conserved among different species. The transcriptional activity of HNF4α is highly stimulated by a co-activator, PGC-1α, which is highly induced during starvation to stimulate gluconeogenesis and energy metabolism in mitochondria. Several cell-signalling pathways have been implicated to inhibit CYP7A1 gene transcription in bile acid feedback regulation and also under pathological conditions such as cholestasis, acute phase response to lipopolysaccharides, liver injury, and partial hepatectomy, to inhibit bile acid synthesis. These signalling pathways converge to regulate HNF4α and affect its *trans*-activation of the CYP7A1 gene. Our current research focuses on the mechanisms of cytokines, glucagon, insulin and hepatocyte growth factor (HGF) regulation of CYP7A1 gene expression in primary human hepatocytes.

BILE ACIDS AND CYTOKINES INHIBIT CYP7A1 GENE EXPRESSION

It has been reported that CYP7A1 mRNA expression remains to be inhibited by bile acids in the liver of Shp knockout mice[3]. This suggests that FXR/SHP-independent mechanisms may play critical roles in bile acid feedback inhibition of CYP7A1 gene transcription. Several cell-signalling pathways have been

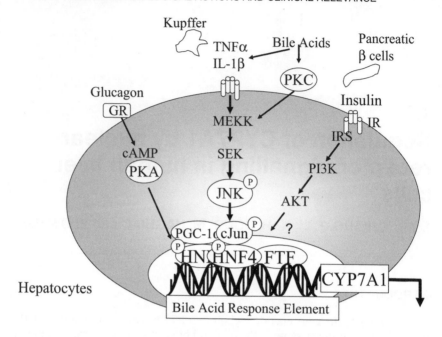

Figure 1 Cell-signalling pathways regulation of CYP7A1 gene transcription. CYP7A1 gene transcription is regulated by nuclear receptors HNF4α and FTF that bind to an overlapping site in the bile acid response element. PGC-1α is an important co-activator of HNF4α. Bile acids and proinflammatory cytokines activate the MAPK pathways ERK1/2 and JNK1/2. JNK phosphorylates cJun to inhibit HNF4α and PGC-1α *trans*-activation of the CYP7A1 gene. JNK also directly phosphorylates HNF4α and reduces its DNA-binding and *trans*-activating activity. Glucagon induces cAMP levels, which activate PKA. PKA phosphorylates HNF4α and decreases its binding to BARE and inhibits CYP7A1 gene transcription. The insulin signalling activates PI3K and AKT pathway and other pathways to regulate CYP7A1

implicated in mediating bile acid inhibition of CYP7A1 (Figure 1)[2]. The best-characterized SHP-independent mechanism is the cytokine-signalling pathway. In cholestasis or acute-phase response to inflammatory agents such as lipopolysaccharides, bile acids are accumulated to stimulate the release of proinflammatory cytokines such as TNF-α and IL-1β from Kupffer cells. These cytokines may cross sinusoid membrane, enter hepatocytes and activate the MAPK pathways. Both CDCA and IL-1β activate a MAPK/JNK signalling pathway that phosphorylates and activates cJun to inhibit CYP7A1 and CYP8B1 gene transcription[4,5]. JNK is able to phosphorylate HNF4α and reduce its DNA-binding and *trans*-activation activity. The cJun interacts with HNF4α and block its interaction with PGC-1α and results in inhibiting CYP7A1 and CYP8B1 gene transcription.

GLUCAGON INHIBITS CYP7A1 GENE TRANSCRIPTION

A recent report shows that cAMP stimulates CYP7A1 mRNA expression in HepG2 cells and fasting increases CYP7A1 mRNA expression in mice in parallel with the increase of PEPCK and PGC-1α mRNA levels[6,7]. Glucagon stimulates cAMP levels in the fasted state and during starvation. It was suggested that bile acid synthesis and gluconeogenesis are coordinately regulated via the fasted-to-fed cycle[6]. These observations are in contrast to earlier reports that CYP7A1 activity is repressed by cAMP and decreased in fasted rats[8,9]. We thus studied the effect of glucagon and cAMP on CYP7A1 expression in human primary hepatocytes. Glucagon (100 nM) strongly and rapidly reduced CYP7A1 mRNA levels. As a positive control, glucagon strongly induced PEPCK mRNA expression as expected. PGC-1α mRNA expression was rapidly induced by glucagon in 1–3 h, and declined after 6–24 h. PGC-1α is highly induced in starvation by glucagon and cAMP. These data suggest that the inhibitory effect of glucagon and cAMP on CYP7A1 mRNA expression dominates over PGC-1α induction. The cAMP activates the protein kinase A pathway to induce PEPCK and gluconeogenesis during starvation. A PKA-specific inhibitor H-89 prevented glucagon inhibition of CYP7A1 mRNA expression. Inhibitors for PKC, ERK, p38 kinase and JNK pathways had no effect. An expression plasmid for the catalytic subunit of PKA strongly inhibited CYP7A1-luciferase reporter activity, but stimulated PEPCK-Luc reporter activity. A mutant PKA plasmid had no effect on these reporters. In-vitro phosphorylation assay showed that glucagon and cAMP were able to phosphorylate HNF4α. Chromatin immunoprecipitation (ChIP) assay showed that glucagon and cAMP decreased the amount of CYP7A1 chromatin precipitated by an antibody against HNF4α. These results suggest that glucagon and cAMP activate PKA, which phosphorylated HNF4α and reduced its recruitment to CYP7A1 chromatin, resulting in inhibition of CYP7A1 gene transcription[10]. These data suggest a discordant regulation of CYP7A1 and PEPCK by glucagon and cAMP.

INSULIN SIGNALLING REGULATION OF CYP7A1 GENE TRANSCRIPTION

Bile acid pool and excretion increase in diabetic patients[11] and in diabetic animal models[12,13]. Insulin restores bile acid pool and rate of bile acid synthesis to normal levels. It has been reported that insulin inhibits CYP7A1[14,15], CYP8B1[16] and CYP27A1[14] activity and mRNA levels in mice and rats. However, the mechanism by which insulin regulates CYP7A1 remains unclear. We studied the effect of insulin on CYP7A1 mRNA expression levels in human primary hepatocytes[17]. It was surprising that insulin rapidly and strongly induced CYP7A1 mRNA levels in a dose-dependent manner with a maximal induction at 10 nM. Extended treatment at higher concentrations modestly reduced CYP7A1 mRNA levels by about 50%. Insulin is known to inhibit PEPCK and other gluconeogenic genes through insulin response elements (IRE), T(G/A)TTT(T/G)(G/T)[18]. It is well established that insulin signalling causes phosphorylation of FoxO1 and phosphorylated FoxO1 is excluded from the nucleus and degraded by the ubiquitin–proteasome system in cytosol. Insulin signalling stimulates SREBP-1c, which is a key regulator of lipogenesis and insulin action[19]. Insulin also activates LXR, which induces SREBP-1c expression and cleavage. Human CYP7A1 promoter does not contain IRE or SRE/E box sequences. FoxO1 and SREBP-1c can act as DNA-binding independent co-repressors by interacting with the DNA-binding domain and ligand-binding domain, respectively, and inhibits HNF4α/PGC-1α *trans*-activation of the PEPCK gene[20,21]. Reporter assays showed that FoxO1 and SREBP-1c strongly inhibited human CYP7A1 reporter activity stimulated by HNF4α and PGC-1α. We performed a ChIP assay using human primary hepatocytes. Without insulin treatment, HNF4α recruits FoxO1 to CYP7A1 chromatin. When treated with insulin (10 nM), FoxO1 is released to allow PGC-1α to be recruited to chromatin. After longer treatment, for 6–24 h, SREBP-1c expression is increased and recruited to chromatin and PGC-1α is released. These data suggest that physiological concentrations of insulin rapidly inhibit FoxO1 activity and allow HNF4α to recruit PGC-1α to stimulate CYP7A1 gene transcription. Extended insulin treatment at concentrations found in insulin resistance induce SREBP-1c and its recruitment to CYP7A1 chromatin to block PGC-1α interaction with HNF4α and results in inhibition of CYP7A1 gene transcription.

SUMMARY

Cell-signalling pathways play critical roles in mediating bile acids, cytokines, and glucagon inhibition of CYP7A1 gene transcription. These signalling pathways converge to regulate the downstream target HNF4α, block its interaction with PGC-1α, and *trans*-activation of the CYP7A1 gene (Figure 1). Glucagon rapidly inhibits the CYP7A1 gene by activating PKA, which phosphorylates HNF4α and reduces its *trans*-activation of the CYP7A1 gene. Our results suggest a discordant regulation of CYP7A1 and PEPCK gene by glucagons and cAMP, and that bile acid synthesis is reduced during starvation. On the other hand, the insulin signalling phosphorylates and inactivates FoxO1 and results in blocking FoxO1 inhibition of CYP7A1 gene transcription. Extended insulin treatment at non-physiological concentration inhibits CYP7A1 by inducing SREBP-1c, which blocks HNF4α and PGC-1α interaction. These two signalling pathways may play key roles in regulation of bile acid synthesis and gluconeogenesis in diabetes. In type I diabetes, insulin deficiency activates FoxO1 activity, which stimulates gluconeogenesis but inhibits bile acid synthesis and lipogenesis to cause hyperglycaemia and hyperlipidaemia respectively. In type II diabetes, insulin resistance increases FoxO1 nuclear retention and SREBP-1c synthesis to stimulate gluconeogenesis but decreases bile acid synthesis and lipogenesis. This also led to hyperglycaemia and hyperlipidaemia, respectively. Activation of bile acid receptor FXR may reduce SREBP-1c and improve insulin sensitivity and the diabetic condition.

Acknowledgement

This research was supported by NIH grants DK44442 and DK58379.

References

1. Chiang JY. Bile Acid regulation of gene expression: roles of nuclear hormone receptors. Endocrinol Rev. 2002;23:443–63.
2. Chiang JY. Regulation of bile acid synthesis: pathways, nuclear receptors, and mechanisms. J Hepatol. 2004;40:539–51.
3. Wang L, Lee YK, Bundman D et al. Redundant pathways for negative feedback regulation of bile acid production. Dev Cell. 2002;2:721–31.
4. Jahan A, Chiang JY. Cytokine regulation of human sterol 12α-hydroxylase (CYP8B1) gene. Am J Physiol Gastrointest Liver Physiol. 2004;288:G685–95.
5. Li T, Jahan A, Chiang JY. Bile acids and cytokines inhibit the human cholesterol 7α-hydroxylase gene via the JNK/c-jun pathway in human liver cells. Hepatology. 2006;43:1202–10.
6. De Fabiani E, Mitro N, Gilardi F, Caruso D, Galli G, Crestani M. Coordinated control of cholesterol catabolism to bile acids and of gluconeogenesis via a novel mechanism of transcription regulation linked to the fasted-to-fed cycle. J Biol Chem. 2003;278:39124–32.
7. Shin DJ, Campos JA, Gil G, Osborne TF. PGC-1a activates CYP7A1 and bile acid biosynthesis. J Biol Chem. 2003;278:50047–52.
8. Noshiro M, Nishimoto M, Okuda K. Rat liver cholesterol 7α-hydroxylase. Pretranslational regulation for circadian rhythm. J Biol Chem. 1990;265: 10036–41.
9. Pandak WM, Hylemon PB, Ren S et al. Regulation of oxysterol 7α-hydroxylase (CYP7B1) in primary cultures of rat hepatocytes. Hepatology. 2002;35:1400–8.
10. Song KH, Chiang JY. Glucagon and cAMP inhibit cholesterol 7α-hydroxylase (CYP7a1) gene expression in human hepatocytes: discordant regulation of bile acid synthesis and gluconeogenesis. Hepatology. 2006;43:117–25.
11. Bennion LJ, Grundy SM. Effects of diabetes mellitus on cholesterol metabolism in man. N Engl J Med. 1977;296:1365–71.
12. Hassan AS, Subbiah MT. Effect of diabetes during pregnancy on maternal and neonatal bile acid metabolism in the rat. Proc Soc Exp Biol Med. 1980;165:490–5.
13. Villanueva GR, Herreros M, Perez-Barriocanal F, Bolanos JP, Bravo P, Marin JJ. Enhancement of bile acid-induced biliary lipid secretion by streptozotocin in rats: role of insulin deficiency. J Lab Clin Med. 1990;115:441–8.
14. Twisk J, Hoekman MFM, Lehmann EM, Meijer P, Mager WH, Princen HMG. Insulin suppresses bile acid synthesis in cultured rat hepatocytes by down-regulation of cholesterol 7α-hydroxylase and sterol 27-hydroxylase gene transcription. Hepatology. 1995;21:501–10.
15. Wang DP, Stroup D, Marrapodi M, Crestani M, Galli G, Chiang JYL. Transcriptional regulation of the human cholesterol 7α-hydroxylase gene (CYP7A) in HepG2 cells. J Lipid Res. 1996;37:1831–41.
16. Ishida H, Yamashita C, Kuruta Y, Yoshida Y, Noshiro M. Insulin is a dominant suppressor of sterol 12α-hydroxylase P450 (CYP8B) expression in rat liver: possible role of insulin in circadian rhythm of CYP8B. J Biochem (Tokyo). 2000;127:57–64.
17. Li T, Kong X, Owsley E, Ellis E, Strom S, Chiang JY. Insulin regulation of Cholesterol 7α-hydroxylase expression in human hepatocytes: role of forkhead box O1 and sterol regulatory element-binding protein 1c. J Biol Chem. 2006;281:28745–54.
18. O'Brien R M, Streeper RS, Ayala JE, Stadelmaier BT, Hornbuckle LA. Insulin-regulated gene expression. Biochem Soc Trans. 2001;29:552–8.
19. Foufelle F, Ferre P. New perspectives in the regulation of hepatic glycolytic and lipogenic genes by insulin and glucose: a role for the transcription factor sterol regulatory element binding protein-1c. Biochem J. 2002;366:377–91.
20. Hirota K, Daitoku H, Matsuzaki H et al. Hepatocyte nuclear factor-4 is a novel downstream target of insulin via FKHR as a signal-regulated transcriptional inhibitor. J Biol Chem. 2003;278:13056–60.

21. Yamamoto T, Shimano H, Nakagawa Y et al. SREBP-1 interacts with HNF-4α and interferes with PGC-1 recruitment to suppress hepatic gluconeogenic genes. J Biol Chem. 2004;279:12027–35.

16
Regulation of hepatic and intestinal bile acid transport by FXR-controlled pathways

J. J. ELORANTA and G. A. KULLAK-UBLICK

OVERVIEW OF ENTEROHEPATIC BILE ACID TRANSPORTERS

Bile acids are physiological detergents that promote absorption and excretion of cholesterol, lipids, and other hydrophobic compounds in the liver and intestine[1]. Bile acids are synthesized *de novo* in the liver through cholesterol catabolism and stored in the gallbladder, from which they are postprandially released into the intestine. From the ileum bile acids are returned back to the liver via portal blood. The enterohepatic circulation of bile acids is a highly efficient process in healthy individuals, and is of crucial importance for the maintenance of bile flow and hepatic secretory function. The recycling of bile acids between the liver and intestine is mediated by specific transporter proteins, expressed at the plasma membranes of hepatocytes and enterocytes in a polarized manner[2].

The chief transporter responsible for the excretion of bile acids from hepatocytes into bile canaliculi is the bile salt export pump (BSEP, *ABCB11*)[3], which belongs to the ATP-binding cassette (ABC) transporter family[4]. Whereas BSEP exports monovalent bile acids, another ABC transporter at the canalicular membrane of hepatocytes, multidrug resistance-associated protein 2 (MRP2, *ABCC2*), excretes divalent and sulphated/glucuronidated bile acids into bile[5]. While bile acids are the most prominent (60–70%) components of bile, it also contains phospholipids and cholesterol, which form mixed micelles with the bile acids. The latter two components are translocated into bile by further canalicular ABC family transporters, namely the multidrug resistance protein 3 (MDR3, *ABCB4*) and the heterodimeric ABCG5/ABCG8, respectively[4].

After their passage to the intestinal lumen, bile acids are taken up into ileocytes via the apical sodium-dependent transporter (ASBT, *SLC10A2*)[6], the activity of which is coupled with cotransport of sodium. At the basolateral membranes of ileal enterocytes, bile acids are extruded into portal blood by the organic solute transporter heterodimer OSTα/OSTβ[7]. The larger subunit OSTα contains seven predicted transmembrane domains, whereas OSTβ has a single membrane-spanning domain. Coexpression of OSTα and OSTβ polypeptides is required for correct localization of the heterodimer at the cell membrane and for transport activity. In agreement with its role as the intestinal bile acid efflux transporter, relative distribution of the OSTα/OSTβ heterodimer along the intestinal tract is similar to that of the bile acid uptake system ASBT.

To complete their enterohepatic circulation, bile acids are finally taken up from sinusoidal blood back into parenchymal hepatocytes by transport proteins located at the basolateral membrane. The chief hepatic uptake system for bile acids is the sodium taurocholate cotransporting polypeptide (NTCP, *SLC10A1*)[6], which belongs to the same SLC10 transporter family as ASBT. A member of the organic anion transporter family located at the basolateral membrane, OATP1B1 (*SLCO1B1*), may to a smaller degree also contribute to hepatic bile acid extraction from portal blood in a sodium-independent manner[8].

INDUCTION OF HUMAN BILE ACID EFFLUX TRANSPORTERS BY THE BILE ACID RECEPTOR FXR

Due to their detergent properties, bile acids can be intrinsically toxic to cells; hence their intracellular concentration must be tightly controlled. In addition to their role as physiological detergents, bile acids can act as signalling molecules and homeostatic regulators of their own transport and metabolism within the enterohepatic circulation. By controlling their own cellular uptake or efflux via regulation of the expression levels of bile acid transporter genes, bile acids can adjust their own intracellular concentrations.

The chief sensor of intracellular bile acid levels and the main executor of bile acid-induced transcriptional programmes is a transcription factor of the nuclear receptor family, namely the farnesoid X receptor (FXR)[9]. Bile acids directly interact with, and function as agonists ligands of, the ligand-binding domain of FXR. In accordance with its function as the bile acid receptor, FXR is most abundantly expressed in the tissues commonly exposed to bile acids: liver, intestine, and kidneys. The preferred DNA-binding sequence for FXR within its target promoters is the so-called 'inverted repeat-1' motif (IR-1, inverted hexameric repeat separated by one base pair)[10], to which FXR binds as a heterodimer with another nuclear receptor, namely the retinoid X receptor (RXR).

In response to bile acids FXR stimulates BSEP expression via direct interaction of FXR–RXR heterodimers with an IR-1 element located in the proximal promoter of the *ABCB11* gene[11–13]. Thus, excessive levels of bile acids lead to stimulation of their own hepatocanalicular clearance. The FXR–RXR response element is conserved between the human and rodent *ABCB11/Abcb11* promoters, in support of its functional importance. Similarly to the *ABCB11* gene, expression of the *ABCC2* gene encoding MRP2, the transporter for divalent bile acids at the canalicular membrane, can also be activated by bile acids and FXR[14]. In the case of the *ABCC2* promoter, FXR transactivates through an atypical 'everted repeat-8' (ER-8) motif. In addition to the canalicular bile acid transporter genes, bile acid-activated FXR can induce the expression of the *ABCB4* gene encoding MDR3, the phospholipid transporter at the canalicular membrane of hepatocytes[15]. Thus, bile acids, by activating FXR, induce the excretion of both bile acids (BSEP, MRP2) and phospholipids (MDR3) into bile in a coordinated manner.

In an analogous manner to the *ABCB11* gene, expression of the two genes encoding the heterodimeric bile acid efflux system in the intestine, OSTα/OSTβ are induced by bile acids through direct binding of FXR–RXR heterodimers to the two human *OST* promoters[16,17]. While the regulatory regions of the *OSTβ* promoter appear to harbour a single IR-1-like motif that mediates binding by FXR–RXR, the human *OSTα* promoter contains two adjacent IR-1-like FXR response elements, both of which are functional and required for maximal induction by bile acids. In addition to established cell lines, both *OSTα* and *OSTβ* gene expression can be induced by bile acids in short-term tissue culture of human ileal biopsies. Further physiological evidence in support of the induction of *OST* gene expression by bile acids is provided by a study showing that both mRNA and protein levels of OSTα and OSTβ are increased in cholestatic liver tissue of patients suffering from primary biliary cirrhosis[18].

SUPPRESSION OF HUMAN BILE ACID UPTAKE TRANSPORTERS BY THE BILE ACID RECEPTOR FXR

In keeping with the model that the bile acid sensor FXR elicits hepatoprotective mechanisms aiming at decreasing the intracellular bile acid load, activation of FXR by elevated intracellular levels of bile acids also results in down-regulation of genes encoding enterohepatic bile acid uptake sytems. In rodent models of cholestasis, expression of the hepatic bile acid uptake system Ntcp is suppressed at both the protein and mRNA level[19]. Importantly, certain human cholestatic states, such as advanced-stage primary biliary cirrhosis and cholestatic alcoholic hepatitis, are also associated with reduced NTCP expression[20,21]. We have recently shown that the mechanism of down-regulation of the human *SLC10A1* gene, encoding NTCP, in response to bile acids involves a bile acid-inducible repressor of the nuclear receptor family, known as the small heterodimer partner (SHP)[22]. SHP is an unusual member of the nuclear receptor family, since it lacks any direct DNA-binding activity[23]. The promoter of the *SHP* gene is itself a target for transcriptional activation by ligand-bound FXR[24,25]. Thus, in response to elevated bile acids, FXR-induced SHP negatively targets a DNA-binding transactivator of the *SLC10A1* gene, the glucocorticoid receptor (GR). The negative interference of GR by SHP involves direct interaction between the two proteins, which may block the recruitment of the transcriptional coactivator PGC-1α to the human *SLC10A1* promoter[22,26].

The bile acid–FXR–SHP cascade also suppresses transcription of the *SLCO1B1* gene encoding the OATP1B1 transporter, which may contribute to bile acid uptake at the basolateral membranes of hepatocytes[27]. The molecular target of *SLCO1B1* down-regulation by bile acids is the liver-enriched transcription factor HNF-1α, which is a strong DNA-binding transactivator of the *SLCO1B1* promoter. The regulatory region of the *HNF-1α* gene itself contains a DNA-binding motif for the nuclear receptor HNF-4α, the transcriptional activity of which is targeted for negative interference by the SHP protein.

HNF-4α also functions as a common transactivator of hepatic drug transporter genes, such as the human *SLC22A1* and *SLC22A7* genes, which encode polyspecific drug transporters OCT1 and OAT2, respectively, both located at the basolateral membranes of hepatocytes[28,29]. The bile acid-induced transcriptional repressor SHP interferes with transactivation by HNF-4α in the context of both the *SLC22A1* and *SLC22A7* genes. Thus, in conditions of elevated intracellular bile acid concentrations, the expression of two major human drug uptake systems at the basolateral hepatic membranes may be reduced. This could restrict the amount of drugs xenobiotics that enter hepatocytes, when intracellular levels of toxic bile acids are already elevated.

In an analogous manner to NTCP, bile acids also suppress the expression of the intestinal bile acid uptake system ASBT, another member of the SLC10 transporter family in humans[30]. In agreement with this, *SLC10A2* gene expression has been reported to be reduced in patients with obstructive cholestasis[31]. Similarly to the *SLC10A1* gene, the transactivator protein GR is targeted for negative interference by the bile acid-induced transcriptional repressor SHP on the *SLC10A2* promoter[22,32]. Interestingly, while both the *SLC10A1* and *SLC10A2* genes are transactivated by GR, the relative locations and sequence configurations of the GR response elements within the two *SLC10* promoters are not conserved.

CONCLUDING REMARKS

The function of enterohepatic bile acid transporters is vital for the maintenance of bile acid homeostasis in healthy individuals. Furthermore, the importance of these transporter proteins for hepatic and intestinal function is emphasized by recent demonstrations that either hereditary or acquired disturbances in the activity and/or expression of bile acid transporters are associated with cholestatic diseases. Bile acids are capable of regulating the expression of transporters that mediate the enterohepatic circulation of both bile acids and drugs via complex feedforward and feedback mechanisms. The main orchestrator of these transcriptional circuits is the nuclear receptor for bile acids, FXR, which controls the expression levels of genes encoding the major bile acid transporters at all membrane domains of enterohepatic circulation.

References

1. Hofmann AF. The continuing importance of bile acids in liver and intestinal disease. Arch Intern Med. 1999;159:2647–58.
2. Kullak-Ublick GA, Stieger B, Meier PJ. Enterohepatic bile salt transporters in normal physiology and liver disease. Gastroenterology. 2004;126:322–42.
3. Arrese M, Ananthanarayanan M. The bile salt export pump: molecular properties, function and regulation. Pflugers Arch. 2004;449:123–31.

4. Borst P, Elferink RO. Mammalian ABC transporters in health and disease. Annu Rev Biochem. 2002;71:537–92.
5. Kullak-Ublick GA, Stieger B, Hagenbuch B, Meier PJ. Hepatic transport of bile salts. Semin Liver Dis. 2000;20:273–92.
6. Hagenbuch B, Dawson P. The sodium bile salt cotransport family SLC10. Pflugers Arch. 2004;447:566–70.
7. Dawson PA, Hubbert M, Haywood J et al. The heteromeric organic solute transporter alpha-beta, Ostalpha-Ostbeta, is an ileal basolateral bile acid transporter. J Biol Chem. 2005;280:6960–8.
8. Hagenbuch B, Meier PJ. Organic anion transporting polypeptides of the OATP/ SLC21 family: phylogenetic classification as OATP/ SLCO superfamily, new nomenclature and molecular/functional properties. Pflugers Arch. 2004;447:653–65.
9. Kalaany NY, Mangelsdorf DJ. LXRS and FXR: the yin and yang of cholesterol and fat metabolism. Annu Rev Physiol. 2006;68:159–91.
10. Laffitte BA, Kast HR, Nguyen CM, Zavacki AM, Moore DD, Edwards PA. Identification of the DNA binding specificity and potential target genes for the farnesoid X-activated receptor. J Biol Chem. 2000;275:10638–47.
11. Ananthanarayanan M, Balasubramanian N, Makishima M, Mangelsdorf DJ, Suchy FJ. Human bile salt export pump promoter is transactivated by the farnesoid X receptor/bile acid receptor. J Biol Chem. 2001;276:28857–65.
12. Schuetz EG, Strom S, Yasuda K et al. Disrupted bile acid homeostasis reveals an unexpected interaction among nuclear hormone receptors, transporters, and cytochrome P450. J Biol Chem. 2001;276:39411–18.
13. Plass JR, Mol O, Heegsma J et al. Farnesoid X receptor and bile salts are involved in transcriptional regulation of the gene encoding the human bile salt export pump. Hepatology. 2002;35:589–96.
14. Kast HR, Goodwin B, Tarr PT et al. Regulation of multidrug resistance-associated protein 2 (ABCC2) by the nuclear receptors pregnane X receptor, farnesoid X-activated receptor, and constitutive androstane receptor. J Biol Chem. 2002;277:2908–15.
15. Huang L, Zhao A, Lew JL et al. Farnesoid X receptor activates transcription of the phospholipid pump MDR3. J Biol Chem. 2003;278:51085–90.
16. Landrier JF, Eloranta JJ, Vavricka SR, Kullak-Ublick GA. The nuclear receptor for bile acids, FXR, transactivates human organic solute transporter-alpha and -beta genes. Am J Physiol Gastrointest Liver Physiol. 2006;290:G476–85.
17. Lee H, Zhang Y, Lee FY, Nelson SF, Gonzalez FJ, Edwards PA. FXR regulates organic solute transporters alpha and beta in the adrenal gland, kidney, and intestine. J Lipid Res. 2006;47:201–14.
18. Boyer JL, Trauner M, Mennone A et al. Upregulation of a basolateral FXR-dependent bile acid efflux transporter OSTalpha-OSTbeta in cholestasis in humans and rodents. Am J Physiol Gastrointest Liver Physiol. 2006;290:G1124–30.
19. Fickert P, Zollner G, Fuchsbichler A et al. Effects of ursodeoxycholic and cholic acid feeding on hepatocellular transporter expression in mouse liver. Gastroenterology. 2001; 121:170–83.
20. Zollner G, Fickert P, Zenz R et al. Hepatobiliary transporter expression in percutaneous liver biopsies of patients with cholestatic liver diseases. Hepatology. 2001;33:633–46.
21. Zollner G, Fickert P, Silbert D et al. Adaptive changes in hepatobiliary transporter expression in primary biliary cirrhosis. J Hepatol. 2003;38:717–27.
22. Eloranta JJ, Jung D, Kullak-Ublick GA. The human Na$^+$-taurocholate cotransporting polypeptide gene is activated by glucocorticoid receptor and peroxisome proliferator-activated receptor-gamma coactivator-1alpha, and suppressed by bile acids via a small heterodimer partner-dependent mechanism. Mol Endocrinol. 2006;20:65–79.
23. Seol W, Choi HS, Moore DD. An orphan nuclear hormone receptor that lacks a DNA binding domain and heterodimerizes with other receptors. Science. 1996;272:1336–9.
24. Goodwin B, Jones SA, Price RR et al. A regulatory cascade of the nuclear receptors FXR, SHP-1, and LRH-1 represses bile acid biosynthesis. Mol Cell. 2000;6:517–26.
25. Lu TT, Makishima M, Repa JJ et al. Molecular basis for feedback regulation of bile acid synthesis by nuclear receptors. Mol Cell. 2000;6:507–15.

26. Borgius LJ, Steffensen KR, Gustafsson JA, Treuter E. Glucocorticoid signaling is perturbed by the atypical orphan receptor and corepressor SHP. J Biol Chem. 2002;277: 49761–6.
27. Jung D, Kullak-Ublick GA. Hepatocyte nuclear factor 1 alpha: a key mediator of the effect of bile acids on gene expression. Hepatology. 2003;37:622–31.
28. Popowski K, Eloranta JJ, Saborowski M, Fried M, Meier PJ, Kullak-Ublick GA. The human organic anion transporter 2 gene is transactivated by hepatocyte nuclear factor-4 alpha and suppressed by bile acids. Mol Pharmacol. 2005;67:1629–38.
29. Saborowski M, Kullak-Ublick GA, Eloranta JJ. The human organic cation transporter-1 gene is transactivated by hepatocyte nuclear factor-4alpha. J Pharmacol Exp Ther. 2006; 317:778–85.
30. Neimark E, Chen F, Li X, Shneider BL. Bile acid-induced negative feedback regulation of the human ileal bile acid transporter. Hepatology. 2004;40:149–56.
31. Hruz P, Zimmermann C, Gutmann H et al. Adaptive regulation of the ileal apical sodium dependent bile acid transporter (ASBT) in patients with obstructive cholestasis. Gut. 2006; 55:395–402.
32. Jung D, Fantin AC, Scheurer U, Fried M, Kullak-Ublick GA. Human ileal bile acid transporter gene ASBT (SLC10A2) is transactivated by the glucocorticoid receptor. Gut. 2004;53:78–84.

17
Regulation of bile acid homeostasis by the nuclear bile acid receptor FXR and fibroblast growth factor 15

S. R. HOLMSTROM, M. CHOI, T. INAGAKI, D. J. MANGELSDORF and S. A. KLIEWER

FARNESOID X RECEPTOR

The nuclear receptors comprise a superfamily of ligand-activated transcription factors that includes the steroid, thyroid hormone and retinoid receptors as well as receptors for xenobiotics, fatty acids and cholesterol metabolites[1]. The farnesoid X receptor (FXR) is a nuclear receptor that was named based on its weak, non-physiological activation by the terpenoid farnesol[2]. Subsequent studies showed that FXR is activated efficiently by physiological concentrations of the primary bile acids cholic acid and chenodeoxycholic acid[3–5]. FXR is highly expressed in the liver, intestine and kidney, where it coordinates bile acid homeostasis by binding to DNA response elements as a heterodimer with the retinoid X receptor (RXR). The physiological role of FXR as a bile acid receptor was confirmed in FXR-knockout (KO) mice: these animals exhibit dramatic changes in bile acid homeostasis, including a marked increase in bile acid synthesis, an expanded bile acid pool, and changes in the composition of their bile acids[6,7]. They are also hypersensitive to the administration of exogenous cholic acid, which causes elevated serum and hepatic bile acid concentrations and severe liver damage[7].

FXR IN LIVER

In liver, FXR regulates the expression of a programme of genes involved in maintaining bile acids at safe concentrations. These genes include the bile salt export protein, multidrug resistance-associated protein 2, and multidrug resistance protein 2[8]. FXR is also a crucial regulator of the classic feedback regulatory loop whereby bile acids inhibit their own synthesis. FXR represses expression of cholesterol 7α-hydroxylase (CYP7A1) and sterol 12α-hydroxylase (CYP8B1), two key enzymes in the bile acid synthetic pathway[7].

FXR does not repress expression of CYP7A1 and CYP8B1 directly; rather, FXR induces expression of small heterodimer partner (SHP), which then represses expression of CYP7A1 and CYP8B1[9–12]. SHP is an atypical orphan nuclear receptor that lacks the canonical DNA-binding domain. SHP represses CYP7A1 expression by partnering with another orphan nuclear receptor, termed liver receptor homologue 1 (LRH-1), which binds to the CYP7A1 promoter[9,11]. As predicted, disruption of the SHP gene results in increased bile acid synthesis and an expanded bile acid pool[10,12]. Thus, activation of FXR by bile acids initiates a nuclear receptor signalling cascade that culminates in SHP-mediated repression of bile acid synthesis.

FXR IN INTESTINE

In the small intestine, FXR regulates genes involved in the reabsorption and transport of bile acids. These genes include the ileal bile acid-binding protein, the ileal apical sodium-dependent bile acid transporter, and the organic solute transporters alpha and beta[8]. Although most studies addressing the feedback regulation of bile acid synthesis have focused on liver, where bile acid synthesis occurs, there is evidence that the intestine also has an important role in this process beyond bile acid reabsorption. In rodents, blocking the flow of bile acids into the intestine by bile duct ligation increases CYP7A1 expression and activity in liver[13,14]. Since hepatic concentrations of bile acids increase under these conditions, this unexpected result suggests a role for the intestine in feedback repression of bile acid synthesis. Subsequent studies in rats subjected to biliary diversion showed that intraduodenal administration of taurocholic acid inhibits CYP7A1 expression whereas intravenous or portal administration of taurocholic acid does not[15,16]. One possible explanation for these results is that the intestine secretes a factor that is important for feedback regulation of bile acid synthesis in liver.

Our group recently demonstrated that fibroblast growth factor 15 (FGF15) is an intestinally derived signalling molecule that represses bile acid synthesis in liver[17]. The stage for this finding was set by work from two other groups. First, McKeehan and colleagues showed that mice lacking FGF receptor 4 (FGFR4), a cell surface receptor with tyrosine kinase activity, have decreased hepatic c-Jun N-terminal kinase (JNK) activity, increased CYP7A1 expression and a corresponding increase in bile acid pool size[18]. Conversely, transgenic mice expressing a constitutively active form of FGFR4 in liver have increased JNK activity, decreased CYP7A1 expression and a reduced bile acid pool size[12]. Second, Holt et al.[19] showed that FGF19, the human orthologue of FGF15, is induced by FXR in cultured, primary human hepatocytes and represses CYP7A1 expression through a JNK-dependent pathway.

Based on these studies we examined FGF15 regulation in mice, fully expecting that it would be regulated by FXR in liver. However, this turned out not to be the case. Whereas FGF15 is expressed and strongly induced by FXR in small intestine, especially ileum[17,20], we were unable to detect FGF15 mRNA in liver despite using highly sensitive PCR approaches. Notably, mice lacking FGF15 have elevated CYP7A1 expression and a corresponding increase in bile acid synthesis[18]. Moreover, intravenous injection of exogenous FGF15 into mice causes a profound repression of CYP7A1 repression, demonstrating that FGF15 can act as a hormone. FGF15 fails to repress CYP7A1 expression in mice lacking FGFR4, demonstrating that FGFR4 is the receptor for FGF15 in liver. Interestingly, FGF15 also fails to repress CYP7A1 in SHP-KO mice, demonstrating that these two pathways converge to repress bile acid synthesis[17]. Thus, FGF15 serves as an enterohepatic hormone linking bile acids in the ileum to the repression of bile acid synthesis in the liver (Figure 1). It remains to be determined precisely how FGF15 gets from the ileum to the liver. Previous findings suggest that this might occur through its release into either the portal circulation or the lymph[15,21].

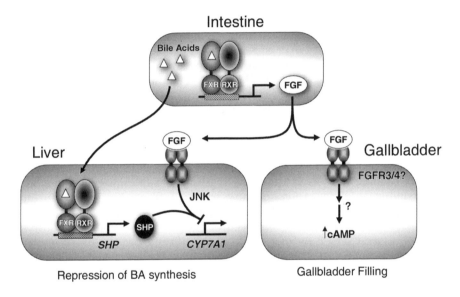

Figure 1 Model for coordinate regulation of bile acid homeostasis by FXR and FGF15. Bile acids activate FXR to induce FGF15 in intestine and SHP in liver. FGF15 acts through FGFR4 in hepatocytes to induce JNK signalling. JNK and SHP cooperate in the repression of CYP7A1 and bile acid synthesis. In gallbladder, FGF15 may act through both FGFR3 and FGFR4 to induce cAMP concentrations and gallbladder filling

A final conundrum: since FGF19 is expressed and induced in response to FXR agonists in cultured human hepatocytes[19], is FGF19 expressed in intact human liver? This appears not to be the case: no FGF19 mRNA was detected by sensitive PCR techniques in human liver samples[22]. Thus, the presence of FGF19 in isolated human hepatocytes appears to be a consequence of culturing them *in vitro*.

FGF15 REGULATES GALLBLADDER FILLING

The gallbladder stores and concentrates bile during fasting and, in response to fat and protein in the diet, releases it into the small intestine to facilitate digestion. The hormone cholecystokinin (CCK), which is secreted postprandially from endocrine cells in the proximal duodenum, is the major determinant of gallbladder emptying. Gallbladder filling is a coordinate response that includes both relaxation of the gallbladder smooth muscle and restriction of bile flow from the common bile duct into the duodenum[23]. The latter process is controlled by contraction of the sphincter of Oddi. While gallbladder contraction and emptying have long been known to be regulated by CCK, it remained unclear whether gallbladder filling is also under endocrine control[23].

Our group recently found that FGF15-KO mice have empty gallbladders even in the fasted state[24]. Intravenous administration of either recombinant FGF15 or FGF19 to FGF15-KO mice causes rapid gallbladder filling and restoration of gallbladder volume to wild-type levels. Notably, in co-injection experiments, FGF15 blocks gallbladder contraction induced by CCK[24]. Thus, FGF15 and CCK have opposing actions on gallbladder contractility. These studies reveal that FGF15 is an essential component of a postprandial feedback loop that stimulates gallbladder filling (Figure 1). Moreover, they suggest a temporal basis for the cycle of gallbladder emptying and filling. Feeding causes CCK secretion from endocrine cells in the proximal duodenum, resulting in gallbladder emptying. The presence of bile acids in the duodenum suppresses further CCK release. After traversing the length of the small intestine, bile acids induce FGF15 expression and secretion from the ileum, causing gallbladder filling. Thus, the differential expression and regulation of CCK and FGF15 in small intestine controls the periodicity of gallbladder motility.

How does FGF15 induce gallbladder filling? *Ex-vivo* tensiometry experiments showed that FGF19 causes a rapid relaxation of gallbladders pre-contracted with CCK[24]. Gallbladder filling correlated with increased concentrations of the second messenger cAMP, which is known to cause smooth muscle relaxation in other contexts. Intravenous injection of forskolin, which stimulates adenylate cyclase activity, caused gallbladder filling in FGF15-KO mice. Taken together, these data indicate that FGF15 causes a cAMP-dependent relaxation of gallbladder smooth muscle. It remains to be determined whether FGF15 causes sphincter of Oddi contraction. It also remains to be determined which FGFR mediates the actions of FGF15 in gallbladder filling. FGFR4-KO mice have small gallbladders[18], but the phenotype is not as severe as that seen in FGF15-KO mice. FGFR3 is the most abundant FGFR in the gallbladder, common bile duct, and sphincter of Oddi[24]. Thus, multiple FGFR may mediate the effects of FGF15 in the gallbladder and biliary tract.

FXR REGULATES INTESTINAL IMMUNE RESPONSE

Bile acids are known to protect the intestinal mucosa. Obstruction of bile flow in rodents causes profound bacterial overgrowth and damage to the epithelium and culminates in bacterial translocation through the intestinal barrier[25–29]. These effects can be reversed by administration of bile acids[30,31]. Similarly, biliary obstruction in humans is associated with bacterial overgrowth and translocation, and bile acid administration can reverse these effects[32–34].

It has been proposed that the detergent properties of bile acids are responsible for their enteroprotective actions. However, a recent study by our group indicates that the effects of bile acids on the intestinal flora are more complex and involve FXR[35]. Microarray experiments were performed using RNA prepared from ileum of mice treated with either vehicle or GW4064, a potent, selective FXR agonist. Among the genes regulated by FXR in ileum were angiogenin, inducible nitric oxide synthase, and interleukin 18. The products of each of these genes have established antimicrobial actions[36–40]. Notably, administration of GW4064 to bile duct-ligated mice resulted in a striking reduction in bacterial overgrowth and translocation[35]. FXR-KO mice had bacterial overgrowth and a deterioration of the mucosal barrier even in the absence of bile duct ligation. Taken together, these results reveal a central role for FXR in controlling bacterial proliferation in the gut. Since elevated concentrations of inducible nitric oxide synthase and interleukin 18 are associated with mucosal damage and inflammatory bowel disease[39,41], regulation of these genes by bile acids, which are released into the small intestine during feeding, may ensure an adequate level of enteroprotection during periods of increased microbial exposure while preventing the overproduction of proteins that can cause inflammation and intestinal disease.

SUMMARY

Recent studies have revealed new and unexpected roles for FXR in regulating bile acid homeostasis. Specifically, the hormone FGF15 has been shown to be selectively induced by FXR in small intestine, to repress hepatic bile acid synthesis and to promote gallbladder filling[17,24]. Thus, FGF15 serves as a hormonal link to coordinate bile acid homeostasis among different tissues. It remains to be seen whether FGF15 emanating from the intestine will exert additional physiological effects. Recent studies have also revealed an unexpected role for FXR in innate immunity in small intestine[35]. Given the broad physiological ramifications of FXR, ligands for this erstwhile orphan receptor may prove useful for treating a variety of diseases ranging from cholestatic liver disease to intestinal disorders.

Acknowledgements

We thank Stacie Cary for assistance with graphics. This work was funded by the Robert A. Welch Foundation (S.A.K. and D.J.M.) and the Howard Hughes Medical Institute (D.J.M.).

References

1. Chawla A, Repa JJ, Evans RM, Mangelsdorf DJ. Nuclear receptors and lipid physiology: opening the X-files. Science. 2001;294:1866–70.
2. Forman BM, Goode E, Chen J et al. Identification of a nuclear receptor that is activated by farnesol metabolites. Cell. 1995;81:687–93.
3. Makishima M, Okamoto AY, Repa JJ et al. Identification of a nuclear receptor for bile acids. Science. 1999;284:1362–5.
4. Parks DJ, Blanchard SG, Bledsoe RK et al. Bile acids: natural ligands for an orphan nuclear receptor. Science. 1999;284:1365–8.
5. Wang H, Chen J, Hollister K, Sowers LC, Forman BM. Endogenous bile acids are ligands for the nuclear receptor FXR/BAR. Mol Cell. 1999;3:543–53.
6. Kok T, Hulzebos CV, Wolters H et al. Enterohepatic circulation of bile salts in farnesoid X receptor-deficient mice: efficient intestinal bile salt absorption in the absence of ileal bile acid-binding protein. J Biol Chem. 2003;278:41930–7.
7. Sinal CJ, Tohkin M, Miyata M, Ward JM, Lambert G, Gonzalez FJ. Targeted disruption of the nuclear receptor FXR/BAR impairs bile acid and lipid homeostasis. Cell. 2000;102: 731–44.
8. Kalaany NY, Mangelsdorf DJ. LXRS and FXR: the yin and yang of cholesterol and fat metabolism. Annu Rev Physiol. 2006;68:159–91.
9. Goodwin B, Jones SA, Price RR et al. A regulatory cascade of the nuclear receptors FXR, SHP-1, and LRH-1 represses bile acid biosynthesis. Mol Cell. 2000;6:517–26.
10. Kerr TA, Saeki S, Schneider M et al. Loss of nuclear receptor SHP impairs but does not eliminate negative feedback regulation of bile acid synthesis. Dev Cell. 2002;2:713–20.
11. Lu TT, Makishima M, Repa JJ et al. Molecular basis for feedback regulation of bile acid synthesis by nuclear receptors. Mol Cell. 2000;6:507–15.
12. Yu C, Wang F, Jin C, Huang X, McKeehan WL. Independent repression of bile acid synthesis and activation of c-Jun N-terminal kinase (JNK) by activated hepatocyte fibroblast growth factor receptor 4 (FGFR4) and bile acids. J Biol Chem. 2005;280: 17707–14.
13. Dueland S, Reichen J, Everson GT, Davis RA. Regulation of cholesterol and bile acid homoeostasis in bile-obstructed rats. Biochem J. 1991;280:373–7.
14. Gustafsson J. Effect of biliary obstruction on 26-hydroxylation of C27-steroids in bile acid synthesis. J Lipid Res. 1978;19:237-43.
15. Nagano M, Kuroki S, Mizuta A et al. Regulation of bile acid synthesis under reconstructed enterohepatic circulation in rats. Steroids. 2004;69:701–9.
16. Pandak WM, Li YC, Chiang JY et al. Regulation of cholesterol 7 alpha-hydroxylase mRNA and transcriptional activity by taurocholate and cholesterol in the chronic biliary diverted rat. J Biol Chem. 1991;266:3416–21.
17. Inagaki T, Choi M, Moschetta A et al. Fibroblast growth factor 15 functions as an enterohepatic signal to regulate bile acid homeostasis. Cell Metab. 2005;2:217–25.
18. Yu C, Wang F, Kan M et al. Elevated cholesterol metabolism and bile acid synthesis in mice lacking membrane tyrosine kinase receptor FGFR4. J Biol Chem. 2000;275:15482–9.
19. Holt JA, Luo G, Billin AN et al. Definition of a novel growth factor-dependent signal cascade for the suppression of bile acid biosynthesis. Genes Dev. 2003;17:1581–91.
20. Li J, Pircher PC, Schulman IG, Westin SK. Regulation of complement C3 expression by the bile acid receptor FXR. J Biol Chem. 2005;280:7427–34.
21. Bjorkhem I, Blomstrand R, Lewenhaupt A, Svensson L. Effect of lymphatic drainage on 7alpha-hydroxylation of cholesterol in rat liver. Biochem Biophys Res Commun. 1978;85: 532–40.
22. Nishimura T, Utsunomiya Y, Hoshikawa M, Ohuchi H, Itoh N. Structure and expression of a novel human FGF, FGF-19, expressed in the fetal brain. Biochim Biophys Acta. 1999; 1444:148–51.
23. Shaffer EA. Review article: Control of gall-bladder motor function. Aliment Pharmacol Ther. 2000;14(Suppl. 2):2–8.
24. Choi M, Moschetta A, Bookout AL et al. Identification of an hormonal basis for gallbladder filling. Nature Med. 2006;12:1253–5.
25. Slocum MM, Sittig KM, Specian RD, Deitch EA. Absence of intestinal bile promotes bacterial translocation. Am Surg. 1992;58:305–10.

26. Ding JW, Andersson R, Soltesz V, Willen R, Bengmark S. Obstructive jaundice impairs reticuloendothelial function and promotes bacterial translocation in the rat. J Surg Res. 1994;57:238–45.

27. Kalambaheti T, Cooper GN, Jackson GD. Role of bile in non-specific defence mechanisms of the gut. Gut. 1994;35:1047–52.

28. Clements WD, Parks R, Erwin P, Halliday MI, Barr J, Rowlands BJ. Role of the gut in the pathophysiology of extrahepatic biliary obstruction. Gut. 1996;39:587–93.

29. Deitch EA, Sittig K, Li M, Berg R, Specian RD. Obstructive jaundice promotes bacterial translocation from the gut. Am J Surg. 1990;159:79–84.

30. Ding JW, Andersson R, Soltesz V, Willen R, Bengmark S. The role of bile and bile acids in bacterial translocation in obstructive jaundice in rats. Eur Surg Res. 1993;25:11–19.

31. Lorenzo-Zuniga V, Bartoli R, Planas R et al. Oral bile acids reduce bacterial overgrowth, bacterial translocation, and endotoxemia in cirrhotic rats. Hepatology. 2003;37:551–7.

32. Cahill CJ. Prevention of postoperative renal failure in patients with obstructive jaundice – the role of bile salts. Br J Surg. 1983;70:590–5.

33. Cahill CJ, Pain JA, Bailey ME. Bile salts, endotoxin and renal function in obstructive jaundice. Surg Gynecol Obstet. 1987;165:519–22.

34. Evans HJ, Torrealba V, Hudd C, Knight M. The effect of preoperative bile salt administration on postoperative renal function in patients with obstructive jaundice. Br J Surg. 1982;69:706–8.

35. Inagaki T, Moschetta A, Lee YK et al. Regulation of antibacterial defense in the small intestine by the nuclear bile acid receptor. Proc Natl Acad Sci USA. 2006;103:3920–5.

36. Biet F, Locht C, Kremer L. Immunoregulatory functions of interleukin 18 and its role in defense against bacterial pathogens. J Mol Med. 2002;80:147–62.

37. Hooper LV, Stappenbeck TS, Hong CV, Gordon JI. Angiogenins: a new class of microbicidal proteins involved in innate immunity. Nat Immunol. 2003;4:269–73.

38. Nathan C. Inducible nitric oxide synthase: what difference does it make? J Clin Invest. 1997;100:2417–23.

39. Reuter BK, Pizarro TT. Commentary: the role of the IL-18 system and other members of the IL-1R/TLR superfamily in innate mucosal immunity and the pathogenesis of inflammatory bowel disease: friend or foe? Eur J Immunol. 2004;34:2347–55.

40. Wallace JL, Miller MJ. Nitric oxide in mucosal defense: a little goes a long way. Gastroenterology. 2000;119:512–20.

41. Alican I, Kubes P. A critical role for nitric oxide in intestinal barrier function and dysfunction. Am J Physiol. 1996;270:G225–37.

18
Bile salts activate endothelial NO synthase in sinusoidal endothelial cells of the liver via the G-protein coupled receptor TGR5

V. KEITEL, R. REINEHR, D. HÄUSSINGER and R. KUBITZ

INTRODUCTION

Over recent years it has become clear that bile salts are not only important for the resorption of dietary lipids and excretion of cholesterol, but that they can act as signalling molecules. Bile salts can bind to nuclear bile salt receptors, such as the farnesoid X receptor (FXR)[1–3], the pregnane X receptor (PXR)[4,5], the vitamin D receptor (VDR)[6], as well as the liver X receptor (LXR)[7] (for reviews see refs 8 and 9). Through activation of FXR, bile salts regulate bile salt synthesis as well as bile salt transport in the gut and liver[3]. Bile salts can not only modulate transcription, but can also activate intracellular protein kinase pathways[10–13]. Recently, the first plasma membrane-bound bile salt receptor, named TGR5[14] or M-BAR[15], has been described. This receptor is coupled to a stimulatory G-protein and bile salts have been identified as the best ligands for this receptor. Expression of TGR5 has been detected in a variety of tissues, including spleen, liver, lung, kidney and placenta[14,15]. On the cellular level TGR5 expression has been demonstrated for CD14 positive monocytes[14], such as alveolar macrophages, an enteroendocrine cell line[16], brown adipocytes, skeletal myofibroblast[17], as well as the gallbladder epithelium[18]. Which of the different cells of the liver express TGR5 remains elusive. This chapter summarizes our recent work on the expression and function of TGR5 in rat liver[19].

LOCALIZATION OF TGR5 IN RAT LIVER

In order to analyse the localization of TGR5 in the liver we developed an antibody against the carboxyterminal 24 amino acids of rat TGR5. The polyclonal anti-TGR5 antisera were evaluated for their specificity on HepG2

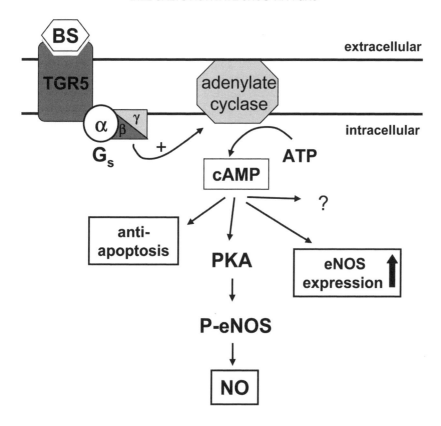

Figure 1 Function of TGR5 in sinusoidal endothelial cells. Bile salts (BS), such as taurolithocholic acid, bind TGR5 from the extracellular space. TGR5 is activated by bile salts, which leads to an activation of adenylate cyclase and an increase in intracellular cyclic AMP. This up-regulates the expression of genes, which contain cAMP-responsive elements in their promoter region, such as the eNOS gene. Protein kinase A is also activated by cAMP and phosphorylates eNOS, leading to an activation of the enzyme and increased NO production. Furthermore, a rise in cAMP leads to a serine phosphorylation of the CD95 receptor, which is an internalization signal, and prevents apoptosis[23]

cells, which were stably transfected with a construct encoding rat TGR5 coupled C-terminally with the yellow fluorescent protein (rTGR5-YFP).

Double-labelling immunofluorescence studies on rat liver slices using the anti-TGR5 antisera and an antibody against rat endothelial antigen-1 (Reca-1) revealed that TGR5 is localized in sinusoidal endothelial cells but not in the endothelial cells of the central vein or in the endothelial cells of any of the vessels in the portal field. Furthermore, we detected a specific staining adjacent to the sinusoidal endothelial cells, which did not co-localize with the Reca-1 fluorescence staining. Using an antibody directed against a Kupffer cell-specific antigen (ED2), we could demonstrate co-localization of this antigen with the anti-TGR5 fluorescence.

FUNCTION OF TGR5 IN SINUSOIDAL ENDOTHELIAL CELLS (SEC)

To assess the function of TGR5 in SEC, we isolated SEC from rat liver by collagenase-pronase perfusion and centrifugal elutriation[20]. Expression of TGR5 in isolated SEC was confirmed by quantitative real-time PCR, Western blotting and immunofluorescence staining. The receptor was localized in the plasma membrane of isolated SEC. Since TGR5 is coupled to a stimulatory G protein we measured intracellular cyclic AMP (cAMP) content after stimulation with different bile salts. Incubation of isolated SEC for 4 min with 25 μM taurolithocholic acid (TLC), taurocholic acid (TC) or taurochenodeoxycholic acid (TCDC) increased intracellular cAMP from 2.1 ± 0.7 pmol/mg protein in unstimulated SEC significantly. TLC led to a 2.9 ± 0.8-fold rise, TC to a 3.2 ± 0.9-fold rise, and TCDC to 2.4 ± 0.9-fold rise in cAMP as compared to controls ($n = 4$). In line with the published data[14,15], TLC was the most potent agonist, increasing intracellular cAMP to a maximum even at a concentration of 10 μM (3.11 ± 0.69-fold). At this concentration (10 μM) TC induced an increase in cAMP of 1.88 ± 0.29-fold as compared to control.

Endothelial nitric oxide synthase (eNOS) is constitutively expressed in endothelial cells. The human eNOS gene contains a cAMP-responsive element (CRE) in its promoter region[21]. Stimulation of SEC for 12 h with taurolithocholic acid (100 μM) or forskolin (10 μM) led to an increase in eNOS mRNA of 1.6 ± 0.1-fold or 1.9 ± 0.3-fold, respectively, as compared to controls ($n = 3$, measured by real-time PCR). ICAM mRNA did not change during the incubation with taurolithocholic acid or forskolin. Nitric oxide (NO) production by eNOS is dependent on the phosphorylation state of eNOS. Phosphorylation of serine residue 1177 leads to an activation of eNOS activity and increased NO production. Using an antibody specific for phosphoserine-1177-eNOS (P-Ser-eNOS) we found that taurolithocholic acid (25 μM, 30 min) induced a 2.4 ± 0.1-fold increase in P-Ser-eNOS as compared to control ($n = 5$). Forskolin led to a similar increase in P-Ser-eNOS (3.3 ± 0.6-fold). The amount of total eNOS did not change during this incubation period. In order to measure NO production we used rat liver slices (400–500 μm thick), which were incubated with the NO-sensitive dye DAF-FM-DA. The dye is taken up into the cells and deacetylated by intracellular esterases into the non-fluorescent DAF-FM. NO rapidly oxidizes DAF-FM into a fluorescent benzotriazole. This increase in fluorescence is detected using an inverted fluorescence microscope and taken as measure for NO production[22]. Incubation of the liver slices with taurolithocholic acid led to an increase in NO production within minutes as measured by DAF-FM fluorescence increase.

Cyclic AMP can inhibit apoptosis in many different cell types. It has recently been shown that cAMP through activation of PKA leads to a serine phosphorylation of the CD95 receptor, which prevents apoptosis[23]. In isolated SEC, incubation with TLC (25 μM, 30 min) induced a significant increase in serine phosphorylation of the CD95 receptor as compared to controls. This may be an important mechanism to protect SEC from bile salt-induced injury.

CONCLUSION

Our data indicate that TGR5 is expressed in sinusoidal endothelial cells and Kupffer cells of rat liver. Bile salts, such as taurolithocholic acid and taurocholic acid, bind and activate TGR5 which leads to an increase in intracellular cAMP in isolated SEC. Rise in cAMP up-regulates mRNA expression of eNOS. Furthermore, through activation of protein kinase A, cAMP promotes phosphorylation of eNOS at position 1177, which leads to an activation of eNOS and increased NO production. Therefore bile salts may modulate hepatic microcirculation directly through the TGR5-cAMP-eNOS-NO pathway.

Acknowledgements

Our studies are supported by grants from the Sonderforschungsbereich 575 Düsseldorf 'Experimentelle Hepatologie' and the Forschungskommission Düsseldorf.

References

1. Makishima M, Okamoto AY, Repa JJ et al. Identification of a nuclear receptor for bile acids. Science. 1999;284:1362–65.
2. Parks DJ, Blanchard SG, Bledsoe RK et al. Bile acids: natural ligands for an orphan nuclear receptor. Science. 1999;284:1365–8.
3. Sinal CJ, Tohkin MM, Miyata M, Ward JM, Lambert G, Gonzalez FJ. Targeted disruption of the nucelar receptor FXR/BAR impairs bile acid and lipid homeostasis. Cell. 2000;102:731–44.
4. Staudinger JL, Goodwin B, Jones SA et al. The nuclear receptor PXR is a lithocholic acid sensor that protects against liver toxicity. Proc Natl Acad Sci USA. 2001;98:3369–74.
5. Jones SA, Moore LB, Shenk JL, Wisely GB, Hamilton GA, McKee DD. The pregnane X receptor: a promiscuous xenobiotic receptor that has diverged during evolution. Mol Endocrinol. 2000;14:27–39.
6. Makishima M, Lu TT, Xie W et al. Vitamin D receptor as an intestinal bile acid sensor. Science. 2002;296:1313–16.
7. Song C, Hiipakka RA, Liao S. Selective activation of liver X receptor alpha by 6 alpha-hydroxy bile acids and analogs. Steroids. 2000;65:423–7.
8. Chiang Y. Bile acid regulation of gene expression: roles of nuclear hormone receptors. Endocrinol Rev. 2002;23:443–63.
9. Zollner G, Marschall HU, Wagner M, Trauner M. Role of nuclear receptors in the adaptive response to bile acids and cholestasis: pathogenetic and therapeutic considerations. Mol Pharm. 2006;3:231–51.
10. Schliess F, Kurz AK, vom Dahl S, Haussinger D. Mitogen-activated protein kinases mediate the stimulation of bile acid secretion by tauroursodeoxycholate in rat liver. Gastroenterology. 1997;113:1306–14.
11. Kurz AK, Graf D, Schmitt M, vom Dahl S, Schliess F, Haussinger D. Tauroursodesoxycholate-induced choleresis involves p38 (MAPK) activation and translocation of the bile salt export pump in rats. Gastroenterology. 2001;121:407–19.
12. Gupta S, Stravitz RT, Dent P, Hylemon PB. Down-regulation of cholesterol 7alpha-hydroxalase (CYP7A1) gene expression by bile acids in primary rat hepatocyte is mediated by the c-Jun N-terminal kinase pathway. J Biol Chem. 2001;276:15816–22.
13. Qiao L, Han SI, Fang Y et al. Bile acid regulation of C/EBPbeta, CREB and c-Jun function, via the extracellular signal-regulated kinase and c-Jun NH2-terminal kinase pathways, modulates the apoptotic response of hepatocytes. Mol Cell Biol. 2003;23:3052–66.

14. Kawamata Y, Fujii R, Hosoya M et al. A G protein-coupled receptor responsive to bile acids. J Biol Chem. 2003;278:9435–40.
15. Maruyama T, Miyamoto Y, Nakamura T et al. Identification of a membrane-type receptor for bile acids (M-BAR). Biochem Biophys Res Commun. 2002;298:714–19.
16. Katsuma S, Hirasawa A, Tsujimoto G. Bile acids promote glucagon-like peptide-1 secretion through TGR5 in a murine enteroendocrine cell line STC-1. Biochem Biophys Res Commun. 2005;329:386–90.
17. Watanabe M, Houten SM, Mataki C et al. Bile acids induce energy expenditure by promoting intracellular thyroid hormone activation. Nature. 2006;439:484–9.
18. Vassileva G, Golovko A, Markowitz I et al. Targeted deletion of Gpbar1 protects mice from cholesterol gallstone formation. Biochem J. 2006;398:423–30.
19. Keitel V, Reinehr R, Gatsios P et al. The G-protein coupled bile salt receptor TGR5 is expressed in liver sinusoidal endothelial cells. Hepatology. 2007;45:695–704.
20. Bode JG, Peters-Regehr T, Kubitz R, Haussinger D. Expression of glutamine synthetase in macrophages. J Histochem Cytochem. 2000;48:415–22.
21. Niwano K, Arai M, Tomaru K, Uchiyama T, Ohyama Y, Kurabayashi M. Transcriptional stimulation of the eNOS gene by the stable prostacyclin analogue beraprost is mediated through cAMP responsive element in vascular endothelial cells: close link between PGI2 signal and NO pathways. Circ Res. 2003;93:523–30.
22. Kojima H, Urano Y, Kikuchi K, Higuchi T, Hirata Y, Nagano T. Fluorescent indicators for imaging nitric oxide production. Angew Chem Int Ed Engl. 1999;38:3209-12.
23. Reinehr R, Haussinger D. Inhibition of bile salt-induced apoptosis by cyclic AMP involves serine/threonine phosphorylation of CD95. Gastroenterology. 2004;126:249–62.

12. Bacq Y, Sapey T, Brechot MC, Pierre F, Fignon A, Dubois F. Intrahepatic cholestasis of pregnancy: a French prospective study. Hepatology. 1997;26:358–64.
13. Axelson M, Graham CE, Sjovall J. Identification and quantitation of steroids in sulfate fractions from plasma of pregnant chimpanzee, orangutan, and rhesus monkey. Endocrinology. 1984;114:337–44.
14. Baillie TA, Curstedt T, Sjovall K, Sjovall J. Production rates and metabolism of sulphates of 3 beta-hydroxy-5 alpha-pregnane derivatives in pregnant women. J Steroid Biochem. 1980;13:1473–88.
15. Anderson RA, Baillie TA, Axelson M, Cronholm T, Sjovall K, Sjovall J. Stable isotope studies on steroid metabolism and kinetics: sulfates of 3 alpha-hydroxy-5 alpha-pregnane derivatives in human pregnancy. Steroids. 1990;55:443–57.
16. Marschall HU, Wagner M, Zollner G et al. Complementary stimulation of hepatobiliary transport and detoxification systems by rifampicin and ursodeoxycholic acid in humans. Gastroenterology. 2005;129:476–85.
17. Jacquemin E, Cresteil D, Manouvrier S, Boute O, Hadchouel M. Heterozygous non-sense mutation of the MDR3 gene in familial intrahepatic cholestasis of pregnancy. Lancet. 1999; 353:210–11.
18. Jacquemin E, De Vree JM, Cresteil D et al. The wide spectrum of multidrug resistance 3 deficiency: from neonatal cholestasis to cirrhosis of adulthood. Gastroenterology. 2001;120:1448–58.
19. Wasmuth HE, Glantz A, Keppeler H et al. Intrahepatic cholestasis of pregnancy: the severe form is associated with common variants of the hepatobiliary phospholipid transporter gene ABCB4. Gut. 2007;56:265–70.
20. Poupon RE, Lindor KD, Cauch-Dudek K, Dickson ER, Poupon R, Heathcote EJ. Combined analysis of randomized controlled trials of ursodeoxycholic acid in primary biliary cirrhosis. Gastroenterology. 1997;113:884–90.
21. Lindor KD. Ursodiol for primary sclerosing cholangitis. Mayo Primary Sclerosing Cholangitis–Ursodeoxycholic Acid Study Group. N Engl J Med. 1997;336:691–5.
22. Olsson R, Boberg KM, de Muckadell OS et al. High-dose ursodeoxycholic acid in primary sclerosing cholangitis: a 5-year multicenter, randomized, controlled study. Gastroenterology. 2005;129:1464–72.
23. Mela M, Mancuso A, Burroughs AK. Review article: Pruritus in cholestatic and other liver diseases. Aliment Pharmacol Ther. 2003;17:857–70.
24. Lammert F, Marschall HU, Matern S. Intrahepatic cholestasis of pregnancy. Curr Treat Options Gastroenterol. 2003;6:123–32.
25. Kondrackiene J, Beuers U, Kupcinskas L. Efficacy and safety of ursodeoxycholic acid versus cholestyramine in intrahepatic cholestasis of pregnancy. Gastroenterology. 2005; 129:894–901.

22
Adolf Windaus Prize Lecture: Primary biliary cirrhosis: from ursodeoxycholic acid towards targeting strategies for therapies

R. POUPON

INTRODUCTION

I am deeply honoured to receive this award from the Falk Foundation and I would like to thank the members of the jury, and especially Professor Gustav Paumgartner, for their support. I am conscious that this award is given to a clinician. As a clinician I have tried to translate into clinical practice some of the advances made in the field of cholanology. I congratulate and thank Dr H. Falk, Ms H. Falk, and Martin Falk for the superb organization of these symposia. May I also thank some of my colleagues, particularly Renée Eugénie Poupon who shifted from biochemistry to clinical epidemiology in order to design and carry out clinical trials, and who has done so much in the collection and interpretation of data; and Y. Chretien, C. Corpechot, O. Chazouillères, C. Housset, P Podevin and Y. Calmus for their collaboration. As previously mentioned by Professor Gustav Paumgartner, Professor J.P. Benhamou asked me to join him when he was appointed head of the department of Hepatology at Beaujon Hospital. He asked me to work with Serge Erlinger, in the field of bile secretion and biliary function. Because I had to infuse bile acids into several species in order to study bile acid kinetics and biliary lipid secretion, it very quickly became apparent to me that the concept of bile acid toxicity which was emerging in the 1970s was real.

Indeed, in 1960, in a short paper in *Nature*, Holsti[1] reported that instillation of bile in the rabbit produced cirrhosis. In 1969 Schaffner and Popper[2] put forward the hypothesis of the role of bile acid (BA) accumulation in liver injury during prolonged cholestasis Following the observations from Japan that ursodeoxycholic acid (UDCA) could dissolve gallstones without any toxicity, S. Erlinger and his group in Beaujon described its unique choleretic properties[3].

Hatoff and Hardison[4], by performing experimental manipulations on hepatic BA concentrations and enzyme activities, concluded that the hepatic response to acute cholestasis is influenced by the composition of the intrahepatic BA pool and that various BA have different effects on this response. Thereafter the concept of BA toxicity was confirmed by several studies showing that BA, depending on their structure, number of OH groups, and amidation, could produce organelle stress, free radical injury, DNA breaks and apoptosis.

This background led to the hypothesis that UDCA, a non-toxic BA could replace endogenous BA when given to patients, and thus could produce improvement in chronic cholestatic diseases. Primary biliary cirrhosis (PBC) was chosen to test this hypothesis because it is a relatively stable and slowly progressive cholestatic process. So we started an open trial in St-Antoine Hospital. We observed striking changes in liver biochemistries, changes suggesting not only that PBC was the result of an immune aggression of the liver, but it also results to some extent from BA toxicity[5].

So, the question raised was: could UDCA be an effective treatment for PBC, or in other words were these effects only cosmetic? To answer this question, we carried out a 2-year double-blind trial followed by a 2-year open trial[6].

LESSONS FROM UDCA THERAPY FOR PBC: EXTENT AND LIMITS OF UDCA TREATMENT

Figure 1 shows some of the results. Considering serum bilirubin levels, UDCA produced two kinds of effects. First, it produced a significant decrease in serum bilirubin during the first 6 months with no further decrease. Thereafter UDCA prevented the increase in serum bilirubin observed in patients receiving placebo, suggesting that UDCA had first a functional effect and thereafter an effect on the pathobiological event(s) leading to cholestasis and increased serum bilirubin.

An unexpected and striking effect were the changes in the two immune hallmarks of PBC, IgM and mitochondrial antibody titre. The falls in IgM levels, as well as the M2 antibody titre, have been confirmed in subsequent studies.

Serum BA decreased in both early and late stages[7]. Meanwhile urinary BA elimination decreased[8], indicating that UDCA acts primarily on hepatic BA secretion and intestinal BA conservation rather that on the cyto-450 pathway of bile acid detoxification.

In parallel with these changes UDCA prevented the aggravation of liver lesions observed in patients receiving placebo, in particular piecemeal necrosis and ductular proliferation, the two features of interface hepatitis[6].

Regarding the hard endpoints, the proportion of failures was significantly reduced in the 4-year study[9]. A similar observation was reported soon after by K. Lindor[10].

To support these observations we collected the individual data of the French, US and Canadian trials, and demonstrated that UDCA reduced by 35% the risk of liver transplantation or death, mostly in patients with advanced disease[11]. This combined analysis led the FDA to approve the drug as medical treatment for PBC.

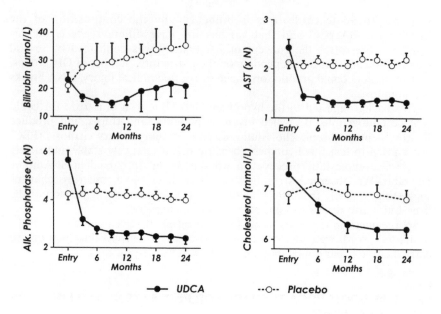

Figure 1   Time course of biochemistries in placebo and UDCA-treated patients

Because 2 or 4 years is too short a period to assess the influence of a drug on a disease with a natural course lasting on average 15 years, we developed a Markov model to assess more accurately the impact of UDCA on liver fibrosis progression and survival. We found that UDCA produced a five-fold reduction of extensive fibrosis development when compared to patients receiving a placebo or D-penicillamine. However, and this is a weakness of UDCA, UDCA was not shown to produce liver fibrosis regression[12].

When Markov modelling was used to study the long-term survival in PBC, we found that UDCA was able to normalize the long-term survival of PBC patients with early-stage disease[13,14].

How does UDCA work to improve cholestasis, and more specifically PBC? How can we improve UDCA efficacy? To answer these questions, an initial factor is what really is PBC in terms of pathophysiological events? Following an insult it is anticipated that, in some cases, due to special host genetic background, the inflammatory response does not resolve, leading to cholestasis.

We have assessed the host genetic background by comparing allelic variation in biliary transporter genes, nucleoreceptor (FXR, PXR, LXR) genes and some candidate genes controlling immunity in 253 French PBC patients and controls. No evidence for a role of the genes controlling biliary function was found, while significant differences were disclosed regarding the CTLA4 gene, which controls duration and intensity of the immune adaptive response, a finding common to some autoimmune disorders.

PBC: AN INFLAMMATORY AND CHOLESTATIC DISEASE

What is inflammation, what is cholestasis in PBC?

In PBC inflammation targets mainly cholangiocytes. The process involved mainly T cells, CD40 activation and IFN-γ, but also many other cells, such as macrophages, polymorphonuclears and fibroblasts, and is characterized by intense crosstalk between all these cells[15]. Because of the multiple players involved, and because of our ignorance of the primary and main insult, it may be anticipated that anti-inflammatory drugs with broad specificity should be more appropriate that specific targeted drugs.

The second major event in PBC is cholestasis. In PBC, cholestasis is primarily a ductal cholestasis and secondarily a canalicular cholestasis as the consequence of the outflow blockade.

Figure 2 shows a simplified view of the signalling events leading to the formation of ductal bile. One the of main features of this signalling pathway it its ability to induce a choleresis rich in bicarbonates.

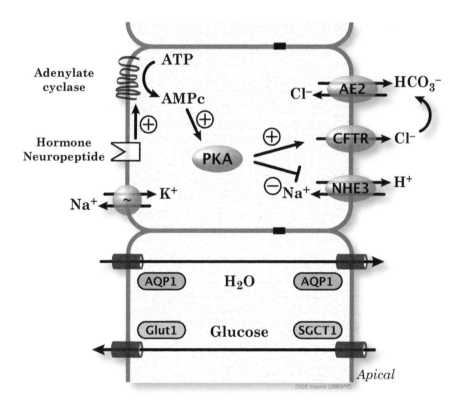

Figure 2 Simplified view of signalling events leading to the formation of ductal bile

This signalling pathway is markedly impaired by a series of mediators and cytokines. All these mediators and cytokines are present around the injured bile ducts in PBC and are associated with a marked reduction in transporter activities and expression[16–19].

In PBC, UDCA restores anion exchanger 2 activity, and as a consequence the response of the pathway to secretin, as elegantly shown by the PET scan imaging studies before and after treatment with UDCA[20].

Occult or overt biliary infections are key features of PBC and primary sclerosing cholangitis respectively. Enteric bacteria and endotoxin escaping from the gut are normally at least in part processed by Kupffer cells and then eliminated and inactivated in bile. In PBC a large amount of endotoxins and other pathogen-associated molecular patterns (PAMP) accumulate in the interlobular bile duct, leading to granuloma[21–24]. PBC patients have very high levels of antibodies against lipid A, the active moiety of endotoxin, as well as antibodies against many bacteria crossreacting with mitochondrial antibodies. We have shown that lipid A antibody titres correlated tightly with IgM levels and inflammatory bile duct lesions. UDCA reduced or suppressed endotoxin accumulation in bile ducts[21,22,25]. Because of the paramount importance of endotoxins in triggering innate, adaptive immune response and autoimmunity, how can we imagine the link between ductal cholestasis and accumulation of endotoxin? The following scenario could be proposed. Alkaline choleresis may protect the biliary epithelium from endotoxin for the following reasons: bile contains alkaline phosphatase, alkaline phosphatase has full activity at pH8 or above, alkaline phosphatase dephosphorylates lipopolysaccharide (LPS) and makes it inactive[26], diluted bile and low salt concentration optimize the activity of anti-microbial peptides[27,28], active reabsorption of glucose and IgA transport from blood to bile may also prevent bacterial overgrowth; both processes are probably impaired in cholestasis due to bile duct injury.

It is thus anticipated that failure to dilute and alkalinize bile should promote cholangitis and accumulation of PAMP. Accordingly drugs which are inducers of ductal choleresis should improve cholangiopathies. Chronic inflammation and cholestasis are responsible for three secondary events: cell death, cholangitis, stellate cell and fibroblast proliferation and activation responsible for fibrosis. Cholangitis and accumulation of LPS are associated with chronic stimulation of the innate immune system. Microbial induction of the Toll pathway blocks the suppressive effect of CD4 CD25 regulatory T cells, allowing activation of pathogen-specific immune reponses and autoimmunity. Apoptosis in general, and specifically of cholangiocytes, may contribute to the generation of autoimmunity.

MECHANISMS OF ACTION OF UDCA

UDCA has multiple biological effects. When given to PBC patients UDCA is metabolized into a series of compounds, the major one being the 3-sulpho-glyco-UDCA and 3-sulpho-7-keto-lithocholate. Currently the *in-vitro* effects of these compounds are unknown, and at least in part for this reason, we ignore the subtle mechanisms of action of UDCA. Nonetheless the following scenario is the most probable according to the present state of knowledge. UDCA relieves cholestasis by several means: as previously mentioned it relieves ductal cholestasis; subsequently canalicular cholestasis is relieved and also because UDCA promotes the targeting of biliary transporters to the canaliculus[29–31] and induced ATP canalicular secretion[32]; finally, intestinal bile acid reabsorption is inhibited[33,34]. The resulting combination of stimulation of biliary secretion together with biliary diversion has multiple consequences that tend to restore the normal physiological patterns by reducing immune activation, apoptosis and fibrogenesis. In addition, UDCA by itself directly abrogates IFN-γ-induced HLA class II hyperexpression[35] and inhibits cytokine-induced apoptosis[36].

TARGETING STRATEGIES TO IMPROVE UDCA ACTION

Theoretically many pathomechanisms could be targeted to improve UDCA action; I will comment on three of them: (1) blockers of the immune activation, (2) inducers of ductal choleresis, (3) NR modulators.

As mentioned previously, the inflammatory process involves many players. Therefore my belief is that we have to use anti-inflammatory drugs with broad specificity rather than specific targeted weapons. Two studies[37,38] have shown that budesonide combined with UDCA is superior to UDCA alone for treating PBC with non-cirrhotic PBC. The combination is better in terms of biochemistries, immune parameters and very importantly in terms of grade of inflammation and fibrosis. This is an important step forward. The next step is to demonstrate that this combination is equally efficient in the subset of patients not responding adequately to UDCA alone.

A second approach is represented by inducers of ductal choleresis. Glybenclamide[39], Sulindac[40] and nor-UDCA[41] belong to this class of drugs. Nor-UDCA is the C23 homologue of UDCA. Nor-UDCA does not undergo significant conjugation and generates a bicarbonate-rich choleresis. In mdr2 knockout mice nor-UDCA markedly improved liver tests and histology, significantly reduced fibrosis and proliferating cholangiocytes and was far more effective than UDCA[42].

A third approach is represented by the nucleoreceptor modulators. The main aim of the biliary function is to irreversibly eliminate from the body a series of harmful lipophilic substances. The export of the compounds is determined by canalicular transporters which are transcriptionally regulated by nucleoreceptors.

When BA concentrations increase in hepatocytes, BA bind to FXR and PXR. Subsequently transcription of a series of gene products aimed to extrude BA from the cell are activated (Figure 3). Accordingly, hepatocytes adapt by reducing import, increasing efflux, decreasing synthesis and increasing biotransformation of BA.

Target genes and inducers of nucleoreceptors are shown in Table 1. UDCA is not an agonist of these receptors *in vitro*; moreover UDCA behaves as an antagonist *in vivo*. Accordingly it is very tempting to imagine that some

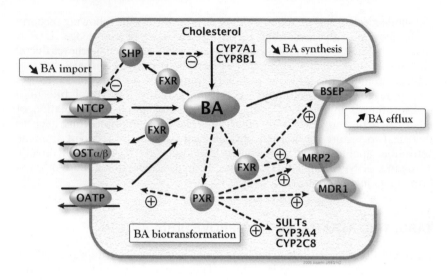

Figure 3 The adaptive response of hepatocytes to bile acid overload

Table 1

	FXR	*PXR*	*LXR*	*PPAR*
Targets	CYP3A4	CYP3A4	Reverse chol tpt	Fatty acid oxidation
	BSEP	MDR3	Inflammation	Inflammation
	MDR3	MRP2		
	MRP2		ABCG5/8	MDR3
Inducers	CDCA	RIF	Oxysterols	Fatty acids
	GW4064	Statin		Eicosanoids
	6ECDCA	Dexa		Fibrates
	Fexaramine	Troglitazone		Statin
		LCA		Thiazolidinediones

agonists of the nucleoreceptors could augment the therapeutic effect of UDCA. PPAR agonists might be of use in cholestasis for two reasons: first, PPARγ is down-regulated in cholangiocytes in PBC[43]; second, PPARγ agonists inhibit stellate cell activation and may counteract liver fibrosis[44].

Rifampicin, a PXR agonist, is widely used for the treatment of cholestasis, in particular in childhood, mainly because of its beneficial effect on pruritus. Very rare cases of side-effects have been reported. There are no data assessing the effects of a UDCA–rifampicin combination in adulthood or childhood; however, in my experience the vast majority of PBC patients presenting with pruritus respond completely with this combination.

This may be explained by the study of Marschall et al.[45] carried out in patients with gallstones. Indeed they found that rifampicin, unlike UDCA, has the unique property to markedly stimulate CYP3A activity and the formation of hydroxylated bile salts, an effect not shared by UDCA. Another argument suggesting that rifampicin could have a long-term benefit is that PXR is expressed not only in hepatocytes but also in human stellate cells, and inhibits the expression of several fibrosis-related genes as well as proliferation-related genes[46].

The potential utility of FXR agonist therapy in cholestasis is based on the fact that the expression of most of the major enzymes and membrane transporters that control the synthesis and enterohepatic circulation of BA are regulated by FXR. GW-4014 and 6 ECDCA are 50–100-fold more potent than UDCA in transactivating FXR. Both have been shown to protect the hepatocyte during BA accumulation induced experimentally[47,48]. GW4064 affords marked protection against α-naphtyl isothiocyanate (ANIT). ANIT-treated rats show large areas of parenchymal necrosis; this was reduced but still noticeable in TUDCA/ANIT-treated rats and absent in rats receiving the agonist. In these rats serum BA and bilirubin were markedly reduced when compared to sham animals or TUDCA-treated rats. Analysis of gene expression in livers from GW4064-treated cholestatic rats revealed decreased expression of BA biosynthetic genes and increased genes involved in BA transport, including mdr2.

It should however be noted that FXR-mediated stimulation of canalicular bile flow via induction of BSEP could aggravate liver injury, as observed in UDCA-fed mice with obstructive cholestasis[49]. Adult cholangiopathies, PBC in advanced stage, i.e. with marked ductopenia and primary sclerosing cholangitis, have a significant obstructive component implying cautious use of an FXR agonist in advanced disease stages.

FXR ligands have in addition recently been demonstrated to have antifibrotic properties through the FXR/SHP cascade that regulates negatively hepatic stellate cell activation, and also through activation of PPARγ[50].

In summary, many novel therapies based on a strong rationale could be available in the next few years; however, it remains to be seen if they are free of side-effects. As in other clinical situations, and because of the number of genes and pathomechanisms involved in cholangiopathies, we can also imagine targeted combination therapies based on liver genetic background characterization and molecular profiling using microarray technologies.

References

1. Holsti P. Cirrhosis of the liver induced in rabbits by gastric instillation of 3-monohydroxycholanic acid. Nature. 1960;186:250.
2. Schaffner F, Popper H. Cholestasis is the result of hypoactive hypertrophic smooth endoplasmic reticulum in the hepatocyte. Lancet. 1969;2:355–9.
3. Dumont M, Erlinger S, Uchman S. Hypercholeresis induced by ursodeoxycholic acid and 7-ketolithocholic acid in the rat: possible role of bicarbonate transport. Gastroenterology. 1980;79:82–9.
4. Hatoff DE, Hardison WG. Bile acids modify alkaline phosphatase induction and bile secretion pressure after bile duct obstruction in the rat. Gastroenterology. 1981;80:666–72.

5. Poupon R, Chretien Y, Poupon RE, Ballet F, Calmus Y, Darnis F. Is ursodeoxycholic acid an effective treatment for primary biliary cirrhosis? Lancet. 1987;1:834–36.

6. Poupon RE, Balkau B, Eschwege E, Poupon R. A multicenter, controlled trial of ursodiol for the treatment of primary biliary cirrhosis. UDCA-PBC Study Group. N Engl J Med. 1991;324:1548–54.

7. Poupon RE, Chretien Y, Poupon R, Paumgartner G. Serum bile acids in primary biliary cirrhosis: effect of ursodeoxycholic acid therapy. Hepatology. 1993;17:599–604.

8. Batta AK, Arora R, Salen G, Tint GS, Eskreis D, Katz S. Characterization of serum and urinary bile acids in patients with primary biliary cirrhosis by gas–liquid chromatography–mass spectrometry: effect of ursodeoxycholic acid treatment. J Lipid Res. 1989;30:1953–62.

9. Poupon RE, Poupon R, Balkau B. Ursodiol for the long-term treatment of primary biliary cirrhosis. The UDCA–PBC Study Group. N Engl J Med. 1994;330:1342–7.

10. Lindor KD, Dickson ER, Baldus WP et al. Ursodeoxycholic acid in the treatment of primary biliary cirrhosis. Gastroenterology. 1994;106:1284–90.

11. Poupon RE, Lindor KD, Cauch-Dudek K, Dickson ER, Poupon R, Heathcote EJ. Combined analysis of randomized controlled trials of ursodeoxycholic acid in primary biliary cirrhosis. Gastroenterology. 1997;113:884–90.

12. Corpechot C, Carrat F, Bonnand AM, Poupon RE, Poupon R. The effect of ursodeoxycholic acid therapy on liver fibrosis progression in primary biliary cirrhosis. Hepatology. 2000;32:1196–9.

13. Poupon RE, Bonnand AM, Chretien Y, Poupon R. Ten-year survival in ursodeoxycholic acid-treated patients with primary biliary cirrhosis. The UDCA–PBC Study Group. Hepatology. 1999;29:1668–71.

14. Corpechot C, Carrat F, Bahr A, Chretien Y, Poupon RE, Poupon R. The effect of ursodeoxycholic acid therapy on the natural course of primary biliary cirrhosis. Gastroenterology. 2005;128:297–303.

15. Fava G, Glaser S, Francis H, Alpini G. The immunophysiology of biliary epithelium. Semin Liver Dis. 2005;25:251–64.

16. Spirli C, Nathanson MH, Fiorotto R et al. Proinflammatory cytokines inhibit secretion in rat bile duct epithelium. Gastroenterology. 2001;121:156–69.

17. Spirli C, Fabris L, Duner E et al. Cytokine-stimulated nitric oxide production inhibits adenylyl cyclase and cAMP-dependent secretion in cholangiocytes. Gastroenterology. 2003;124:737–53.

18. Medina JF, Martinez A, Vazquez JJ, Prieto J. Decreased anion exchanger 2 immunoreactivity in the liver of patients with primary biliary cirrhosis. Hepatology. 1997;25:12–17.

19. Melero S, Spirli C, Zsembery A et al. Defective regulation of cholangiocyte Cl–/HCO3(–) and Na+/H+ exchanger activities in primary biliary cirrhosis. Hepatology. 2002;35:1513–21.

20. Prieto J, Garcia N, Marti-Climent JM, Penuelas I, Richter JA, Medina JF. Assessment of biliary bicarbonate secretion in humans by positron emission tomography. Gastroenterology. 1999;117:167–72.

21. Sasatomi K, Noguchi K, Sakisaka S, Sata M, Tanikawa K. Abnormal accumulation of endotoxin in biliary epithelial cells in primary biliary cirrhosis and primary sclerosing cholangitis. J Hepatol. 1998;29:409–16.

22. Ide T, Sata M, Nakano H, Suzuki H, Tanikawa K. Increased serum IgM class anti-lipid A antibody and therapeutic effect of ursodeoxycholic acid in primary biliary cirrhosis. Hepatogastroenterology. 1997;44:1569–73.

23. Harada K, Tsuneyama K, Sudo Y, Masuda S, Nakanuma Y. Molecular identification of bacterial 16S ribosomal RNA gene in liver tissue of primary biliary cirrhosis: is Propionibacterium acnes involved in granuloma formation? Hepatology. 2001;33:530–6.

24. Tsuneyama K, Harada K, Kono N et al. Scavenger cells with gram-positive bacterial lipoteichoic acid infiltrate around the damaged interlobular bile ducts of primary biliary cirrhosis. J Hepatol. 2001;35:156–63.

25. Ballot E, Bandin O, Chazouilleres O, Johanet C, Poupon R. Immune response to lipopolysaccharide in primary biliary cirrhosis and autoimmune diseases. J Autoimmun. 2004;22:153–8.

26. Poelstra K, Bakker WW, Klok PA, Hardonk MJ, Meijer DK. A physiologic function for alkaline phosphatase: endotoxin detoxification. Lab Invest. 1997;76:319–27.

27. Chen H, Xu Z, Peng L et al. Recent advances in the research and development of human defensins. Peptides. 2006;27:931–40.
28. Bals R, Wang X, Wu Z et al. Human beta-defensin 2 is a salt-sensitive peptide antibiotic expressed in human lung. J Clin Invest. 1998;102:874–80.
29. Beuers U, Bilzer M, Chittattu A et al. Tauroursodeoxycholic acid inserts the apical conjugate export pump, Mrp2, into canalicular membranes and stimulates organic anion secretion by protein kinase C-dependent mechanisms in cholestatic rat liver. Hepatology. 2001;33:1206–16.
30. Kurz AK, Graf D, Schmitt M, Vom Dahl S, Haussinger D. Tauroursodeoxycholate-induced choleresis involves p38(MAPK) activation and translocation of the bile salt export pump in rats. Gastroenterology. 2001;121:407–19.
31. Dombrowski F, Stieger B, Beuers U. Tauroursodeoxycholic acid inserts the bile salt export pump into canalicular membranes of cholestatic rat liver. Lab Invest. 2006;86:166–74.
32. Nathanson MH, Burgstahler AD, Masyuk A, Larusso NF. Stimulation of ATP secretion in the liver by therapeutic bile acids. Biochem J. 2001;358:1–5.
33. Marteau P, Chazouilleres O, Myara A, Jian R, Rambaud JC, Poupon R. Effect of chronic administration of ursodeoxycholic acid on the ileal absorption of endogenous bile acids in man. Hepatology. 1990;12:1206–8.
34. Chazouilleres O, Marteau P, Haniche M, Jian R, Poupon R. Ileal absorption of bile acids in patients with chronic cholestasis: SeHCAT test results and effect of ursodeoxycholic acid (UDCA). Dig Dis Sci. 1996;41:2417–22.
35. Tanaka H, Makino Y, Miura T et al. Ligand-independent activation of the glucocorticoid receptor by ursodeoxycholic acid. Repression of IFN-gamma-induced MHC class II gene expression via a glucocorticoid receptor-dependent pathway. J Immunol.1996;156:1601–8.
36. Rodrigues CM, Fan G, Ma X, Kren BT, Steer CJ. A novel role for ursodeoxycholic acid in inhibiting apoptosis by modulating mitochondrial membrane perturbation. J Clin Invest. 1998;101:2790–9.
37. Leuschner M, Maier KP, Schlichting J et al. Oral budesonide and ursodeoxycholic acid for treatment of primary biliary cirrhosis: results of a prospective double-blind trial. Gastroenterology. 1999;117:918–25.
38. Rautiainen H, Karkkainen P, Karvonen AL et al. Budesonide combined with UDCA to improve liver histology in primary biliary cirrhosis: a three-year randomized trial. Hepatology. 2005;41:747–52.
39. Nathanson MH, Burgstahler AD, Mennone A, Dranoff JA, Rios-Velez L. Stimulation of bile duct epithelial secretion by glybenclamide in normal and cholestatic rat liver. J Clin Invest. 1998;101:2665–76.
40. Bolder U, Trang NV, Hagey LR et al. Sulindac is excreted into bile by a canalicular bile salt pump and undergoes a cholehepatic circulation in rats. Gastroenterology. 1999;117:962–71.
41. Yoon YB, Hagey LR, Hofmann AF, Gurantz D, Michelotti EL, Steinbach JH. Effect of side-chain shortening on the physiologic properties of bile acids: hepatic transport and effect on biliary secretion of 23-nor-ursodeoxycholate in rodents. Gastroenterology. 1986; 90:837–52.
42. Fickert P, Wagner M, Marschall HU et al. 24-norUrsodeoxycholic acid is superior to ursodeoxycholic acid in the treatment of sclerosing cholangitis in Mdr2 (Abcb4) knockout mice. Gastroenterology. 2006;130:465–81.
43. Harada K, Isse K, Kamihira T, Shimoda S, Nakanuma Y. Th1 cytokine-induced downregulation of PPARgamma in human biliary cells relates to cholangitis in primary biliary cirrhosis. Hepatology. 2005;41:1329–38.
44. Fiorucci S, Rizzo G, Antonelli E et al. Cross-talk between farnesoid X-receptor (FXR) and peroxisome proliferator-activated receptor gamma contributes to the antifibrotic activity of FXR ligands in rodent models of liver cirrhosis. J Pharmacol Exp Ther. 2005;315:58–68.
45. Marschall HU, Wagner M, Zollner G et al. Complementary stimulation of hepatobiliary transport and detoxification systems by rifampicin and ursodeoxycholic acid in humans. Gastroenterology. 2005;129:476–85.
46. Haughton EL, Tucker SJ, Marek CJ et al. Pregnane X receptor activators inhibit human hepatic stellate cell transdifferentiation in vitro. Gastroenterology. 2006;131:194–209.
47. Liu Y, Binz J, Numerick MJ et al. Hepatoprotection by the farnesoid X receptor agonist GW4064 in rat models of intra- and extrahepatic cholestasis. J Clin Invest. 2003;112:1678–87.

48. Fiorucci S, Rizzo G, Antonelli E et al. A farnesoid X receptor-small heterodimer partner regulatory cascade modulates tissue metalloproteinase inhibitor-1 and matrix metalloprotease expression in hepatic stellate cells and promotes resolution of liver fibrosis. J Pharmacol Exp Ther. 2005;314:584–95.
49. Fickert P, Zollner G, Fuchsbichler A et al. Ursodeoxycholic acid aggravates bile infarcts in bile duct-ligated and Mdr2 knockout mice via disruption of cholangioles. Gastroenterology. 2002;123:1238–51.
50. Fiorucci S, Antonelli E, Rizzo G et al. The nuclear receptor SHP mediates inhibition of hepatic stellate cells by FXR and protects against liver fibrosis. Gastroenterology. 2004; 127:1497–512.

Section VI
Bile acids, cellular injury, and hepatic fibrosis

Chair: D HÄUSSINGER and PLM JANSEN

23
Bile acids and liver fibrosis – causative agent and therapeutic tool

P. FICKERT, A. FUCHSBICHLER, T. MOUSTAFA, E. HALILBASIC, C. LANGNER, H. DENK and M. TRAUNER

INTRODUCTION

Depending on the cause of liver injury hepatic fibrosis can present as biliary-type fibrosis with portal-portal septa (e.g. cholangiopathies), bridging fibrosis including portal-central septa (e.g. viral and autoimmune hepatitis), pericellular/sinusoidal fibrosis (e.g. ASH/NASH), and centrolobular fibrosis (e.g. venous-outflow obstruction). This chapter focuses on the pathogenesis of biliary-type fibrosis.

Current concepts of the pathogenesis of biliary-type fibrosis include: (a) the formation of a reactive phenotype of cholangiocytes (e.g. the production of proinflammatory and profibrogenic cytokines and chemokines and their respective receptors), (b) ductular proliferation (as possible pacemaker of biliary fibrosis) with subsequent epithelial–mesenchymal interactions (e.g. activation and proliferation of periductal myofibroblasts), and (c) accumulation and cross-linkage of extracellular matrix products. Bile acids have been suggested to play a key role in each of these individual pathogenetic steps. As such lithocholic acid feeding in mice leads to pronounced periductal fibrosis due to proliferation and activation of portal myofibroblasts within days as a direct result of bile acid toxicity. Feeding of the porphyrogenic substance diethoxycarbonyl dihydrocollidine (DDC) (serving as a model system for xenobiotic-induced cholangiopathies) results in activation of cholangiocytes (i. e. overexpression of VCAM) and pericholangitis within a few days, followed by periductal and portal–portal bridging fibrosis. Proinflammatory and profibrogenic cytokine expression in injured hepatocytes along the portal tract interface and in proliferating cholangiocytes may play a key role in the pathogenesis of biliary fibrosis in these models. Absence of biliary phospholipids in Mdr2$^{-/-}$ mice causes sclerosing cholangitis and biliary-type fibrosis as a result of toxic bile lacking formation of mixed micelles between phospholipids and bile acids. Side chain-modified *nor*UDCA and – to a lesser extent – UDCA reduces ductular proliferation and consequently biliary-type fibrosis in Mdr2$^{-/-}$ mice. Despite these recent findings several key questions remain unresolved: (a) What drives ductular proliferation? (b) Is ductular proliferation a prerequisite for portal–portal bridging? (c) Are bile acids participating in the activation and proliferative response of portal myofibroblasts? (d) Finally, the antifibrotic mechanisms of *nor*UDCA require further detailed mechanistic studies to develop novel potent antifibrotic agents.

BACKGROUND

Cholangiopathies, associated with the retention of potentially toxic bile acids and biliary-type fibrosis, are now recognized as an important group of liver diseases[1,2]. They cause significant morbidity, mortality and the need for liver transplantation[1,3]. Several key questions arise in regard (a) to the current understanding of their pathobiology and (b) to the development of novel treatment strategies:

- Are there different types of liver fibrosis?

- What are the current concepts of the biliary type of liver fibrosis?

- What have we learned from mouse models?

- How could bile acids be a therapeutic tool in liver fibrosis?

THE DIFFERENT TYPES OF LIVER FIBROSIS

Liver fibrosis is currently viewed as the result of a dynamic process with progressive accumulation of fibrillar extracellular matrix (ECM) in the liver as the consequence of a perpetual wound-healing process in response to different stimuli (e.g. viral or autoimmune hepatitis, toxic/drug-induced liver injury, cholestasis)[4,5]. In the biliary type of liver fibrosis co-proliferation of bile ductules together with (myo)fibroblast-like cells is characteristically observed along the margins of the liver acinus leading to portal–portal fibrous septa (for comprehensive review see ref. 6). In contrast, patients suffering from (non)-alcoholic steatohepatitis develop pericellular fibrosis with deposition of the ECM along the sinusoids mainly formed by activated stellate cells (for different histological patterns of liver fibosis see also Figure 1). However, we do not know whether the distinct types of fibrosis observed in different liver diseases are related to the kind of trigger or the cell types involved (e.g. hepatic stellate cells vs myofibroblasts). The following considerations are restricted to the biliary type of liver fibrosis.

CURRENT PATHOPHYSIOLOGICAL CONCEPTS OF THE BILIARY TYPE OF LIVER FIBROSIS

An emerging concept in the pathobiology of cholangiopathies is that cholangiocytes are active participants in their pathogenesis by transformation

Silver Stain   Sirius red

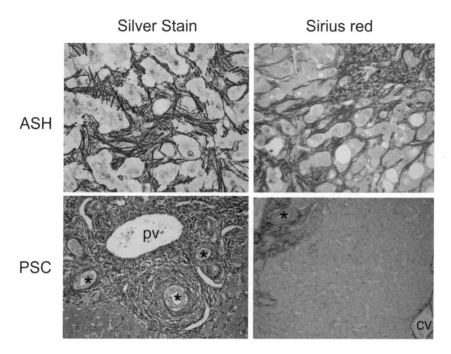

Figure 1 Different types of liver fibrosis. Liver biopsy from a patient with alcoholic steatohepatis (ASH, upper panel) showing characteristic paracellular fibrosis mainly due to activated stellate cells with ECM depositions in the space of Disse. In contrast, in primary sclerosing cholangitis (PSC, lower panel) the fibrotic process is almost limited to the portal field primarily related to activated portal myofibroblasts (lower left), whereas stellate cells are activated only near the portal field (lower right). pv, portal vein; cv, central vein. Asterisks indicate bile ducts

into a reactive phenotype[1,2]. This phenotype is characterized by secretion of proinflammatory (e.g. TNF-α, MCP-1), chemotactic (e.g. VCAM, ICAM), and profibrotic chemokines and cytokines (e.g. TGF-β, PDGF) (Figure 2). In addition, portal inflammation with more or less pronounced infiltration by neutrophils and lymphocytes is a frequent finding[1,2]. Furthermore, the activation of portal (myo)fibroblasts is believed to play a key role in the pathogenesis of biliary-type fibrosis since these cells may represent the main source of collagen and of other components of the extracellular matrix in portal fibrosis. However, we know neither the nature of the initiating trigger (e.g. bile acids, cytokines, reactive oxygen species, growth factors) nor the sequence of these events. Preliminary results in our own laboratory suggest that bile acids (e.g potentially toxic cholic acid) may not represent the main trigger for the activation of bile duct epithelial cells (Halilbasic et al., unpublished observation) and periductal myofibroblasts (Fickert et al., unpublished observation).

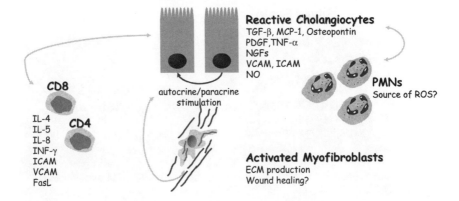

Figure 2   Model of the pathobiology of biliary fibrosis. The reactive phenotype of bile duct epithelial cells is characterized by secretion of proinflammatory (e.g. TNF-α, MCP-1), chemotactic (VCAM, ICAM), and profibrotic chemokines and cytokines (TGF-β, PDGF). Portal inflammation with more or less pronounced infiltration by neutrophils (probably representing the main source for ROS) and lymphocytes is a frequent finding in cholangiopathies. Activation of portal (myo)fibroblasts is believed to play a key role in the pathogenesis of biliary fibrosis since these cells may represent the main source of collagen and other components of the extracellular matrix in portal fibrosis

LESSONS FROM MOUSE MODELS FOR BILIARY FIBROSIS

Despite common bile duct-ligated rodents several well-characterized mouse models for cholestatic liver diseases and resulting biliary fibrosis have been studied over recent years. We have shown that sclerosing cholangitis and biliary-type fibrosis in *Mdr2* knockout (Mdr2$^{-/-}$) mice is a multi-step process with: (a) regurgitation of bile from leaky ducts into the portal tracts leading to (b) induction of periductal inflammation, followed by (c) activation of periductal fibrogenesis and finally (d) causing obliterative cholangitis due to atrophy and death of bile duct epithelial cells[7]. In a longitudinal study feeding the porphyrinogenic substance DDC up to 8 weeks in mice we found a reactive bile duct epithelial cell phenotype which correlated well with the recruitment of neutrophils in the portal fields (Fickert et al., unpublished observation). Ductular reaction was paralleled by the formation of portal–portal bridges and periductal fibrosis. We also demonstrated proliferation of periductal myofibroblasts together with ductular reaction leading to biliary fibrosis in lithocholic acid-fed mice[8]. The availability of several mouse models for biliary fibrosis (e.g. common bile duct-ligated, lithocholic acid-fed, DDC-fed mice, Mdr2$^{-/-}$ mice) will hopefully lead to novel mechanistic insights. However, currently we know little about causes and consequences of bile duct epithelial cell/myofibroblast activation and the specific role of bile acids, cytokines/ chemokines and inflammatory cells in these *in-vivo* models. Moreover, the critical issue has to be resolved how far the lessons learned from these mouse models will be able to extrapolate to the pathobiology of human cholangiopathies. Cross validation of the available mouse models with prototypic cholestatic liver diseases (e.g. PSC, PBC) and non-cholestatic liver diseases represents a mandatory direction for future research strategies in the field of biliary fibrosis.

BILE ACIDS AS THERAPEUTIC TOOL IN LIVER FIBROSIS

Ursodeoxycholic acid was previously shown to have antifibrotic properties[9]. We have recently demonstrated that *nor*UDCA is superior to UDCA in regard to its antifibrotic effects in the Mrd2 knockout mouse model[10]. Currently we are not able to answer the questions as to whether the superior effects of *nor*UDCA are related to possible direct antifibrotic properties or due to the rescue of the reactive phenotype of bile duct epithelial cells. Detailed *in-vitro* studies using the different cell types (e.g. bile duct epithelial cells, myofibroblasts, endothelial cells, mononuclear/Kupffer cells) engaged in the complicated pathophysiology of cholangiopathies will be necessary to obtain deeper insights into these processes.

PROBLEMS TO BE RESOLVED – FUTURE RESEARCH DIRECTIONS

Most of our present knowledge of the mechanisms of liver fibrosis is based on *in-vitro* studies using cultured and activated hepatic stellate cells isolated from rodents (reasoned in the possibility of isolating them from liver tissue with high purity) or human liver and *in-vivo* studies with bile duct-ligated or carbon tetrachloride (CCl_4)-intoxicated rodents[4,11]. We do not know how far findings obtained in these undoubtedly helpful but still artificial systems (e.g. isolated stellate cells activated by growth on plastic dishes) mirror the pathophysiological processes in real life (e.g. human cholestatic liver diseases). The orchestrated interplay between activated proliferating cholangiocytes (bile duct epithelial cells), extracellular matrix-producing cells (e.g. periductal/portal myofibroblasts, bone marrow-derived fibrocytes, stellate cells), inflammatory cells (e.g. neutrophils, macrophages/Kupffer cells, lymphocytes), and smooth muscle cells localized in vessel walls may be pivotal in the pathogenesis of cholangiopathy-related biliary fibrosis[1,2]. However, the precise mechanisms by which cholangiopathies – irrespective of their aetiology – drive biliary fibrosis are still poorly understood. This, at least in part, reflects the previous lack of well-defined, highly reproducible and easy-to-perform animal models allowing detailed longitudinal long-term studies. Despite increasing knowledge on the pathogenesis of hepatic fibrosis several key questions are still, at least in part, unresolved:

● What drives ductular proliferation?

● Is ductular reaction a prerequisite for portal–portal bridging/biliary type of liver fibrosis?

- How do activated myofibroblasts influence ductular reaction?

- Are bile acids engaged in the activation and proliferative response of myofibroblasts?

- Are findings obtained in animal models relevant for human cholestatic liver disease?

References

1. Lazaridis KN, Strazzabosco M, LaRusso NF. The cholangiopathies: disorders of biliary epithelia. Gastroenterology. 2004;127:1565–77.
2. Strazzabosco M, Fabris L, Spirli C. Pathophysiology of cholangiopathies. J Clin Gastroenterol. 2005;39(Suppl. 2):S90–102.
3. Talwalkar JA, Lindor KD. Primary sclerosing cholangitis. Inflamm Bowel Dis. 2005;11:62–72.
4. Bataller R, Brenner DA. Liver fibrosis. J Clin Invest. 2005;115:209–18.
5. Friedman SL. Liver fibrosis – from bench to bedside. J Hepatol. 2003;38(Suppl. 1):S38–53.
6. Pinzani M. Cholestasis and fibrogenesis. In: Alpini G, Alvaro D, Marzioni M, LeSage G, La Russo N, eds. The Pathophysiology of Biliary Epithelia. Landes Bioscience. 2004.
7. Fickert P, Fuchsbichler A, Wagner M et al. Regurgitation of bile acids from leaky bile ducts causes sclerosing cholangitis in Mdr2 (Abcb4) knockout mice. Gastroenterology. 2004;127:261–74.
8. Fickert P, Fuchsbichler A, Marschall HU et al. Lithocholic acid feeding induces segmental bile duct obstruction and destructive cholangitis in mice. Am J Pathol. 2006;168:410–22.
9. Paumgartner G, Beuers U. Mechanisms of action and therapeutic efficacy of ursodeoxycholic acid in cholestatic liver disease. Clin Liver Dis. 2004;8:67–81.
10. Fickert P, Wagner M, Marschall HU et al. 24-norUrsodeoxycholic acid is superior to ursodeoxycholic acid in the treatment of sclerosing cholangitis in Mdr2 (Abcb4) knockout mice. Gastroenterology. 2006;130:465–81.
11. Rippe RA, Brenner DA. From quiescence to activation: gene regulation in hepatic stellate cells. Gastroenterology. 2004;127:1260–2.

24
Mechanisms of bile acid-induced cell death *in vivo* and *in vitro*

H. MOSHAGE

INTRODUCTION

Many liver diseases are accompanied by elevated levels of bile acids, in particular cholestatic disorders. The consequences of the exposure to elevated bile acid levels is dependent on the specific liver cell type: in cholestatic conditions the hepatocytes perish, whereas the hepatic stellate cells (HSC) florish. Both effects are undesirable: excessive hepatocyte death leads to diminished functional liver mass and eventually liver failure, whereas increased numbers of activated HSC contribute to excessive matrix deposition, culminating in fibrosis and cirrhosis and portal hypertension. Detailed knowledge of the response of hepatocytes and HSC to bile acids is therefore essential for the development of strategies that interfere with bile acid-induced processes.

BACKGROUND

In acute and chronic liver diseases, hepatocytes are exposed to increased levels of reactive oxygen species (ROS), cytokines (e.g. tumour necrosis factor-alpha (TNF-α) and bile acids[1]. Exposure to these compounds results in cell death of hepatocytes and proliferation of hepatic stellate cells[1]; therefore it is important to know the mechanisms leading to hepatocyte cell death and stellate cell proliferation, because a more complete understanding of the cellular response to bile acids and ROS will be of significant relevance to understand and treat liver diseases.

Two distinct modes of cell death are known[1-3]: necrosis and apoptosis. However, features characteristic of both necrotic and apoptotic cell death can occur in the same tissue and even the same cell simultaneously. Necrosis is passive and associated with adenosine triphosphate (ATP) depletion, rupture of the plasma membrane and spilling of the cellular content eliciting inflammation. In contrast, apoptosis, or programmed cell death, is an active process characterized by cell shrinkage, chromatin condensation, formation of apoptotic bodies (small membrane-surrounded cell fragments) and activation of caspases. Apoptosis represents a regulated form of cell death and it is important in many physiological processes such as cell selection in development and immunological responses and homeostasis. Deregulated apoptosis contributes to pathological states and many diseases. The strict regulation of apoptotic cell death allows therapeutic intervention strategies.

EFFECTS OF BILE ACIDS ON HEPATOCYTES

The effect of bile acids on primary cultured hepatocytes is dependent on the type of bile acid: hydrophobic bile acids such as glycochenodeoxycholic acid (GCDCA) induce apoptosis in primary hepatocytes, whereas others such as tauroursodeoxycholic acid (TUDCA) are anti-apoptotic, or have no effect on cell death, such as taurochenodeoxycholic acid (TCDC)[4]. The pro- and anti-apoptotic effects of the bile acids GCDCA and TUDCA are absolutely dependent on the uptake of bile acids via the bile acid importer NTCP. The exact difference between different bile acids with respect to the activation of signal transduction pathways is not completely elucidated: all three bile acids activate survival pathways such as the MAP-kinases ERK, p38 and phosphoinositide-3-kinase (PI-3-K)/Akt. The protective effect of the PI-3-K/Akt pathway appears to be more important than the survival pathways p38 and ERK, since inhibition of the PI-3-K/Akt pathway increases GCDCA-induced apoptosis, whereas inhibition of the p38 and ERK pathways has little effect. However, inhibition of both the PI-3-K/Akt and p38 or ERK pathways synergistically increases apoptosis, indicating the importance of all three pathways in the protection against GCDCA-induced apoptosis[4]. In contrast, the JNK pathway activated by GCDCA is pro-apoptotic and inhibition of this pathway completely prevents GCDCA-induced apoptosis. The NF-κB pathway is involved in protection against bile acid-induced apoptosis: activation of NF-κB results in increased expression of genes encoding anti-inflammatory and anti-apoptotic proteins, limiting bile acid-induced apoptosis[5]. Many elegant and excellent studies by Professor Haussinger's group have elucidated in great detail the mechanisms leading to bile acid-induced cell death[6–8]. In these studies it is proposed that hydrophobic bile acids activate hepatocytic NADPH-oxidase followed by phosphorylation and activation of the Src-family member Yes and the EGF receptor. This is followed by heterodimerization of the EGF-R with the Fas receptor CD95. Subsequent translocation of CD95 to the plasma membrane leads to DISC formation and activation of the apoptosis pathway.

It should be noted that in all the discussed studies normal primary cultured hepatocytes were used. In experimental models of cholestasis the predominant mode of cell death appears to be necrosis, rather than apoptosis, although this matter is still subject of intense debate and investigation[2,3,9,10]. Although initially it was believed that apoptotic cell death is the dominant mode of cell death in chronic cholestatic conditions, this view has now been challenged by at least three independent groups using a variety of approaches[5,11,12]. The outcome of this controversy will be important for the design of future therapeutic interventions, since the mode of cell death will determine to a large extent the therapeutic strategies aimed to intervene with cell death. The lack of apoptotic cell death despite exposure to elevated bile acid levels in chronic experimental cholestasis may be due to different mechanisms. (1) It is not known whether the serum bile acid composition in chronic cholestasis is actually pro-apoptotic, necrotic or non-apoptotic. All experiments performed so far on primary cultured hepatocytes have used single bile acids (e.g. GCDCA), whereas the bile acid mixture in cholestatic serum contains many different bile acids. In addition, the mode of cell death of hepatocytes may be dependent on the concentration of bile acids in cholestatic patients. Apoptosis may prevail at low concentrations, whereas higher concentrations may induce necrosis. In this respect it is interesting to note that, in the bile duct ligation model in the rat, the serum concentrations of bile acids are much higher (> 500 µmol/L) than the apoptosis-inducing concentrations used in primary cultures of hepatocytes (50–100 µmol/L). (2) Hepatocytes may also adapt to chronic apoptotic stress. We and others have reported that bile acids activate survival mechanisms. In addition, in experimental cholestasis, inflammation is present, leading to activation of the transcription factor NF-κB. Activation of NF-κB protects against bile acid-induced apoptosis. Recently Black et al. reported that hepatocytes isolated from cholestatic rats are more resistant to transforming growth factor beta-induced cell death than normal hepatocytes[13]. We hypothesize that chronic exposure to bile acids will adapt hepatocytes by inducing an anti-apoptotic phenotype[14]. Elucidation of the mechanisms determining the mode of cell death of hepatocytes in cholestasis and the differential effects of pro- and anti-apoptotic bile acids will remain an important research focus.

EFFECTS OF BILE ACIDS ON HSC

In chronic cholestatic conditons hepatocytes die, whereas the HSC become activated and start to proliferate and produce excessive amounts of connective tissue components such as collagens, fibronectin, laminin and proteoglycans. Exposure of HSC to bile acids does not induce cell death because HSC are not able to import bile acids, since they lack the relevant bile acid importers like NTCP[15]. In contrast, all bile acids induce proliferation of HSC, although to a lesser extent than known potent mitogens for stellate cells such as platelet-derived growth factor (PDGF)[15]. Bile acid-induced proliferation is dependent on phosphorylation and activation of the EGF receptor and subsequent ERK activation in stellate cells[15].

SUMMARY AND CONCLUSION

In chronic cholestatic conditions hepatocytes die and stellate cells proliferate. We have shown that one class of compounds, present at elevated levels in chronic cholestatic conditions, contribute to explain these findings: bile acids induce cell death in hepatocytes and proliferation of stellate cells. Similar results have been demonstrated for ROS[16]: ROS induce cell death of hepatocytes via either apoptosis (superoxide anions) or necrosis (hydrogen peroxide), whereas ROS exposure has also been associated with stellate cell proliferation[16].

The elucidation of the mechanisms involved in hepatocyte cell death and stellate cell proliferation is essential in order to direct therapeutic interventions to the relevant targets. Several key issues to be resolved include the discrepancy between the effects of bile acids on hepatocytes *in vivo* and *in vitro* and the relevance of bile acid-induced stellate cell proliferation compared to other mitogens such as PDGF and reactive oxygen species.

References

1. Schoemaker MH, Moshage H. Defying death: the hepatocyte's survival kit. Clin Sci. 2004;107:13–25.
2. Schulze-Bergkamen H, Schuchmann M, Fleischer B, Galle PR. The role of apoptosis versus oncotic necrosis in liver injury: facts or faith? J Hepatol. 2006;44:984–93.
3. Jaeschke H, Gujral JS, Bajt ML. Apoptosis and necrosis in liver disease. Liver Int. 2004;24:85–9.
4. Schoemaker MH, Conde de la Rosa L, Homan M et al. TUDCA protects rat hepatocytes from bile acid-induced apoptosis via activation of survival pathways. Hepatology. 2004;39:1563–73.
5. Schoemaker MH, Gommans WM, Conde de la Rosa L et al. Resistance of rat hepatocytes against bile acid-induced apoptosis in cholestatic liver injury is due to NF-κB activation. J Hepatol. 2003;39:153–61.
6. Reinehr R, Graf D, Haussinger D. Bile salt-induced hepatocyte apoptosis involves epidermal growth factor receptor-dependent CD95 tyrosine phosphorylation. Gastroenterology. 2003;125:839–53.
7. Reinehr R, Becker S, Wettstein M, Haussinger D. Involvement of the Src family kinase Yes in bile salt-induced apoptosis. Gastroenterology. 2004;127:1540–57.
8. Reinehr R, Becker S, Keitel V, Eberle A, Grether-Beck S, Haussinger D. Bile salt-induced apoptosis involves NADPH oxidase isoform activation. Gastroenterology. 2005;129:2009–31.
9. Malhi H, Gores GJ, Lemasters JJ. Apoptosis and necrosis in the liver: a tale of two deaths? Hepatology. 2006;43:S31–44.
10. Guicciardi ME, Gores GJ. Cholestatic hepatocellular injury: what do we know and how should we proceed. J Hepatol. 2005;42:297–300.
11. Gujral JS, Liu J, Farhood A, Jaeschke H. Reduced oncotic necrosis in Fas receptor-deficient C57BL/6J-lpr mice after bile duct ligation. Hepatology. 2004;40:998–1007.
12. Fickert P, Trauner M, Fuchsbichler A et al. Oncosis represents the main type of cell death in mouse models of cholestasis. J Hepatol. 2005;42:378–85.
13. Black D, Bird MA, Samson CM et al. Primary cirrhotic hepatocytes resist TGFβ-induced apoptosis through a ROS-dependent mechanism. J Hepatol. 2004;40:942–51.
14. Moshage H. The cirrhotic hepatocyte: navigating between Scylla and Charybdis. J Hepatol. 2004;40:1027–9.
15. Svegliati-Baroni G, Ridolfi F, Hannivoort R et al. Bile acids induce hepatic stellate cell proliferation via activation of the EGF-receptor. Gastroenterology. 2005;128:1042–55.
16. Conde de la Rosa L, Schoemaker MH, Vrenken TE et al. Superoxide anions and hydrogen peroxide induce hepatocyte death by different mechanisms: involvement of JNK and ERK MAP kinases. J Hepatol. 2005;44:918–29.

25
Bile acids enhance cellular motility of the hepatic myofibroblast-like cell through the regulation of p38/JNK signalling

Y. ZHANG, T. IKEGAMI, A. HONDA, B. BOUSCAREL and Y. MATSUZAKI

INTRODUCTION

Hepatic fibrosis is a wound-healing process in the liver with acute and chronic injury and is characterized by the excess production and deposition of extracellular matrix (ECM) components[1]. Hepatic mesenchymal cells, such as stellate cell as well as hepatic myofibroblasts, play a pivotal role in liver fibrogenesis as the main source of the ECM. Among the fibrogenic mesenchymal cells in the liver, the best-studied subpopulation is a hepatic stellate cell[2]. Hepatic stellate cells (HSC, also known as lipocytes, fat-storing cells, or Ito cells), reside in the perisinusoidal area in the subendothelial space between hepatocytes and sinusoidal endothelial cells (space of Disse). In response to a variety of liver injuries, HSCs undergo a phenotypic change into highly-proliferative myofibroblast-like cells (a process termed 'activation') and synthesis fibrotic matrix rich in type I collagen, which leads to the formation of scar tissue and, ultimately, liver cirrhosis.

It has been well documented that elevated bile acid (BA) concentration (whether in intrahepatic cholestasis or in extrahepatic cholestasis) leads to hepatocyte[3,4] and cholangiocyte damage[5]. These sustained injuries of parenchymal cells have been thought to be a cause of hepatic fibrosis in cholestatic liver diseases. On the other hand, the direct role of BA on mesenchymal cells, including myofibroblast/HSC, has not yet been fully elucidated .

Svegliati-Baroni et al. indicated that HSC are resistant to BA-induced cell apoptosis and can survive even in the presence of toxic concentrations of BA[6]. Moreover, they found that GCDCA can induce HSC proliferation via activation of the epidermal growth factor receptor (EGFR), thus aiding in the development of the hepatic fibrosis[7].

Besides its proliferative character the activated HSC shows several different behaviours in the process of hepatic fibrosis. These include: (1) enhanced contractility which promotes portal hypertension, and (2) increased cell motility which contributes to the effective distribution of HSC at the injured sites. The effect of BA on these characters in the individual cells has not yet been clarified; therefore we focused on the effect of BA in the motility of activated HSC in the present study.

MATERIALS AND METHODS

We employed the rat liver hepatic stellate cell line (CFSC-2G), which was derived from a rat treated with CCl_4. As for BA, 50 μM glycocheno-deoxycholic acid (GCDCA), a non-toxic concentration confirmed by MTT assay, was used throughout the following study. The proliferation of CFSC-2G was determined by BrdU assay. The phosphorylation of p38 and JNK was determined with Western blotting. The F-actin organization in CFSC-2G cell was visualized by staining with Alexa 448 phalloidin.

RESULTS

GCDCA induced cell proliferation in the presence of 10% serum, but this proliferative effect of GCDCA was not seen in the cells preincubated over 24 h with 1% fetal calf serum (FCS)-containing medium. To exclude the influence on cell proliferation, the cells preincubated with 1% FCS-containing medium for 24 h were used in the following experiments.

To determine the effect of GCDCA on cellular motility the wound-healing assay was performed. The monolayer cell sheet on a plastic dish was wounded by using a pipette tip, then cultured in the presence or absence of 50 μM of GCDCA. The closure of the wound was monitored over time. The wound closure was enhanced by the presence of GCDCA (Figure 1). To investigate the possible mechanisms of action we then focused on MAP kinase signalling, since previous studies have demonstrated the alteration of MAP kinase signalling by BA. Especially in the MAP kinase family members, we focused on p38 as well as JNK, namely stress-activate protein kinase, since their involvement in the cellular motility has been suggested. After 1 h exposure to 50 μM of GCDCA, the phosphorylation of p38 augmented dramatically. This pattern of phosphorylation was also observed by the presence of TGF-β_1, which has been considered a most potent fibrogenic cytokine (Figure 2). Likewise, the phosphorylation of JNK in the presence of GCDCA was also determined. Although TGF-β induced JNK phosphorylation slightly and transiently, the effect of GCDCA on it was significantly greater than that of TGF-β_1 and remained until 24 h after exposure (Figure 2). Furthermore, both the p38 and JNK inhibitor partially inhibited the enhancement of the wound closure by GCDCA (Figure 3).

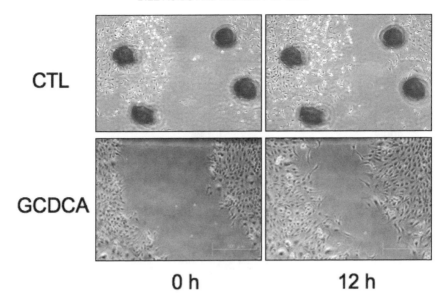

Figure 1 GCDCA can facilitate wound closure. The wound closure was monitored over time in the presence or absence of 50 μM GCDCA. The presence of cells in the wound site was confirmed by haematoxylin–eosin staining after fixation of the cell monolayer with 4% paraformaldehyde containing 0.01% Triton X100. A representative image of three independent assays is shown

DISCUSSION

Cell migration is a key aspect of many physiological and pathological processes[8,9]. In response to a variety of stimuli the activated HSC migrates to the injured area and releases ECM[10–12]. It is generally accepted that the driving force for cell movement is provided by the dynamic reorganization of the cytoskeleton, directing protrusion at the front of the cell and retraction at the rear. Meanwhile, the complicated network which drives cells to move also depends on the cooperation of intermediate filaments, adhesion molecules, and accessory proteins[13,14]. In our experiment, compared with the control group, the greater number of HSC exposed to GCDCA presented a phenotype with lamellipodia, a sheet-like protrusive structure found at the leading edge consisting of a crosslinked meshwork of actin filaments (data not shown). Furthermore, we also demonstrated that GCDCA facilitated wound closure by the HSC cell line. These characteristics induced by GCDCA are independent from the proliferative effect of BA in our experimental condition. The report by Yang et al. mentioned that the migration induced by PDGF-BB was associated with increased proliferation, whereas TGF-β_1/EGF-induced migration was proliferation-independent[11]. Therefore, it is possible that the BA can facilitate HSC activation in both a proliferation-dependent and -independent way. Our data showed that BA could enhance HSC proliferation

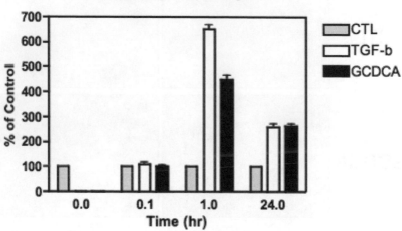

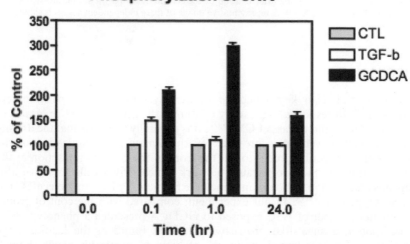

Figure 2 GCDCA can facilitate phosphorylation of p38 and JNK. Expression of total and phosphorylated p38 and JNK in CFSC-2G cells treated either with 50 μM GCDCA or 10 nM TGF-β₁ were determined by Western blotting. The mean ± SEM obtained from three independent experiments is shown in the graph

0 h **12 h**

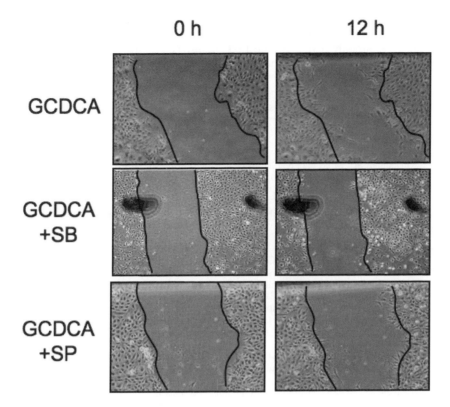

Figure 3 Specific inhibitor of p38 and JNK can partially block the effect of GCDCA. The effect of GCDCA on wound closure was monitored in the co-presence either of p38-specific or JNK-specific inhibitor. A representative image of three independent assays is shown. SB: SB239063, a specific p38 inhibitor, SP: SP600125, a specific JNK inhibitor

only in the case of the presence of 10% FCS. This suggests that some factors in the FCS are necessary for the proliferative effect of GCDCA, while the factors in the FCS are not prerequisite for the migratory effect of GCDCA. Although the synthetic FXR ligand can regulate the progression of hepatic fibrosis through the suppression of HSC activation[15], no confirmed evidence has demonstrated that the uptake of BA in HSC is available. Instead, various receptors as well as a second messenger localized near the plasma membrane have been considered as the target molecules of BA in HSC[7]. In the present study involvement of p38 and JNK in the enhancement of cellular motility by BA was revealed. In a bile duct ligation model the synthesis of TGF-β, especially of TGF-β_1, was found to be increased dramatically only in HSC in liver tissue[16]. Since TGF-β is a most potent profibrogetic cytokine which induces HSC activation, the idea of the modulation of TGF-β signalling by BA merits discussion. Moreover, the p38, as well as JNK, have been identified as the molecules under the control of the TGF-β signalling pathway. However, the direct enhancement of TGF-β$_1$ expression by BA is unlikely, since Svegliati et al. have already demonstrated that the mRNA expression level of TGF-β$_1$ was not altered by the presence of GCDCA[7]. We should further identify the 'real' target of BA in order to understand the pathological mechanism of cholestatic fibrosis, which may lead to the future development of new therapeutic concepts of the diseases.

References

1. Friedman SL. Molecular regulation of hepatic fibrosis, an integrated cellular responseto tissue injury. J Biol Chem. 2000;275:2247–50.
2. Reeves HL, Friedman SL. Activation of hepatic stellate cells – a key issue in liver fibrosis. Front Biosci. 2002;7:d808–26.
3. Rodrigues CM, Fan G, Ma X, Kren BT, Steer CJ. A novel role for ursodeoxycholic acid in inhibiting apoptosis by modulating mitochondrial membrane perturbation. J Clin Invest. 1998;101:2790–9.
4. Reinehr R, Becker S, Wettstein M, Haussinger D. Involvement of the Src family kinase yes in bile salt-induced apoptosis. Gastroenterology. 2004;127:540–57.
5. Fickert P, Fuchsbichler A, Marschall HU et al. Lithocholic acid feeding induces segmental bile duct obstruction and destructive cholangitis in mice. Am J Pathol. 2006;168:410–22.
6. Svegliati-Baroni G, Ridolfi F, Caradonna Z et al. Regulation of ERK/JNK/p70S6K in two rat models of liver injury and fibrosis. J Hepatol. 2003;39:528–37.
7. Sveghati-Baroni G, Ridolfi F, Hannivoort R et al. Bile acids induce hepatic stellate cell proliferation via activation of the epidermal growth factor receptor. Gastroenterology. 2005;128:1042–55.
8. Nodder S, Martin P. Wound healing in embryos: a review. Anat Embryol. 1997;195:215–28.
9. Larsson C. Protein kinase C and the regulation of the actin cytoskeleton. Cell Signal. 2006; 1:276–84.
10. Yanase M, Ikeda H, Ogata I et al. Functional diversity between Rho-kinase- and MLCK-mediated cytoskeletal actions in a myofibroblast-like hepatic stellate cell line. Biochem Biophys Res Commun. 2003;305:223–8.
11. Yang C, Zeisberg M, Mosterman B et al. Liverfibrosis: insights into migration of hepatic stellate cells in response to extracellularmatrix and growth factors. Gastroenterology. 2003; 124:147–59.
12. Park S, Koch D, Cardenas R, Kas J, Shih CK. Cell motility and local viscoelasticity of fibroblasts. Biophys J. 2005;89:4330–42.
13. Juliano RL. Signal transduction by cell adhesion receptors and the cytoskeleton: functions of integrins, cadherins, selectins, and immunoglobulin-superfamily members. Annu Rev Pharmacol Toxicol. 2002;42:283–323.
14. Reddig PJ, Juliano RL. Clinging to life: cell to matrix adhesion and cell survival. Cancer Metastasis Rev. 2005;24:425–39.
15. Fiorucci S, Antonelli E, Rizzo G et al. The nuclear receptor SHP mediates inhibition of hepatic stellate cells by FXR and protects against liver fibrosis. Gastroenterology. 2004;27: 1497–512.
16. Bissell DM, Wang SS, Jarnagin WR, Roll FJ. Cell-specific expression of transforming growth factor-beta in rat liver. Evidence for autocrine regulation of hepatocyte proliferation. J Clin Invest. 1995;96:447–55.

Section VII
Bile acids as therapeutic agents: mechanisms and actions

Chair: GP VAN BERGE HENEGOUWEN and A STIEHL

26
Side-chain-shortened bile acids for the treatment of cholestasis: lessons from *nor*-ursodeoxycholic acid

M. TRAUNER, T. MOUSTAFA, P. FICKERT, E. HALILBASIC,
C. GUELLY, A. FUCHSBICHLER, H. DENK, K. ZATLOUKAL,
M. WAGNER and G. ZOLLNER

INTRODUCTION

Current pharmacological treatment for chronic cholangiopathies such as primary sclerosing cholangitis (PSC) needs improvement[1,2]. A major drawback for the development of novel therapeutic strategies for cholangiopathies has been the lack of easily reproducible animal models[1]. Mice with targeted disruption of the *Mdr2* (*Abcb4*) gene encoding a canalicular phospholipid flippase represent a highly reproducible cholangiopathy model which may be suitable for testing novel therapies for cholestasis[3-6].

The 'ideal' drug for cholangiopathies such as PSC should be specifically targeted to the bile duct epithelium and have bile duct-protective, anticholestatic, antifibrotic and antineoplastic properties. Ursodeoxycholic acid (UDCA) shows some of these properties, but is of limited efficacy in the treatment of PSC[7,8]. Side-chain shortening of bile acids could increase their therapeutic efficacy since this modification significantly alters the physiological properties and pharmacological profile of bile acids[9-12].

nor-URSODEOXYCHOLIC ACID (*nor*UDCA)

*nor*UDCA is a side-chain-shortened C_{23} homologue of UDCA possessing one less methylene group in its side-chain (Figure 1)[9,10]. As a result of this chemical modification *nor*UDCA is more resistant to conjugation with taurine or glycine than UDCA, but instead is secreted into bile mostly in unchanged form[9,10]. The secreted *nor*UDCA undergoes absorption by cholangiocytes, returns to the liver and is resecreted into bile[9,10]. Such cholehepatic shunting leads to a

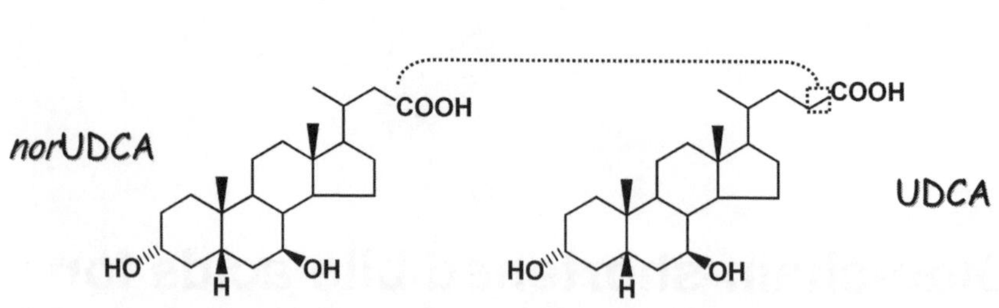

Figure 1 Chemical structure of *nor*UDCA and UDCA. *nor*UDCA (left) is a side-chain-shortened C_{23} homologue of UDCA (right) and possesses one less methylene group in its side-chain (dotted box)

bicarbonate-rich hypercholeresis[9,10] and may also result in improved targeting to the injured bile duct epithelium and liver. These unique mechanisms make *nor*UDCA an attractive candidate drug for the treatment of cholangiopathies.

Mdr2 KNOCKOUT MOUSE (*Mdr2$^{-/-}$*) CHOLANGIOPATHY MODEL WITH FEATURES OF SCLEROSING CHOLANGITIS

The canalicular phospholipid floppase (Mdr2 in rodents/MDR3 in humans; gene name *Abcb4/ABCB4*) mediates translocation of phosphatidylcholine (PC) into the outer leaflet of the canalicular cell membrane, thus facilitating their subsequent extraction by bile acids and excretion into bile[13,14]. *Mdr2 (Abcb4)* knockout mice (*Mdr2/Abcb4$^{-/-}$*) are not capable of excreting PC into bile[13]. Abnormal PC excretion in *Mdr2$^{-/-}$* mice can be rescued by transgenic overexpression of the human *ABCB4* gene, indicating that these two orthologous genes have the same physiological function[14]. In addition, *Mdr2$^{-/-}$* mice have reduced cholesterol excretion, indicating that BA/PC micelles are important in facilitating biliary excretion of cholesterol[14].

  Mdr2$^{-/-}$ spontaneously develop full-blown sclerosing cholangitis within 2 months with macroscopic and microscopic features closely resembling those observed in human sclerosing cholangitis (e.g. PSC)[5,6]. Bile duct injury in these mice is linked to defective biliary phospholipid secretion, resulting in an increased concentration of free non-micellar bile acids which subsequently cause bile duct epithelial cell (cholangiocyte) injury, pericholangitis, periductal fibrosis with ductular proliferation and finally sclerosing cholangitis[5] (Figure 2). Gene expression profiling has revealed remarkable similarities between *Mdr2$^{-/-}$* and human PSC (Moustafa and Trauner, unpublished). In addition, *Mdr2$^{-/-}$* spontaneously develop cholesterol cholecystolithiasis and hepatolithiasis as a result of impaired cholesterol solubility in PC-deficient bile and hepatocellular carcinomas[15–17].

  Hereditary *MDR3* defects result in bile duct injury and liver disease ranging from progressive familial intrahepatic cholestasis subtype 3 (PFIC-3) in infants to adult biliary cirrhosis[18–20]. Moreover, reduced biliary phospholipid

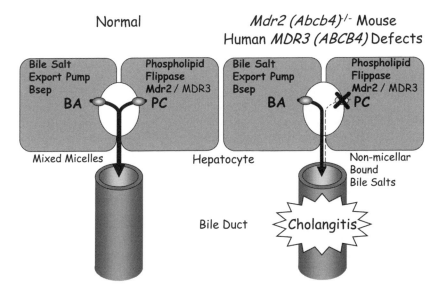

Figure 2 Mechanisms of bile duct injury in the *Mdr2* (*Abcb4*)$^{-/-}$ mouse cholangiopathy model. *Left:* Under normal conditions bile acids (BA) are excreted into bile via the canalicular bile salt export pump (Bsep). Phosphatidylcholine (PC) is exported via the phospholipid flippase (Mdr2; MDR3 in humans). Following their excretion into bile, BA normally form mixed biliary micelles with PC and cholesterol, which prevents BA toxicity. *Right: Mdr2* (*Abcb4*)$^{-/-}$ mice lack biliary excretion of PC, resulting in 'toxic' bile and bile duct injury with development of sclerosing cholangitis. Bile duct injury appears to be linked to an increased concentration of free non-micellar BA which cause cholangiocyte injury, pericholangitis and periductal fibrosis. The *Mdr2*$^{-/-}$ mouse model has important implications for understanding the pathophysiology of human diseases resulting from *MDR3* defects

excretion (in relation to bile salt excretion) has been demonstrated following liver transplantation where it has also been linked to bile duct injury[21,22]. Apart from the experimental evidence in *Mdr2*$^{-/-}$ mice, *MDR3* variants could play a role in the pathogenesis of various cholangiopathies such as PSC, primary biliary cirrhosis (PBC) and adulthood idiopathic ductopenia/biliary fibrosis. Considering the complex pathophysiology of PSC, a *causative* role for any single gene mutation would come as a surprise. A heterozygous *MDR3* mutation was found to be specific to PSC and one *MDR3* haplotype was encountered more frequently in PSC patients[23]. Inherited or acquired (e.g. cytokine- and drug-induced) *MDR3* defects could play a role as *modifyer* gene in subgroups of PSC patients[23]. Such possible scenarios could include female PSC patients with stones, small duct PSC, or paediatric PSC.

Irrespective of the underlying cause of sclerosing cholangitis, the *Mdr2*$^{-/-}$ model has *face validity* since it reliably reproduces the final common pathways of bile duct injury and (peri)biliary fibrosis which could be targeted by pharmacological strategies. Thus the *Mdr2*$^{-/-}$ model provides the unique opportunity to study novel treatments for chronic cholangiopathies (e.g. sclerosing cholangitis/PSC). In addition, this model has *construct validity* for the wide spectrum of human liver diseases resulting from *MDR3* mutations, ranging from neonatal cholestasis/cholangiopathy to adult liver disease (see above). Apart from hereditary or acquired Mdr2/MDR3 transport defects, the $Mdr2^{-/-}$ model may have general validity as a model for cholangiopathies resulting from bile toxicity with a deranged biliary phospholipid/bile salt equilibrium. Finally, the $Mdr2^{-/-}$ mouse model may be important for testing novel therapeutic approaches to sclerosing cholangitis and biliary fibrosis[3]. However, one has to be aware of considerable species differences in transporter regulation, bile acid pool toxicity and immune/inflammatory response between humans and mice that may dramatically influence the cholestatic phenotype.

*nor*UDCA IN THE *Mdr2*$^{-/-}$ MODEL

*nor*UDCA (but not 'conventional' UDCA) reverses sclerosing cholangitis in the $Mdr2^{-/-}$ cholangiopathy model within 4 weeks of treatment[3]. Its therapeutic mechanisms include: (a) amelioration of bile hydrophobicity by biliary enrichment with hydrophilic *nor*UDCA and its metabolites; (b) flushing of injured bile ducts by stimulation of bile flow and bicarbonate-rich choleresis, which dilutes toxic biliary content; (c) induction of alternative bile acid detoxification (phase I and II enzymes) and elimination routes for bile acids (multidrug-resistance associated proteins 3 and 4); and (d) direct anti-inflammatory and antifibrotic properties[3] (Figure 3). Microarray gene expression profiling in *nor*UDCA-treated $Mdr2^{-/-}$ mice showed normalization of several genes including pro-collagen family members, chemokine ligands, TGF-β, PDGF and integrin signalling pathways known to promote liver fibrosis, hepatic stellate cell activation and the pathogenesis of PSC (Moustafa and Trauner, unpublished data). Interestingly, *nor*UDCA had profound effects on the neurotrophic tyrosine kinase receptor-2 and its ligand, both induced in PSC and the corresponding $Mdr2^{-/-}$ model, osteopontin and the VCAM-1 (Moustafa and Trauner, unpublished data). Osteopontin and VCAM-1 are of particular interest since both genes act as ligands for integrin receptors and are expressed on epithelial cells and neutrophils which contribute to bile duct injury in $Mdr2^{-/-}$ mice. *nor*UDCA also reduced hepatocyte and cholangiocyte proliferation. Future studies will show whether *nor*UDCA is capable of preventing development of hepatocellular carcinomas in $Mdr2^{-/-}$ mice. These effects make *nor*UDCA an attractive candidate drug for the treatment of cholangiopathies, in particular of PSC. Other modified bile acids and non-bile acid compounds which also undergo cholehepatic shunting (e.g. sulindac) may also be explored for the treatment of cholangiopathies in the future[24,25].

EXPERIENCE WITH *nor*UDCA IN HUMANS

Of note, metabolism and biological effects of *nor*UDCA show important parallels between mice and men[10]. Both men and mice show considerable renal excretion of *nor*UDCA. In line with the findings in mice the major metabolites of *nor*UDCA in humans are also glucuronides and sulphates. Last

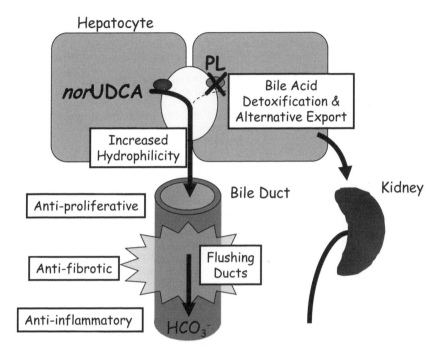

Figure 3 Proposed mechanisms of action of *nor*UDCA in the *Mdr2* (*Abcb4*)$^{-/-}$ mouse cholangiopathy model. The biliary enrichment of hydrophilic *nor*UDCA and its metabolites increases the hydrophilicity of bile. Moreover, *nor*UDCA stimulates bile flow with flushing of injured ducts with a hydrophilic alkalinized (bicarbonate-rich) bile. *nor*UDCA also induces bile acid and bilirubin detoxification via phase I and II enzymes and alternative export pumps at the sinusoidal membrane of hepatocytes, thus permitting their renal elimination. These mechanisms together with *nor*UDCA's anti-inflammatory, antifibrotic and antiproliferative effects result in healing of sclerosing cholangitis

but not least, *nor*UDCA is also capable of inducing a bicarbonate-rich hypercholeresis in humans[10]. Future clinical studies will have to demonstrate whether *nor*UDCA is suitable for the treatment of PSC and other cholangiopathies such as PBC.

Acknowledgements

This work was supported by grant P19118-B05 from the Austrian Science Fund and a GEN-AU grant from the Austrian Ministry for Science (to M.T. and K.Z.).

References

1. LaRusso NF, Shneider BL, Black D et al. Primary sclerosing cholangitis: summary of a workshop. Hepatology. 2006;44:746–64.
2. Cullen SN, Chapman RW. The medical management of primary sclerosing cholangitis. Semin Liver Dis. 2006;26:52–61.
3. Fickert P, Wagner M, Marschall HU et al. 24-*nor*Ursodeoxycholic acid is superior to ursodeoxycholic acid in the treatment of sclerosing cholangitis in Mdr2 (Abcb4) knockout mice. Gastroenterology. 2006;130:465–81.
4. Popov Y, Patsenker E, Fickert P, Trauner M, Schuppan D. Mdr2 (Abcb4)$^{-/-}$ mice spontaneously develop severe biliary fibrosis via massive dysregulation of pro- and antifibrogenic genes. J Hepatol. 2005;43:1045–54.
5. Fickert P, Fuchsbichler A, Wagner M et al. Regurgitation of bile acids from leaky bile ducts causes sclerosing cholangitis in Mdr2 (Abcb4) knockout mice. Gastroenterology. 2004;127: 261–74.
6. Fickert P, Zollner G, Fuchsbichler A et al. Ursodeoxycholic acid aggravates bile infarcts in bile duct-ligated and Mdr2 knockout mice via disruption of cholangioles. Gastroenterology. 2002;123:1238–51.
7. Beuers U. Drug insight: mechanisms and sites of action of ursodeoxycholic acid in cholestasis. Nat Clin Pract Gastroenterol Hepatol. 2006;3:318–28.
8. Paumgartner G, Beuers U. Mechanisms of action and therapeutic efficacy of ursodeoxycholic acid in cholestatic liver disease. Clin Liver Dis. 2004;8:67–81.
9. Yoon YB, Hagey LR, Hofmann AF, Gurantz D, Michelotti EL, Steinbach JH. Effect of side-chain shortening on the physiologic properties of bile acids: hepatic transport and effect on biliary secretion of 23-nor-ursodeoxycholate in rodents. Gastroenterology. 1986; 90:837–52.
10. Hofmann AF, Zakko SF, Lira M et al. Novel biotransformation and physiological properties of norursodeoxycholic acid in humans. Hepatology. 2005;42:1391–8.
11. Hofmann AF. The continuing importance of bile acids in liver and intestinal disease. Arch Intern Med. 1999;159:2647–58.
12. Hofmann AF. Bile acids as drugs: principles, mechanisms of action and formulations. Ital J Gastroenterol. 1995;27:106–13.
13. Smit JJ, Schinkel AH, Oude Elferink RP et al. Homozygous disruption of the murine mdr2 P-glycoprotein gene leads to a complete absence of phospholipid from bile and to liver disease. Cell. 1993;75:451–62.
14. Oude Elferink RP, Paulusma CC, Groen AK. Hepatocanalicular transport defects: pathophysiologic mechanisms of rare diseases. Gastroenterology. 2006;130:908–25.
15. Mauad TH, van Nieuwkerk CM, Dingemans KP et al. Mice with homozygous disruption of the mdr2 P-glycoprotein gene. A novel animal model for studies of nonsuppurative inflammatory cholangitis and hepatocarcinogenesis. Am J Pathol. 1994;145:1237–45.
16. Pikarsky E, Porat RM, Stein I et al. NF-kappaB functions as a tumour promoter in inflammation-associated cancer. Nature. 2004;431:461–6.
17. Lammert F, Wang DQ, Hillebrandt S et al. Spontaneous cholecysto- and hepatolithiasis in Mdr2$^{-/-}$ mice: a model for low phospholipid-associated cholelithiasis. Hepatology. 2004; 39:117–28.
18. Jansen PL, Sturm E. Genetic cholestasis, causes and consequences for hepatobiliary transport. Liver Int. 2003;23:315–22.
19. Pauli-Magnus C, Stieger B, Meier Y, Kullak-Ublick GA, Meier PJ. Enterohepatic transport of bile salts and genetics of cholestasis. J Hepatol. 2005;43:342–57.
20. Jacquemin E, De Vree JM, Cresteil D et al. The wide spectrum of multidrug resistance 3 deficiency: from neonatal cholestasis to cirrhosis of adulthood. Gastroenterology. 2001; 120:1448–58.
21. Geuken E, Visser D, Kuipers F et al. Rapid increase of bile salt secretion is associated with bile duct injury after human liver transplantation. J Hepatol. 2004;41:1017–25.
22. Hoekstra H, Porte RJ, Tian Y et al. Bile salt toxicity aggravates cold ischemic injury of bile ducts after liver transplantation in Mdr2$^{+/-}$ mice. Hepatology. 2006;43:1022–31.
23. Pauli-Magnus C, Kerb R, Fattinger K et al. BSEP and MDR3 haplotype structure in healthy Caucasians, primary biliary cirrhosis and primary sclerosing cholangitis. Hepatology. 2004;39:779–91.

24. Bolder U, Trang NV, Hagey LR et al. Sulindac is excreted into bile by a canalicular bile salt pump and undergoes a cholehepatic circulation in rats. Gastroenterology. 1999;117:962–71.
25. Leuschner M, Holtmeier J, Ackermann H, Leuschner U. The influence of sulindac on patients with primary biliary cirrhosis that responds incompletely to ursodeoxycholic acid: a pilot study. Eur J Gastroenterol Hepatol. 2002;14:1369–76.

27
Ursodeoxycholic acid-disulphate (SUDCA) – a potent chemopreventive agent against colon cancer

K. D. R. SETCHELL, N. M. BROWN and K. BOVE

INTRODUCTION

Ursodeoxycholic acid (UDCA) has now been in clinical use for several decades. This hydrophilic bile acid was first approved for the dissolution of cholesterol gallstones and later found to benefit patients with cholestatic liver diseases[1,2]. It was ultimately approved for the treatment of primary biliary cirrhosis where it has been shown to improve serum liver function tests and to prolong transplant-free survival time[3]. The mechanism of action of UDCA in cholestatic liver is probably multifactorial. The earliest mechanism proposed was that the hydrophilic properties of UDCA protected hepatocytes from the membrane-damaging effects of more hydrophobic bile acids that accumulate in cholestastic liver disease[4]. UDCA, however, has since been found to exhibit many other actions, including immunomodulatory, anti-inflammatory, antiproliferative, and antioxidant effects, and to influence cell-signalling pathways involved in apoptosis[5]. Based on some of these properties the potential use of UDCA in colon cancer prevention has more recently been studied, stimulated by a report that UDCA exhibited chemopreventive actions in the azoxymethane-induced animal model of colon cancer[6]. Bile acids, particularly hydrophobic secondary bile acids, have long been implicated in the aetiology of colon cancer[7] and in animal models of colon cancer, deoxycholic and lithocholic acids promote the growth of colonic tumours[8–11]. There is consequently good rationale for reducing or displacing intraluminal hydrophobic bile acids with a hydrophilic bile acid such as UDCA. However, several clinical studies of UDCA have now been performed with variable findings related to the ability of UDCA to reduce the extent of colonic dysplasia or risk of colon cancer[12–15].

The major drawback of UDCA for application to colon disease is that it is relatively efficiently absorbed in the small intestine and undergoes extensive biotransformation to the secondary bile acid lithocholic[1,2], which is known to promote colon cancer in animal models of colon cancer. It is therefore probable that these deficiencies impair the real potential of UDCA for chemoprevention.

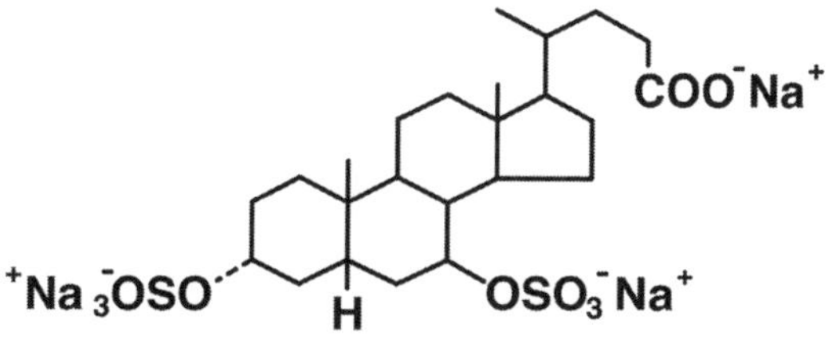

Ursodeoxycholic acid-disulfate sodium salt

Figure 1 Chemical structure of the highly hydrophilic bile acid, sodium salt of ursodeoxycholic acid

In an attempt to overcome these limitations we synthesized sulphate analogues of UDCA[16], because insertion of a functional group at the C-7 position serves several purposes (Figure 1). First, it greatly increases the hydrophilicity of UDCA. Secondly, it prevents absorption of the molecule in the proximal small bowel, thereby permitting complete delivery of a highly hydrophilic bile acid to the colon. Thirdly, it completely blocks biotransformation by intestinal bacteria to the hydrophobic bile acids, chenodeoxycholic and lithocholic acid. In principle these features suggest that ursodeoxycholic acid disulphate (SUDCA) may have chemopreventive action. We have therefore investigated the chemopreventive action of SUDCA in the classical animal model of azoxymethane (AOM)-induced colon cancer and have compared it with UDCA that has previously been reported to be chemopreventive in this same animal model[6].

STUDY DESIGN

Two hundred and forty male Fisher 344 adult rats were divided into six groups as indicated in Figure 2. Animals were fed an AIN-93 standard diet alone, an AIN-93 diet supplemented with 0.4% UDCA, or an AIN-93 diet supplemented with 0.4% SUDCA. After feeding these diets for 1–2 weeks, azoxymethane (15 mg/kg body weight in saline, once each week for 2 weeks) was injected subcutaneously into 60 animals from each diet group, while 20 animals were injected with saline. All animals were weighed weekly and maintained on their respective diets for 28 weeks.

After 28 weeks all animals were sacrificed and the caecum and colon were removed from each, the intraluminal contents were collected and the bowel was washed with saline, cut lengthwise, and examined macroscopically for tumours. All tumours were excised, weighed, and fixed overnight, sectioned for H&E staining and classified as either benign or malignant based on histological evaluation. The intraluminal colonic contents were collected and bile acids extracted, isolated into unconjugated and sulphated fractions, hydrolysed and

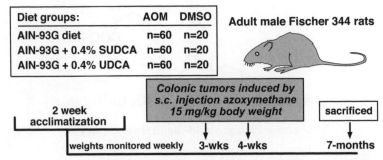

Figure 2   Study design to determine the chemopreventive actions of SUDCA and UDCA

derivatized, and then analysed by gas chromatography and mass spectrometry (GC/MS) using previously described methods[17]. The concentrations of individual bile acids identified by mass spectrometry were quantified, and the relative percentage bile acid composition was calculated.

EFFECT OF SUDCA IN THE AZOXYMETHANE-INDUCED ANIMAL MODEL OF COLON CANCER

The mean body weight of the SUDCA-treated and UDCA-treated animals was not significantly different throughout the experiment with growth curves that were essentially identical. Dietary SUDCA was well tolerated by the animals and did not affect the growth of animals. No tumours were found in any of the animals that were injected with saline (i.e. in the absence of carcinogen induction), indicating that neither SUDCA nor UDCA causes colonic tumour formation. Histological examination of the animals given AOM revealed lesions ranging from atypical hyperplasia to micro- and macro-adenomas, but the majority of lesions were found to be adenocarcinomas. There was no significant difference in the distribution of tumours along the length of the colon among the three AOM-treated groups. However, there was a statistically significant reduction in the numbers of tumours/animal in those animals fed SUDCA when compared with controls. This was not the case for the animals in the UDCA-treated group, which showed a slight but non-significant reduction in the number of tumours (Figure 3). In the control group 73% of the animals exposed to AOM developed tumours, whereas in animals fed UDCA or SUDCA only 57% and 45%, respectively, of the animals developed tumours. Thus, 55% of the animals fed SUDCA did not develop colonic tumours. These findings are consistent with a potent chemopreventive action of SUDCA. The

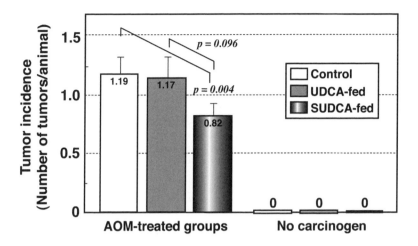

Figure 3 Comparison of the effect of SUDCA and UDCA on tumour burden, expressed as mean ($\pm$SEM) number of tumours/animal in the AOM chemically induced animal model of colon cancer

previously reported chemopreventive effects of UDCA[6] were not evident when tumour burden was expressed as number of tumours/animal. However, the lower proportion of animals with tumours that were fed UDCA compared with controls is suggestive of a modest chemopreventive action for UDCA, although this bile acid is less effective than SUDCA in preventing tumour formation. Overall, our data for UDCA are consistent in trends with the study published by Earnest et al.[6], although a major difference was the finding of a tumour incidence for all groups that was twice that found in this previous study. Nevertheless, our study clearly shows SUDCA to be superior to UDCA in its chemopreventive actions in the AOM chemically induced animal model of colon cancer.

INTRALUMINAL BILE ACID COMPOSITION AND BIOTRANSFORMATION OF SUDCA AND UDCA

GC/MS analysis of the intraluminal colonic contents collected at the time of sacrifice revealed distinct qualitative and quantitative differences among the three groups of animals (Table 1). In the control group hyodeoxycholic, hyocholic, β-muricholic, ω-muricholic acids, and deoxycholic acid with its isomers, were the major bile acid species identified, and these were predominantly found in the unconjugated bile acid fraction. By contrast, when UDCA was fed, the colonic bile acid profile was significantly changed. Specifically, the intraluminal total bile acid concentration increased markedly

Table 1 Summary of typical bile acid concentrations (μg/g wet weight) in Fischer F44 rats with azoxymethane chemically induced colon cancer fed a control AIN-93G diet, and the same diet supplemented with 0.4% UDCA, or 0.4% SUDCA

	Control group (n = 7)	UDCA-treated group (n = 7)	SUDCA-treated group (n = 7)
Total bile acids (mg/g)	4884 ± 1339	11 803 ± 4166	5091 ± 1513
Lithocholic (LCA)	177 ± 48	4900 ± 517	124 ± 35
Deoxycholic (DCA)	425 ± 25	456 ± 99	192 ± 2
Ursodeoxycholic (UDCA)	n.d.	668 ± 197	1480 ± 191*
Ratio LCA/DCA	0.41	10.75	0.64
Percentage unconjugated bile acids	69.2	69.3	25.4
Percentage conjugated bile acids	30.8	30.7	74.6

*Exclusively in the sulphate fraction in SUDCA-treated animals (i.e. as unchanged SUDCA).

compared with that of the control animals and there was a vast increase in the colonic concentrations of lithocholic acid and its isomers, allo-lithocholic and iso-lithocholic acids, secondary bile acids that are normally present in relatively low concentrations in control animals. UDCA was not detected in the colonic contents of the control animals, but was present in the colon of UDCA-treated animals, although it was not a major bile acid. These findings confirm extensive biotransformation of UDCA to hydrophobic bile acids that are known to promote tumour growth in this experimental animal model of colon cancer[8–11], and show that, despite feeding large concentrations of UDCA (approximately 80 mg/day orally), only a small proportion of the ingested dose remains intact by the time it reaches the colon. It is our contention that this extensive biotransformation is a key factor in limiting the efficacy of UDCA for chemoprevention in humans[12–15].

In SUDCA-fed animals the qualitative profile of endogenous bile acids was largely unchanged, except for the presence of relatively high concentrations of UDCA, exclusively found in the sulphate fraction and indicating lack of biotransformation of SUDCA. A significant reduction in the colonic concentration of deoxycholic acid and its isomers was observed. These findings indicate that orally fed SUDCA was delivered unchanged to the colon and led to a marked reduction in the concentration of the secondary bile acid, deoxycholic acid. High levels of deoxycholic acid, because of its apoptotic action on colonic cells[18–22], are postulated to play a key role in risk for colon cancer, and any reduction in the intraluminal deoxycholic acid concentration would be considered a benefit. The lithocholic acid/deoxycholic acid ratio, proposed many years ago as a risk marker for colon cancer if elevated[23,24], was relatively unchanged in SUDCA-fed animals, while by contrast this ratio was greatly increased in UDCA-fed animals. The proportion of bile acids identified in the conjugated bile acid fraction of the colonic contents of SUDCA-fed animals was high, reflecting a marked shift towards a hydrophilic milieu within the colonic lumen. The major bile acid present in the sulphate fraction was unchanged SUDCA.

Since displacement of hydrophobic secondary bile acids from the colon is probably beneficial in protecting mucosal membranes, SUDCA feeding accomplishes this goal, and this we propose may explain in part its greater chemopreventive effect when compared with UDCA. Further studies are ongoing to elucidate other potential mechanisms for the chemopreventive action of SUDCA in this animal model of colon cancer.

In conclusion, we report a potent chemopreventive effect of the highly hydrophilic bile acid SUDCA in the classical rodent model of azoxymethane chemically induced colon cancer. This new non-absorbable bile acid is now in phase 1 clinical studies and under development as a potential chemopreventive agent in humans.

Acknowledgements

These studies were first presented at the Digestive Disease Week (DDW), May 2004 in New Orleans, MS. This work was supported by Axcan Pharma in licensing agreements with Cincinnati Children's Hospital Medical Center for US Patents 5 763 435 and 6 251 884 .

References

1.   Hofmann AF. Pharmacology of ursodeoxycholic acid, an enterohepatic drug. Scand J Gastroenterol Suppl. 1994;204:1–15.
2.   Crosignani A, Setchell KDR, Invernizzi P, Larghi A, Rodrigues CM, Podda M. Clinical pharmacokinetics of therapeutic bile acids. Clin Pharmacokinet. 1996;30:333–58.
3.   Poupon RE, Lindor KD, Cauch-Dudek K, Dickson ER, Poupon R, Heathcote EJ. Combined analysis of randomized controlled trials of ursodeoxycholic acid in primary biliary cirrhosis. Gastroenterology. 1997;113:884–90.
4.   Paumgartner G, Beuers U. Ursodeoxycholic acid in cholestatic liver disease: mechanisms of action and therapeutic use revisited. Hepatology. 2002;36:525–31.
5.   Paumgartner G, Beuers U. Mechanisms of action and therapeutic efficacy of ursodeoxycholic acid in cholestatic liver disease. Clin Liver Dis. 2004;8:67–81, vi.
6.   Earnest DL, Holubec H, Wali RK et al. Chemoprevention of azoxymethane-induced colonic carcinogenesis by supplemental dietary ursodeoxycholic acid. Cancer Res. 1994; 54:5071–4.
7.   Hill MJ, Drasar BS, Williams RE et al. Faecal bile-acids and clostridia in patients with cancer of the large bowel. Lancet. 1975;1:535–9.
8.   Narisawa T, Magadia NE, Weisburger JH, Wynder EL. Promoting effect of bile acids on colon carcinogenesis after intrarectal instillation of N-methyl-N'-nitro-N-nitrosoguanidine in rats. J Natl Cancer Inst. 1974;53:1093–7.
9.   Reddy BS, Narisawa T, Maronpot R, Weisburger JH, Wynder EL. Animal models for the study of dietary factors and cancer of the large bowel. Cancer Res. 1975;35:3421–6.
10. Reddy BS, Watanabe K, Weisburger JH, Wynder EL. Promoting effect of bile acids in colon carcinogenesis in germ-free and conventional F344 rats. Cancer Res. 1977;37:3238–42.
11. Narisawa T, Reddy BS, Weisburger JH. Effect of bile acids and dietary fat on large bowel carcinogenesis in animal models. Gastroenterol Jpn. 1978;13:206–12.
12. Tung BY, Emond MJ, Haggitt RC et al. Ursodiol use is associated with lower prevalence of colonic neoplasia in patients with ulcerative colitis and primary sclerosing cholangitis. Ann Intern Med. 2001;134:89–95.
13. Pardi DS, Loftus EV Jr, Kremers WK, Keach J, Lindor KD. Ursodeoxycholic acid as a chemopreventive agent in patients with ulcerative colitis and primary sclerosing cholangitis. Gastroenterology. 2003;124:889–93.

14. Serfaty L, De Leusse A, Rosmorduc O et al. Ursodeoxycholic acid therapy and the risk of colorectal adenoma in patients with primary biliary cirrhosis: an observational study. Hepatology. 2003;38:203–9.
15. Alberts DS, Martinez ME, Hess LM et al. Phase III trial of ursodeoxycholic acid to prevent colorectal adenoma recurrence. J Natl Cancer Inst. 2005;97:846–53.
16. Rodrigues CM, Kren BT, Steer CJ, Setchell KDR. The site-specific delivery of ursodeoxycholic acid to the rat colon by sulfate conjugation. Gastroenterology. 1995;109: 1835–44.
17. Setchell KDR, Lawson AM, Tanida N, Sjovall J. General methods for the analysis of metabolic profiles of bile acids and related compounds in feces. J Lipid Res. 1983;24:1085–100.
18. Rodrigues CM, Fan G, Ma X, Kren BT, Steer CJ. A novel role for ursodeoxycholic acid in inhibiting apoptosis by modulating mitochondrial membrane perturbation. J Clin Invest. 1998;101:2790–9.
19. Martinez JD, Stratagoules ED, LaRue JM et al. Different bile acids exhibit distinct biological effects: the tumor promoter deoxycholic acid induces apoptosis and the chemopreventive agent ursodeoxycholic acid inhibits cell proliferation. Nutr Cancer. 1998;31:111–18.
20. Im E, Martinez JD. Ursodeoxycholic acid (UDCA) can inhibit deoxycholic acid (DCA)-induced apoptosis via modulation of EGFR/Raf-1/ERK signalling in human colon cancer cells. J Nutr. 2004;134:483–6.
21. Im E, Akare S, Powell A, Martinez JD. Ursodeoxycholic acid can suppress deoxycholic acid-induced apoptosis by stimulating Akt/PKB-dependent survival signaling. Nutr Cancer. 2005;51:110–16.
22. Shiraki K, Ito T, Sugimoto K et al. Different effects of bile acids, ursodeoxycholic acid and deoxycholic acid, on cell growth and cell death in human colonic adenocarcinoma cells. Int J Mol Med. 2005;16:729–33.
23. Owen RW, Dodo M, Thompson MH, Hill MJ. Fecal steroids and colorectal cancer. Nutr Cancer. 1987;9:73–80.
24. Owen RW, Henly PJ, Thompson MH, Hill MJ. Steroids and cancer: faecal bile acid screening for early detection of cancer risk. J Steroid Biochem. 1986;24:391–4.

28
Prevention of cholesterol gallstones by the potent cholesterol absorption inhibitor ezetimibe in gallstone-susceptible C57L/J mice

H. H. WANG, P. PORTINCASA and D. Q.-H. WANG

INTRODUCTION

Cholesterol gallstone formation represents a failure of biliary cholesterol homeostasis in which the physical–chemical balance of cholesterol solubility in bile is disturbed[1,2]. The liver is the only substantial excretory route for cholesterol and its catabolic products, the bile salts from the body. The *primum movens* in cholesterol gallstone formation is the persistent hepatic hypersecretion of biliary cholesterol (both hepatic and small intestinal components), causing a lithogenic bile. Evidently, in an animal receiving no dietary cholesterol, all biliary cholesterol must ultimately be derived from *de novo* synthesis. It has been found that the contribution of *de novo* cholesterol synthesis to biliary cholesterol secretion is likely to be small, possibly less than 15%[3]. The small intestine is a unique organ providing dietary and re-absorbed biliary cholesterol to the body. Under high dietary cholesterol conditions, the metabolism of exogenous chylomicrons (i.e. lipoproteins of intestinal origin) plays a major regulatory role in the response of biliary cholesterol secretion to high dietary cholesterol and greatly contributes to the formation of cholesterol gallstones[4]. We observed recently that there is a significant and positive correlation between the efficiency of intestinal cholesterol absorption and the prevalence of cholesterol gallstone formation in 15 strains of inbred male mice, suggesting that high efficiency of intestinal cholesterol absorption and high dietary cholesterol are two independent risk factors for cholesterol gallstone formation[4]. In this study we investigated whether cholesterol gallstones could be prevented by ezetimibe through inhibiting intestinal cholesterol absorption in gallstone-susceptible C57L mice challenged with a lithogenic diet. Ezetimibe belongs to the new class of 2-azetidinones and has recently been found to be a potent inhibitor of intestinal cholesterol absorption by suppressing the Niemann-Pick C1 like 1 (NPC1L1) protein, a putative intestinal sterol influx transporter that facilitates the uptake of cholesterol into the enterocyte[5].

Our preliminary results show that, by effectively curtailing intestinal cholesterol absorption, ezetimibe can prevent not only cholesterol gallstone formation but also deranged gallbladder motility, mostly due to decreased biliary cholesterol content. Our findings point to an efficacious novel approach for preventing or treating cholesterol gallstones by inhibiting intestinal cholesterol absorption in humans.

MATERIALS AND METHODS

Animals and diets

Male C57L/J mice, 6–8-weeks old, were purchased from the Jackson Laboratory (Bar Harbor, ME). The C57L strain is homozygous for susceptible *Lith* alleles[6]. All mice were provided free access to water and normal rodent chow (Harlan Teklad F6 Rodent Diet 8664, Madison, WI) containing trace ($<0.02\%$) cholesterol. For gallstone prevention studies the mice were divided into four groups ($n = 20$ per group) fed 8 weeks with a lithogenic diet (1% cholesterol plus 0.5% cholic acid and 15% butter fat) supplemented with ezetimibe in doses of 0, 2, 10, or 20 µg/day. Since we had previously observed that, at 12 weeks on 2% cholesterol plus 0.5% cholic acid and 15% butter fat, 100% of C57L mice formed cholesterol gallstones[7], for gallstone dissolution experiments, additional groups ($n = 20$ per group) of mice that have formed cholesterol gallstones with this diet, were fed the chow diet supplemented with ezetimibe in doses of 0, 2, 10, or 20 µg/day for 8 weeks.

Microscopic study of gallbladder biles and determination of biliary lipid outputs

At 8 weeks on the lithogenic diet supplemented with various doses of ezetimibe, a cholecystectomy was performed in overnight-fasted mice. Gallbladder volume was determined by weighing the whole gallbladder and equating volume with gallbladder weight. Fresh gallbladder bile was examined for mucin gel, solid and liquid crystals, and gallstones, which were defined according to previously established criteria[6]. Additional groups of mice ($n = 5$ per group) were studied for biliary lipid secretion through the first hour collection of hepatic biles[8]. Total and individual bile salt concentrations, and bile cholesterol, as well as cholesterol content in chow and gallstones, were measured by HPLC[6]. Biliary phospholipids were determined as inorganic phosphorus by the method of Bartlett[9]. Cholesterol saturation indexes (CSI) in gallbladder and hepatic biles were calculated from the critical tables[10]. Faecal neutral steroids were saponified and extracted, as well as being measured by HPLC[11].

Measurement of intestinal cholesterol absorption

Non-fasted and non-anaesthetized mice ($n = 10$ per group) were fed by gavage an intragastric bolus of 150 µl of medium-chain triglyceride containing 1 µCi of

Although we found no significant evidence for influence on overall disease susceptibility from the investigated polymorphisms, median survival was significantly reduced in patients homozygous for the minor allele as compared to patients carrying at least one major allele of the three neighbouring SNP rs6785049 (10.8 vs 14.0 years, $p = 0.01$), rs1054190 (3.6 vs 13.6 years, $p = 0.004$) and rs3814058 (3.5 vs 13.3 years, $p = 0.01$)[15]. In general, these findings are interesting as they point to an important role for genes involved in bile acid detoxification and elimination in influencing disease progression in PSC. Regarding SXR, further studies are needed to characterize the consequences of both coding and non-coding polymorphisms in the SXR gene in relation to its function as a bile acid receptor (Figure 2)[70]. Due to linkage disequilibrium (LD), it should be considered equally plausible that any of the identified polymorphisms, or even another hitherto not genotyped polymorphism in strong LD, is responsible for the observed effects[76].

ONGOING STUDIES AND FUTURE PERSPECTIVE

There is increasing awareness of the importance of interaction between polymorphisms in functionally related genes in complex diseases, i.e. epistasis[77–79]. In some cases, epistatic considerations have proven necessary for the detection of effects from genetic variation on disease susceptibility and disease progression[64,65,80]. It is anticipated that study design may prove crucial in identifying the most critical components in the tangle of NR networks[42]. In future studies in PSC and other human cholestatic conditions, not only the role of polymorphisms in the FXR and CAR genes needs to be addressed alongside SXR[50], but even other NRs and transcription factors with possible importance for the regulation of bile acid homeostasis must be studied (Figure 3)[41,48,51,52].

Disrupted integrity of barrier function plays an important role in the pathogenesis of chronic inflammatory conditions at mucosal surfaces[81]. Given the known influence from bile acids even on intestinal inflammation and carcinogenesis[82,83], genes encoding proteins involved in transepithelial bile acid transport throughout the enterohepatic circulation (Figure 3) serve as an obvious group of candidate genes for PSC. Studies in limited populations ($n < 50$) have interestingly pointed to a non-significant increase of particular multidrug resistance gene 3 (MDR3) variants among PSC patients as compared with healthy controls[84,85]. Possibly due to loss of protection of the biliary epithelium from toxic bile acids, knockout mice for the rodent analogue (*mdr2*) of this phospholipid transporter spontaneously develop hepatic lesions resembling PSC[86], and a well-powered enquiry into the effects of MDR3 polymorphisms in human PSC seems warranted. The speculation that a bile acid-mediated insult in an immunogenetically susceptible individual may be imprinted in the anatomical compartments of the enterohepatic circulation, either primarily or throughout disease course, is worth pursuing experimentally for a disease concomitantly affecting liver, bile ducts and the terminal ileum/colon, i.e. PSC.

References

1. Chapman RW, Arborgh BA, Rhodes JM et al. Primary sclerosing cholangitis: a review of its clinical features, cholangiography, and hepatic histology. Gut. 1980;21:870–7.
2. Schrumpf E, Boberg KM. Epidemiology of primary sclerosing cholangitis. Best Pract Res Clin Gastroenterol. 2001;15:553–62.
3. Loftus EV Jr, Harewood GC, Loftus CG et al. PSC–IBD: a unique form of inflammatory bowel disease associated with primary sclerosing cholangitis. Gut. 2005;54:91–6.
4. Abdelrazeq AS, Wilson TR, Leitch DL, Lund JN, Leveson SH. Ileitis in ulcerative colitis: is it a backwash? Dis Colon Rectum. 2005;48:2038–46.
5. Saarinen S, Olerup O, Broome U. Increased frequency of autoimmune diseases in patients with primary sclerosing cholangitis. Am J Gastroenterol. 2000;95:3195–9.
6. Broome U, Olsson R, Loof L et al. Natural history and prognostic factors in 305 Swedish patients with primary sclerosing cholangitis. Gut. 1996;38:610–15.
7. Cullen S, Chapman R. Aetiopathogenesis of primary sclerosing cholangitis. Best Pract Res Clin Gastroenterol. 2001;15:577–89.
8. Bergquist A, Ekbom A, Olsson R et al. Hepatic and extrahepatic malignancies in primary sclerosing cholangitis. J Hepatol. 2002;36:321–7.
9. Boberg KM, Aadland E, Jahnsen J, Raknerud N, Stiris M, Bell H. Incidence and prevalence of primary biliary cirrhosis, primary sclerosing cholangitis, and autoimmune hepatitis in a Norwegian population. Scand J Gastroenterol. 1998;33:99–103.
10. Kingham JG, Kochar N, Gravenor MB. Incidence, clinical patterns, and outcomes of primary sclerosing cholangitis in South Wales, United Kingdom. Gastroenterology. 2004; 126:1929–30.
11. Bambha K, Kim WR, Talwalkar J et al. Incidence, clinical spectrum, and outcomes of primary sclerosing cholangitis in a United States community. Gastroenterology. 2003;125: 1364–9.
12. Cullen SN, Chapman RW. Review article: Current management of primary sclerosing cholangitis. Aliment Pharmacol Ther. 2005;21:933–48.
13. Brandsaeter B, Friman S, Broome U et al. Outcome following liver transplantation for primary sclerosing cholangitis in the Nordic countries. Scand J Gastroenterol. 2003;38: 1176–83.
14. Talwalkar JA, Lindor KD. Primary sclerosing cholangitis. Inflamm Bowel Dis. 2005;11:62– 72.
15. Karlsen TH, Lie BA, Frey Froslie K et al. Polymorphisms in the steroid and xenobiotic receptor gene influence survival in primary sclerosing cholangitis. Gastroenterology. 2006; 131:781–7.
16. Talwalkar JA, Lindor KD. Natural history and prognostic models in primary sclerosing cholangitis. Best Pract Res Clin Gastroenterol. 2001;15:563–75.
17. Bergquist A, Lindberg G, Saarinen S, Broome U. Increased prevalence of primary sclerosing cholangitis among first-degree relatives. J Hepatol. 2005;42:252–6.
18. Rioux JD, Abbas AK. Paths to understanding the genetic basis of autoimmune disease. Nature. 2005;435:584–9.
19. Donaldson PT, Norris S. Immunogenetics in PSC. Best Pract Res Clin Gastroenterol. 2001; 15:611–27.
20. Bowlus CL, Karlsen TH, Broome U et al. Analysis of MAdCAM-1 and ICAM-1 polymorphisms in 365 Scandinavian patients with primary sclerosing cholangitis. J Hepatol. 2006;45:633–5.
21. Melum E, Karlsen TH, Broome U et al. The 32-base pair deletion of the chemokine receptor 5 gene (CCR5-Delta32) is not associated with primary sclerosing cholangitis in 363 Scandinavian patients. Tissue Ant. 2006;68:78–81.
22. Glazier AM, Nadeau JH, Aitman TJ. Finding genes that underlie complex traits. Science. 2002;298:2345–9.
23. Boberg KM, Lundin KE, Schrumpf E. Etiology and pathogenesis in primary sclerosing cholangitis. Scand J Gastroenterol Suppl. 1994;204:47–58.
24. Cullen S, Chapman R. Primary sclerosing cholangitis. Autoimmun Rev. 2003;2:305–12.
25. Trauner M, Meier PJ, Boyer JL. Molecular pathogenesis of cholestasis. N Engl J Med. 1998;339:1217–27.

26. Wiesner RH. Liver transplantation for primary sclerosing cholangitis: timing, outcome, impact of inflammatory bowel disease and recurrence of disease. Best Pract Res Clin Gastroenterol. 2001;15:667–80.
27. Guicciardi ME, Gores GJ. Cholestatic hepatocellular injury: what do we know and how should we proceed? J Hepatol. 2005;42:297–300.
28. Guicciardi ME, Gores GJ. Apoptosis: a mechanism of acute and chronic liver injury. Gut. 2005;54:1024–33.
29. Gujral JS, Farhood A, Bajt ML, Jaeschke H. Neutrophils aggravate acute liver injury during obstructive cholestasis in bile duct-ligated mice. Hepatology. 2003;38:355–63.
30. Thompson R, Strautnieks S. BSEP: function and role in progressive familial intrahepatic cholestasis. Semin Liver Dis. 2001;21:545–50.
31. Porayko MK, LaRusso NF, Wiesner RH. Primary sclerosing cholangitis: a progressive disease? Semin Liver Dis. 1991;11:18–25.
32. Schrumpf E, Fausa O, Elgjo K, Kolmannskog F. Hepatobiliary complications of inflammatory bowel disease. Semin Liver Dis. 1988;8:201–9.
33. Balasubramaniam K, Wiesner RH, LaRusso NF. Primary sclerosing cholangitis with normal serum alkaline phosphatase activity. Gastroenterology. 1988;95:1395–8.
34. Wiesner RH, Grambsch PM, Dickson ER et al. Primary sclerosing cholangitis: natural history, prognostic factors and survival analysis. Hepatology. 1989;10:430–6.
35. Farrant JM, Hayllar KM, Wilkinson ML et al. Natural history and prognostic variables in primary sclerosing cholangitis. Gastroenterology. 1991;100:1710–17.
36. Dickson ER, Murtaugh PA, Wiesner RH et al. Primary sclerosing cholangitis: refinement and validation of survival models. Gastroenterology. 1992;103:1893–901.
37. Boberg KM, Rocca G, Egeland T et al. Time-dependent Cox regression model is superior in prediction of prognosis in primary sclerosing cholangitis. Hepatology. 2002;35:652–7.
38. Boyer JL. Nuclear receptor ligands: rational and effective therapy for chronic cholestatic liver disease? Gastroenterology. 2005;129:735–40.
39. Trauner M, Boyer JL. Bile salt transporters: molecular characterization, function, and regulation. Physiol Rev. 2003;83:633–71.
40. Francis GA, Fayard E, Picard F, Auwerx J. Nuclear receptors and the control of metabolism. Annu Rev Physiol. 2003;65:261–311.
41. Glass CK, Ogawa S. Combinatorial roles of nuclear receptors in inflammation and immunity. Nat Rev Immunol. 2006;6:44–55.
42. Carlberg C, Dunlop TW. An integrated biological approach to nuclear receptor signaling in physiological control and disease. Crit Rev Eukaryot Gene Expr. 2006;16:1–22.
43. Schuetz E, Strom S. Promiscuous regulator of xenobiotic removal. Nat Med. 2001;7:536–7.
44. Pascussi JM, Gerbal-Chaloin S, Drocourt L, Maurel P, Vilarem MJ. The expression of CYP2B6, CYP2C9 and CYP3A4 genes: a tangle of networks of nuclear and steroid receptors. Biochim Biophys Acta. 2003;1619:243–53.
45. Handschin C, Meyer UA. Induction of drug metabolism: the role of nuclear receptors. Pharmacol Rev. 2003;55:649–73.
46. Chen J, Raymond K. Nuclear receptors, bile-acid detoxification, and cholestasis. Lancet. 2006;367:454–6.
47. Savkur RS, Miller AR. Investigational PPAR-gamma agonists for the treatment of Type 2 diabetes. Expert Opin Investig Drugs. 2006;15:763–78.
48. Wang H, LeCluyse EL. Role of orphan nuclear receptors in the regulation of drug-metabolising enzymes. Clin Pharmacokinet. 2003;42:1331–57.
49. Modica S, Moschetta A. Nuclear bile acid receptor FXR as pharmacological target: Are we there yet? FEBS Lett. 2006;580:5492–9.
50. Guo GL, Lambert G, Negishi M et al. Complementary roles of farnesoid X receptor, pregnane X receptor, and constitutive androstane receptor in protection against bile acid toxicity. J Biol Chem. 2003;278:45062–71.
51. Zollner G, Marschall HU, Wagner M, Trauner M. Role of nuclear receptors in the adaptive response to bile acids and cholestasis: pathogenetic and therapeutic considerations. Mol Pharm. 2006;3:231–51.
52. Zhou C, Tabb MM, Nelson EL et al. Mutual repression between steroid and xenobiotic receptor and NF-kappaB signaling pathways links xenobiotic metabolism and inflammation. J Clin Invest. 2006;116:2280–9.

53. Kullak-Ublick GA, Stieger B, Meier PJ. Enterohepatic bile salt transporters in normal physiology and liver disease. Gastroenterology. 2004;126:322–42.
54. Wagner M, Halilbasic E, Marschall HU et al. CAR and PXR agonists stimulate hepatic bile acid and bilirubin detoxification and elimination pathways in mice. Hepatology. 2005; 42:420–30.
55. Parks DJ, Blanchard SG, Bledsoe RK et al. Bile acids: natural ligands for an orphan nuclear receptor. Science. 1999;284:1365–8.
56. Marschall HU, Wagner M, Zollner G et al. Complementary stimulation of hepatobiliary transport and detoxification systems by rifampicin and ursodeoxycholic acid in humans. Gastroenterology. 2005;129:476–85.
57. Karpen SJ. Exercising the nuclear option to treat cholestasis: CAR and PXR ligands. Hepatology. 2005;42:266–9.
58. Gillespie DA, Vickers CR. Pruritus and cholestasis: therapeutic options. J Gastroenterol Hepatol. 1993;8:168–73.
59. Bachs L, Pares A, Elena M, Piera C, Rodes J. Comparison of rifampicin with phenobarbitone for treatment of pruritus in biliary cirrhosis. Lancet. 1989;1:574–6.
60. Wietholtz H, Marschall HU, Sjovall J, Matern S. Stimulation of bile acid 6 alpha-hydroxylation by rifampin. J Hepatol. 1996;24:713–18.
61. Schuetz EG, Strom S, Yasuda K et al. Disrupted bile acid homeostasis reveals an unexpected interaction among nuclear hormone receptors, transporters, and cytochrome P450. J Biol Chem. 2001;276:39411–18.
62. Pan DH, Chen F, Neimark E, Li X, Shneider BL. FTF and LRH-1, two related but different transcription factors in human Caco-2 cells: their different roles in the regulation of bile acid transport. Biochim Biophys Acta. 2005;1732:31–7.
63. Drumm ML, Konstan MW, Schluchter MD et al. Genetic modifiers of lung disease in cystic fibrosis. N Engl J Med. 2005;353:1443–53.
64. Martin MP, Gao X, Lee JH et al. Epistatic interaction between KIR3DS1 and HLA-B delays the progression to AIDS. Nat Genet. 2002;31:429–34.
65. Khakoo SI, Thio CL, Martin MP et al. HLA and NK cell inhibitory receptor genes in resolving hepatitis C virus infection. Science. 2004;305:872–4.
66. Boberg KM, Spurkland A, Rocca G et al. The HLA-DR3,DQ2 heterozygous genotype is associated with an accelerated progression of primary sclerosing cholangitis. Scand J Gastroenterol. 2001;36:886–90.
67. Valentonyte R, Hampe J, Huse K et al. Sarcoidosis is associated with a truncating splice site mutation in BTNL2. Nat Genet. 2005;37:357–64.
68. van der Linden MW, van der Slik AR, Zanelli E et al. Six microsatellite markers on the short arm of chromosome 6 in relation to HLA-DR3 and TNF-308A in systemic lupus erythematosus. Genes Immun. 2001;2:373–80.
69. Colhoun HM, McKeigue PM, Davey Smith G. Problems of reporting genetic associations with complex outcomes. Lancet. 2003;361:865–72.
70. Orans J, Teotico DG, Redinbo MR. The nuclear xenobiotic receptor PXR: recent insights and new challenges. Mol Endocrinol. 2005;19:2891–900.
71. Staudinger JL, Goodwin B, Jones SA et al. The nuclear receptor PXR is a lithocholic acid sensor that protects against liver toxicity. Proc Natl Acad Sci USA. 2001;98:3369–74.
72. Xie W, Radominska-Pandya A, Shi Y et al. An essential role for nuclear receptors SXR/PXR in detoxification of cholestatic bile acids. Proc Natl Acad Sci USA. 2001;98:3375–80.
73. Stedman CA, Liddle C, Coulter SA et al. Nuclear receptors constitutive androstane receptor and pregnane X receptor ameliorate cholestatic liver injury. Proc Natl Acad Sci USA. 2005;102:2063–8.
74. Zhang J, Kuehl P, Green ED et al. The human pregnane X receptor: genomic structure and identification and functional characterization of natural allelic variants. Pharmacogenetics. 2001;11:555–72.
75. Uno Y, Sakamoto Y, Yoshida K et al. Characterization of six base pair deletion in the putative HNF1-binding site of human PXR promoter. J Hum Genet. 2003;48:594–7.
76. Cardon LR, Abecasis GR. Using haplotype blocks to map human complex trait loci. Trends Genet. 2003;19:135–40.
77. Gregersen JW, Kranc KR, Ke X et al. Functional epistasis on a common MHC haplotype associated with multiple sclerosis. Nature. 2006;443:574–7.

78. Cordell HJ. Epistasis: what it means, what it doesn't mean, and statistical methods to detect it in humans. Hum Mol Genet. 2002;11:2463–8.
79. Gaya DR, Russell RK, Nimmo ER, Satsangi J. New genes in inflammatory bowel disease: lessons for complex diseases? Lancet. 2006;367:1271–84.
80. Brassat D, Motsinger AA, Caillier SJ et al. Multifactor dimensionality reduction reveals gene–gene interactions associated with multiple sclerosis susceptibility in African Americans. Genes Immun. 2006;7:310–15.
81. Schreiber S, Rosenstiel P, Albrecht M, Hampe J, Krawczak M. Genetics of Crohn disease, an archetypal inflammatory barrier disease. Nat Rev Genet. 2005;6:376–88.
82. Kajiura K, Ohkusa T, Okayasu I. Relationship between fecal bile acids and the occurrence of colorectal neoplasia in experimental murine ulcerative colitis. Digestion. 1998;59:69–72.
83. Ung KA, Gillberg R, Kilander A, Abrahamsson H. Role of bile acids and bile acid binding agents in patients with collagenous colitis. Gut. 2000;46:170–5.
84. Pauli-Magnus C, Kerb R, Fattinger K et al. BSEP and MDR3 haplotype structure in healthy Caucasians, primary biliary cirrhosis and primary sclerosing cholangitis. Hepatology. 2004;39:779–91.
85. Rosmorduc O, Hermelin B, Boelle PY, Poupon RE, Poupon R, Chazouilleres O. ABCB4 gene mutations and primary sclerosing cholangitis. Gastroenterology. 2004;126:1220–2; author reply 1222–3.
86. Popov Y, Patsenker E, Fickert P, Trauner M, Schuppan D. Mdr2 (Abcb4)$^{-/-}$ mice spontaneously develop severe biliary fibrosis via massive dysregulation of pro- and antifibrogenic genes. J Hepatol. 2005;43:1045–54.

32
High-dose ursodeoxycholic acid in the treatment of primary sclerosing cholangitis

R. W. CHAPMAN

INTRODUCTION

Primary sclerosing cholangitis (PSC) is a chronic cholestatic liver disease characterized by a progressive obliterating fibrosis of the intrahepatic and extrahepatic bile ducts. The disease in symptomatic patients often progresses to secondary biliary cirrhosis, and premature death from liver failure, hepatobiliary and colon cancer[1]. PSC is closely associated with inflammatory bowel disease (IBD), particularly ulcerative colitis (UC), which is found in approximately two-thirds of patients with PSC of northern European origin. PSC is the most common hepatobiliary disease associated with UC. The prevalence in UC populations of PSC is between 2 and 6%. There are also associations between PSC and other immune-mediated diseases such as coeliac disease and rheumatoid arthritis.

Although the aetiopathogenesis of PSC is poorly understood it is thought to be immune-mediated. The detection of a disease-specific autoantibody (ANCA)[2], the association with the HLA-B8-DR3 haplotype found in other autoimmune diseases, the relationship between HLA status and prognosis[3] and the presence of an organ-specific T-cell infiltrate in PSC[4] provide indirect evidence for the role of genetic and immune mechanisms in the aetiology of PSC. The mechanisms underlying the loss of immune tolerance which allow such 'autoimmune' disease processes to occur have not as yet been defined.

All these studies provide indirect evidence that PSC is an autoimmune disease possibly involving an exaggerated cell-mediated immune response with immunological damage targeted at the biliary epithelial cells. The putative antigens that may set off this immune response have not yet been identified.

An alternative hypothesis has been proposed; i.e. that bacterial cell products ascending in portal venous blood are taken up by hepatic macrophages which in turn set up an immune response leading to peribiliary fibrosis in immunogenetically susceptible hosts.

NATURAL HISTORY AND PROGNOSIS

Unlike primary biliary cirrhosis (PBC), the natural history of PSC is very difficult to predict in an individual patient as the rate of progression of the disease can be highly variable. This clinical variability makes the timing of medical and endoscopic therapy and liver transplantation difficult when compared with other chronic liver disease. Even when the diagnosis is made in the asymptomatic phase PSC can be a progressive disease with the insidious development of biliary cirrhosis and the complications arising from this. The median survival of patients, including those who are symptomatic and at presentation, appears to be about 12 years, although a study from Sweden has suggested a better prognosis in asymptomatic patients with a median survival of 21 years[5].

Prognostic indices or models of the natural history of PSC have proved useful in studying large populations but are generally of less use in predicting the course of an individual patient. This is largely because no markers or risk factors can predict which patients will develop cholangiocarcinoma or progressive jaundice due a dominant biliary stricture, both of which may lead to premature death. Acute bacterial cholangitis is uncommon and usually follows instrumental biliary intervention. It tends also to occur in endstage disease where multiple strictures and biliary sludging can lead to the formation of brown pigment stones intensifying the degree of biliary obstruction[6]. The development of cholangiocarcinoma carries a poor prognosis and precludes orthotopic liver transplant (OLT). In a recent series cholangiocarcinoma has been reported in 14–27% of patients with PSC[7,8]. The annual risk of developing hepatobiliary cancer in PSC has been estimated at 1.5% per year[7].

TREATMENT

At present there is no curative treatment for PSC. Treatments either serve to manage the general and specific complications of the disease or more specifically to retard and reverse the rate of disease progression. The optimal therapy which successfully improves symptoms, delays progression towards liver failure and OLT and prevents the onset of cholangiocarcinoma remains elusive.

Management of complications

As PSC slowly progresses to biliary cirrhosis and portal hypertension. complications may arise from chronic cholestasis or endstage liver failure (as in PBC and other liver diseases) or complications specific to PSC such as biliary strictures, biliary sludge and the development of cholangiocarcinoma. The general management of these complications will not be discussed in this chapter. Endoscopic therapy with balloon dilation and/or biliary stenting is usually reserved for complications such as main duct stricturing causing jaundice, when good short-term relief of symptoms can be achieved. However Stiehl et al.[8] have reported the technique of prospective regular dilation of

Table 1 Controlled studies of ursodeoxycholic acid in PSC

Reference	No. of patients	Study type	Dose	Study duration	LFTs improved				Symptoms improved	Liver histology improved
					Alk P	GGT	Bili	Ast		
Beuers et al. 1992[36]	14	DBPC	13–15 mg/kg daily	12 months	Yes	Yes	Yes	Yes	No	Yes
Lo et al.1992[33]	23	DBPC	10–15 mg/kg daily	24 months	Trend	Trend	No	Trend	No	No
Stiehl et al. 1994[37]	20	DBPC, Unc	750 mg daily	Controlled for 3 months; uncontrolled up to 4 years	Yes	Yes	No	Yes	No	Yes
Mitchell et al.2001[41]	26	DBPC	20–25 mg/kg daily	24 months	Yes	Yes	No	No	No	Yes
van Hoogstraten et al. 1998[53]	48	DB	10 mg/kg daily in single (group 1) or three (group 2) doses	24 months	Yes	Yes	No	Yes	No	NA
Lindor et al. 1997[38]	105	DBPC	13–15 mg/kg daily	Mean 2.9 years	Yes	Yes	Yes	Yes	No	No

Unc, uncontrolled; DB, double-blinded trial; PC, placebo-contolled trial; Alk P, alkaline phosphatase; GGT, γ-glutamyltranspeptidase; Bili, bilirubin; Ast, aspartate transaminase; NA, data not available.

biliary strictures leading to increased survival rates when compared with predicted survival calculated from the Mayo multicentre survival model. These impressive results need to be confirmed by other studies.

Specific medical therapy – the prevention of disease progression

In both PBC and PSC the primary site of inflammation and damage is the biliary epithelium. When severely damaged or destroyed the bile ducts do not have the capacity to regenerate like hepatocytes, which are the primary target for injury in various parenchymal liver diseases. Given the finite number of bile ducts in the liver the natural history of PSC, like PBC, is that of progressive loss of functioning intrahepatic bile ducts (ductopenia). This ductopenia leads to a progressive and irreversible failure of hepatic biliary excretion. To delay and reverse this process physicians have tried a variety of agents but in PSC, in contrast to PBC, few prospective randomized controlled trials have been performed.

Corticosteroids

It is surprising that there have been no long-term studies of the effect of corticosteroid therapy on histological progression and survival in PSC, especially as the disease may be immune-mediated. This may reflect concerns about the long-term side-effect profile of corticosteroids. Systemic and topical corticosteroid therapy has been evaluated in a number of small, often uncontrolled, trials. In an uncontrolled pilot study 10 patients with PSC, selected because they had elevated aminotransferases, were given oral prednisolone and the majority responded with improvement in their biochemistry[10]. In a subsequent study Lindor et al.[11] were unable to confirm these optimistic results. They treated 12 patients with a combination of low-dose prednisone (10 mg daily) and colchicine (0.6 mg twice daily). The clinical course of the treated patients was compared with a control group, but the study was not randomized. After 2 years no significant differences in biochemistry and liver histology were detected between the two groups. In this study treatment did not alter the rate of disease progression or improve survival. The absence of a beneficial response, and the suspicion that corticosteroid therapy enhanced cortical bone loss and hence the risk of developing compression fractures of the spine – even in young male patients, led the authors to advise against empirical corticosteroid therapy in these patients. This conclusion was strengthened by the observation that spontaneous fractures in post-liver transplantation occur almost exclusively in PSC patients who are already osteopenic at the time of transplantation[12].

Topical corticosteroids are usually administered through a nasobiliary drain left *in situ* following endoscopic retrograde cholangiopancreatography (ERCP). Three anecdotal studies[13–15] have reported benefit. The only controlled trial of nasobiliary lavage with corticosteroids from the Royal Free Hospital[16] showed no benefit when compared with a placebo group. Although the numbers were small the bile of all the treated patients became rapidly colonized with enteric bacteria, and a higher incidence of bacterial cholangitis was recorded in the treatment group. Recently a complete therapeutic response to steroids was found retrospectively in only 4.5% of a large group of PSC patients from Norway. Reponse was associated with marked elevations in serum transaminase in a small subgroup of patients[17].

More recent clinical trials have studied the possible benefit of budesonide, a second generation corticosteroid with a high first-pass metabolism and minimal systemic availability. Unfortunately preliminary results, both alone[18] and in combination with ursodeoxycholic acid (UDCA)[19], have been disappointing.

A recent Cochrane review has concluded that there is no direct evidence to suggest that either oral or topical corticosteroids are beneficial in PSC. Indeed when PSC patients with coexistent ulcerative colitis (UC) are given courses of corticosteroids to treat their UC this treatment appears to have little influence on the behaviour of their liver disease. It may be difficult to justify a trial using corticosteroids as monotherapy but a large controlled trial could clarify their role in combination with a choleretic agent. Potentially serious side-effects may be reduced by new agents such as biphosphonates which prevent cortical bone loss.

Methotrexate

After demonstrating a promising response to low-dose oral pulse methotrexate in an open study[20] involving 10 PSC patients without evidence of portal hypertension, Knox and Kaplan[21] performed a prospective double-blind, randomized control trial comparing oral pulse methotrexate at a dose of 15 mg per week with a well-matched placebo group. Twelve patients with PSC were entered into each group. Although each patient was monitored with both liver biopsy and ERCP (at baseline and yearly) and biochemical tests the only significant change was a fall in serum alkaline phosphatase by 31% in those receiving methotrexate.

There was no significant improvement in liver histology, or any differences in outcome of the two groups with regard to treatment failure or death. In a pilot study Lindor et al.[22] found that methotrexate given in combination with UDCA to 19 PSC patients was associated with toxicity (alopecia, pulmonary complications) but no further improvement in liver biochemistries compared with UDCA given alone to a matched group of nine patients.

Other immunosuppressants

Despite the evidence that PSC may be an immune-mediated disease there have been few randomized controlled trials of immunosuppressive agents containing sufficient numbers of patients with early disease. Immunosuppression is unlikely to be effective in patients with advanced liver disease and irreversible bile duct loss, and this may account for the disappointing results so far seen in PSC with these agents. No control trials of azathioprine in PSC have been reported. In one case report[23], two patients improved clinically on azathioprine, but in another[24] the patient deteriorated. The use of cyclosporin in PSC has been evaluated in a randomized controlled trial from the Mayo

Clinic[25] involving 34 patients with PSC and in the majority coexistent UC. Treatment with cyclosporin may help the symptoms of UC[26] but had no effect on the course or prognosis of PSC. Follow-up liver histology after 2 years of treatment revealed progression in 9/10 of the placebo group but only 11/20 of the cyclosporin-treated group[25]. This was not reflected by any beneficial effect on the biochemical tests. The prevalence of side-effects was low; serious renal complications were not reported.

Tacrolimus (FK 506) an immunosuppressive macrolide antibiotic, has been used to treat 10 patients with PSC in an open study[27]. After 1 year of treatment with a twice-daily oral regime all patients experienced an improvement in their liver biochemical tests. For example the median serum bilirubin level was reduced by 75% and the serum alkaline phosphatase was reduced by 70%. No major adverse events were reported in this initial study in PSC. A randomized controlled trial is required to confirm these encouraging preliminary results.

The hepatobiliary injury which occurs in rats with experimental bacterial overgrowth is said to result from peptidoglycan-polysaccharide-mediated activation of Kupffer cells which in turn release cytokines such as tumour necrosis factor (TNF-alpha). In rats the liver injury can be prevented by pentoxifylline. In an open pilot study 20 patients with PSC were treated with pentoxifylline 400 mg q.i.d. for 1 year. In this dose pentoxifylline did not improve symptoms or liver tests[28]. Negative results were also obtained in a open pilot study of 10 PSC patients using etanercept, an anti-TNF antibody, administered twice weekly subcutaneously for 1 year[29]. However, the anti-TNF antibody infliximab which has been shown to be efficacious in the treatment of Crohn's disease, in marked contrast to entanercept which has surprisingly not been studied in the treatment of PSC.

Antifibrogenic agents

In the light of initial reports which suggested a positive trend of the antifibrogenic agent colchicine on survival in PBC and other types of cirrhosis, a randomized trial from Sweden[30] compared colchicine in a dose of 1 mg daily by mouth in 44 patients with PSC with a matched placebo group of 40 patients. At 3-year follow-up there were no differences in clinical symptoms, serum biochemistry, liver histology or survival between the two groups. The absence in this study of any proven effect of colchicine on disease progression, outcome or survival is in keeping with more recent long-term studies of colchicine in PBC and other chronic liver diseases which have failed to confirm the initial reported survival benefits.

Ursodeoxycholic acid (UDCA)

This hydrophilic bile acid has become widely used in the treatment of cholestatic liver of all causes. UDCA appears to exert a number of effects all of which may be beneficial in chronic cholestasis: a choleretic effect by increasing bile flow; a direct cytoprotective effect; an indirect cytoprotective effect by displacement of the more hepatotoxic endogenous hydrophobic bile acids from the bile acid pool; an immunomodulatory effect and finally an inhibitory effect on apoptosis.

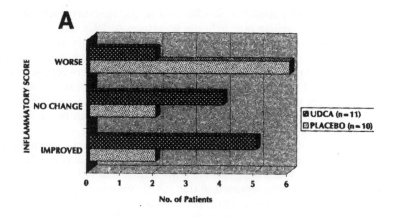

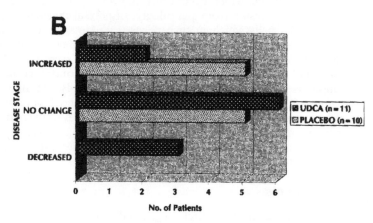

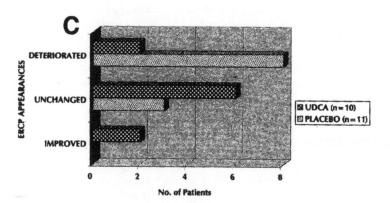

Figure 1 Comparison of (**A**) changes in portal inflammatory score, (**B**) disease progression by staging, and cholangiographic assessment (**C**) in patients treated with high-dose UDCA versus placebo over the 2-year trial (reproduced from ref. 41)

Using a labelled bile acid analogue Jazrawi et al.[31] demonstrated a defect in hepatic bile acid excretion but not in uptake in patients with PBC and PSC resulting in bile acid retention. They observed an improvement of hepatic excretory function with UDCA in patients with PBC, but only a trend towards improvement in the small number of patients with PSC. Not only is hepatic bile acid excretion affected by UDCA but so is ileal reabsorption of endogenous bile acids. The net result is enrichment of the bile acid pool with UDCA. Hydrophobic bile acids are more toxic than UDCA, which can protect and stabilize membranes.

In a recent study Rost et al. determined the biliary acid compositon in patients with PSC treated with various dosages of UDCA. Biliary enrichment increased with increasing dosage and reached a plateau of $58.6 \pm 2.3\%$ at 22–25 mg/kg doses[32]. From this study this dose range appears to be optimal in the treatment of PSC.

Studies have demonstrated that long-term treatment with UDCA decreases aberrant expression of HLA class I on hepatocytes and reduces levels of soluble cell adhesion molecules (sICAM) in PBC patients. *In-vitro* studies have shown that UDCA may alter cytokine production by human peripheral mononuclear cells. In PSC, one study has shown that UDCA has been shown to decrease aberrant HLA DR expression on bile ducts[33]. However, a more recent study could not demonstrate any alteration in expression of either HLA class I and II or ICAM-1 on either biliary epithelial cells or hepatocytes[34]. The body of evidence suggests that UDCA does have some modulatory effects on immune function, but how important these are remains unclear.

Numerous studies have attempted to address the clinical efficacy of UDCA treatment in PSC. The majority have been uncontrolled studies in small numbers of patients. In a pilot study O'Brien et al.[35] treated 12 patients with UDCA on an open basis over 30 months. They documented improvement in fatigue, pruritus and diarrhoea, and significant improvement of all liver biochemical tests, particularly alkaline phosphatase, during the two UDCA treatment periods. Symptoms and liver biochemistry relapsed during a 6-month withdrawal period between treatment phases. During UDCA treatment the amount of cholic acid declined slightly, but the levels of other relatively hydrophobic bile acids did not change significantly.

In the first prospective randomized double-blind controlled trial of UDCA in PSC Beuers et al.[36] compared over a 12-month period six patients who received UDCA 13–15 mg per kg body weight with eight patients who received placebo. The majority of patients had early disease (Ludwig classification stages I and II). After 6 months a significant reduction in alkaline phosphatase and aminotransferases was achieved in the treatment group. A significant fall in bilirubin was only noted after 12 months. Using a multiparametric score the UDCA-treated group showed significant improvement in their liver histology, mainly attributed to decreased portal and parenchymal inflammation. Unfortunately treatment did not ameliorate their symptoms. UDCA-induced diarrhoea was the only important side-effect requiring one patient to withdraw.

Similar results were obtained by Stiehl et al.[37], who randomized 20 patients to either 750 mg daily of UDCA or placebo.

However, in a larger prospective randomized placebo-controlled trial of UDCA in PSC by Lindor et al.[38], no benefit could be demonstrated. In this trial 105 patients were randomized to treatment with UDCA in conventional doses; i.e. 13–15 mg/kg body weight daily, or placebo, and followed up for up to 6 years (mean 2.9 years). Treatment with UDCA had no effect upon the time until treatment failure defined as death, liver transplantation, the development of cirrhosis, quadrupling of bilirubin, marked relapse of symptoms or the development of signs of chronic liver disease. Furthermore the significant improvement in liver biochemical tests seen in the treated group was not reflected by any beneficial changes in liver histology. On the contrary there was a suggestion that the liver histology of patients on UDCA showed a greater tendency to progress towards fibrosis. However, this could also be explained by sampling variability between serial liver biopsies[39].

The failure of standard doses of UDCA to provide clinical benefit led our group to consider the use of higher doses. Our rationale is that, as previously discussed, with increasing cholestasis there is decreasing enrichment of the bile acid pool with UDCA and higher doses are required to achieve the same level of enrichment[32]. Furthermore the *in-vitro* immunomodulatory effects of UDCA are enhanced with increasing UDCA concentrations[40].

In a pilot study we evaluated 26 patients with PSC who were randomized to either high-dose (20–25 mg/kg) UDCA or placebo[41] for 2 years. High-dose UDCA had no effect on symptoms but, as expected, there was a significant improvement in liver biochemistry. More importantly we found a significant reduction in cholangiographic appearances and liver fibrosis. In the treatment group bile acid saturation with UDCA >70% confirmed patient compliance. No significant side-effects were reported; in particular no worsening of colitis was seen.

These encouraging results were confirmed by an open study in 30 patients with PSC treated for 1 year[42]. When compared with historical controls a significant improvement in projected survival using the Mayo risk score was observed with high-dose UDCA but not with the conventional dose (13–15 mg/kg per day) of UDCA.

In the light of these promising data, a large controlled trial of a moderately high dose of UDCA (17–22 mg/kg) has been completed in Scandinavia. The provisional results have shown no significant differences between the two groups, although there was a strong trend in favour of improved survival in the UDCA group. Moreover the study was probably underpowered to show a positive result, as the endpoints of death or transplant were lower than expected in both groups[43].

In a recent pilot study from Oxford and Munich[44], the effects of very high-dose UDCA (25–30 mg/kg body weight) were compared with a medium dose of 20–25 mg/kg and a low-dose group of 10–15 mg/kg. Over a 2-year period a possible effect of prolonged survival was indicated by the Mayo risk score, which was significantly reduced in the 25–30 mg/kg body weight group. In addition there was a trend towards a greater improvement in liver histology using the Ludwig score. No side-effects were observed.

It is established that patients with UC with PSC have a higher rate of colonic dysplasia and cancer than patients with PSC alone[45]. Recent studies have suggested that treatment with UDCA reduces the rate of colonic dysplasia and cancer[46,47]. Whether UDCA reduces the high rate of cholangiocarcinoma in PSC remains to be established, although UDCA appeared to be protective against the development of cholangicarcinoma in a study in PSC transplant patients from the Nordic countries[48].

MISCELLANEOUS TREATMENTS

In keeping with UC, there is a strong inverse relationship between PSC and cigarette smoking. This led Angulo et al.[49] to test the hypothesis that oral nicotine might have a beneficial effect in PSC. Eight non-smoking patients with PSC were treated with nicotine 6 mg q.i.d. for up to 1 year. Side-effects were high, requiring cessation in three patients, and no beneficial effects were seen,

COMBINED THERAPY

In an important pilot study the potential of combination therapy was explored by Schramm et al.[50], who treated 15 patients with PSC. All patients received low-dose UDCA (500–750 mg daily), prednisolone 1 mg/kg daily and azathioprine 1–1.5 mg/kg daily. After a median follow-up period of 41 months, all patients showed a significant improvement in liver function tests. Seven patients had been previously treated with UDCA but liver enzymes improved only after immunosuppressive therapy was added. More importantly, six of 10 with follow-up biopsies showed histological improvement, and significant radiological deterioration was seen only in in one of 10 patients who had ERCP.

In a prospective trial Stiehl et al.[8,51] studied the survival of 106 patients with PSC for up to 13 years, treated with 750 mg UDCA daily and by endoscopic balloon dilation of major dominant stenoses whenever necessary. Some of the patients developed dominant strictures during the trial, and UDCA did not prevent such stricture formation. This combined approach of UDCA and endoscopic intervention significantly improved survival compared with predicted survival rates. This was an uncontrolled study and it is therefore difficult to ascertain whether UDCA or endoscopic therapy, if either, prolonged survival, although the results are promising.

CONCLUSION

There is no established effective medical treatment for PSC. However, promising recent studies suggest that high-dose UDCA may have a role in at least slowing disease progression, and reduces the rate of colonic dysplasia and cancer, although larger long-term studies are awaited. The chemoprotective effect of UDCA on the colon and possibly the bile ducts probably means that all PSC patients with inflammatory bowel disease should be treated with UDCA. Randomized controlled trials of combination therapy in early PSC are needed, possibly high-dose UDCA in combination with immunosuppressant agents and/or antibiotics. With the identification of T cell subsets involved in PSC and the cytokines they produce, it may be possible to use particular recombinant cytokines or antibodies to specific cytokines such as anti-TNF antibody (infliximab) to manipulate the immune response in PSC and alter disease progression. Greater insight into the pathogenetic mechanisms involved in PSC would enable therapy to be targeted more specifically at the area of initial damage, namely the biliary epithelium.

Liver transplantation remains the mainstay of treatment for patients with endstage disease[52].

References

1. Chapman RW, Arborgh BA, Rhodes JM et al. Primary sclerosing cholangitis: a review of its clinical features, cholangiography, and hepatic histology. Gut. 1980;21:870–7.
2. Lo SK, Fleming KA, Chapman RW. Prevalence of anti-neutrophil antibody in primary sclerosing cholangitis and ulcerative colitis using an alkaline phosphatase technique. Gut. 1992;33:1370–5.
3. Chapman R. Does HLA status influence prognosis in primary sclerosing cholangitis? Gastroenterology. 1995;108:937–40.
4. Martins E, Graham AK, Chapman RW, Fleming KA. Elevation of gamma delta T lymphocytes in peripheral blood and livers of patients with primary sclerosing cholangitis and other autoimmune liver diseases. Hepatology. 1996;23:988–93.
5. Broome U, Olsson R, Loof L et al. Natural history and prognostic variables in 305 Swedish patients with primary sclerosing cholangitis. Gut. 1996;38:610–15.
6. Pokorny CS, McCaughan GW, Gallagher ND, Selby WS. Sclerosing cholangitis and biliary tract calculi – primary or secondary? Gut. 1992;33:1376–80.
7. Bergquist A, Ekbom A, Olsson R et al. Hepatic and extrahepatic malignancies in primary sclerosing cholangitis. J Hepatol. 2002;36:321–7.
8. Stiehl A, Rudolph G, Kloters-Plachy P, Sauer P, Walker S. Development of dominant bile duct stenoses in patients with primary sclerosing cholangitis treated with ursodeoxycholic acid:outcome after endoscopic treatment. J Hepatol. 2002;36:151–6.
9. Sivak M Jr, Farmer RG, Lalli AF. Sclerosing cholangitis: its increasing frequency of recognition and association with inflammatory bowel disease. J Clin Gastroenterol. 1981;3:261–6.
10. Burgert SL, Brown BP, Kirkpatrick RB, LaBrecque DR. Positive corticosteroid response in early primary sclerosing cholangitis. Gastroenterology. 1984;86:1037 (Abstract).
11. Lindor KD, Wiesner RH, Colwell LJ et al. The combination of prednisone and colchicine in patients with primary sclerosing cholangitis. Am J Gastroenterol. 1991;86:57–61.
12. Porayko MK, Wiesner RH, Hay JE et al. Bone disease in liver transplant recipients: incidence, timing and risk factors. Transplant Proc. 1991;23:1462–5.
13. Grijm R, Huibregtse K, Bartelsman J et al. Therapeutic investigations in primary sclerosing cholangitis. Dig Dis Sci. 1986;31:792–8.
14. Jeffrey GP, Reed WD, Laurence BH, Shilkin KB. Primary sclerosing cholangitis: clinical and immunopathological review of 21 cases. J Gastroenterol Hepatol. 1990;5:135–40.
15. Craig PI, Williams SJ, Hatfield ARW, Ng M, Cotton PB. Endoscopic management of primary sclerosing cholangitis. Gut. 1990;31:1182a (Abstract).
16. Allison MC, Burroughs AK, Noone P, Summerfield JA. Biliary lavage with corticosteroids in primary sclerosing cholangitis. A clinical, cholangiographic and bacteriological study. J Hepatol. 1986;3:118–22.
17. Boberg KM, Egeland T, Schrumpf E. Long term corticosteroid treatment in PSC. Scand J Gastroenterol. 2003;38:991–5.
18. Angulo P, Batts KP, Jorgensen A, Lindor KD. Budesonide in the treatment of primary sclerosing cholangitis: a pilot study. Hepatology. 1999;30:477 (Abstract).

19. van Hoogstraten HJF, Vieggar FP, Boland GI et al. Budesonide or prednisone in combination with ursodeoxycholic acid in primary sclerosing cholangitis: a randomized double-blind pilot study. Am J Gastroenterol. 2000;95:2015–22.
20. Knox TA, Kaplan MM. Treatment of primary sclerosing cholangitis with oral methotrexate. Am J Gastroenterol. 1991;86:546–52.
21. Knox TA, Kaplan MM. A double-blind controlled trial of oral-pulse methotrexate therapy in the treatment of primary sclerosing cholangitis. Gastroenterology. 1994;106:494–9.
22. Lindor KD, Jorgensen RA, Anderson ML et al. Ursodeoxycholic acid and methotrexate for primary sclerosing cholangitis: a pilot study. Am J Gastroenterol. 1996;91:511–15.
23. Javett SL. Azathioprine in primary sclerosing cholangitis. Lancet. 1971;i:810–11.
24. Wagner A. Azathioprine treatment in primary sclerosing cholangitis. Lancet. 1971;2:663–4.
25. Wiesner RH, Steiner B, LaRusso NF, Lindor KD, Baldus WP. A controlled clinical trial evaluating cyclosporine in the treatment of primary sclerosing cholangitis. Hepatology. 1991;14:63A (Abstract).
26. Sandborn WJ, Wiesner RH, Tremaine WJ, Larusso NF. Ulcerative colitis disease activity following treatment of associated primary sclerosing cholangitis with cyclosporin. Gut. 1993;34:242–6.
27. Van-Thiel DH, Carroll P, Abu-Elmagd K et al. Tacrolimus (FK 506), a treatment for primary sclerosing cholangitis: results of an open-label preliminary trial. Am J Gastroenterol. 1995;90:455–9.
28. Harucha AE, Jorgensen R, Lichtman SN, La RussoNF, Lindor KD. A pilot study of pentoxifylline for the treatment of primary sclerosing cholangitis. Am J Gastroenterol. 2000;95:2338–42.
29. Epstein MP, Kaplan MM. Pilot study of etanercept in the treatment of PSC. Dig Dis Sci. 2004;49:1–4.
30 Olsson R, Broome U, Danielsson A et al. Colchicine treatment of primary sclerosing cholangitis. Gastroenterology. 1995;108:1199–203.
31. Jazrawi RP, de-Caestecker JS, Goggin PM et al. Kinetics of hepatic bile acid handling in cholestatic liver disease: effect of ursodeoxycholic acid. Gastroenterology. 1994;106:134–42.
32. Rost D, Rudolph G, Kloeters-Planchky P, Stiehl A. Effect of high dose ursodeoxycholic acid on its biliary enrichment in primary sclerosing cholangitis. Hepatology. 2004;50:693–8.
33. Lo SK, Hermann R, Chapman RW et al. Ursodeoxycholic acid in primary sclerosing cholangitis; a double blind controlled trial. Hepatology. 1992:14:16A.
34. van Milligen de Wit AW, Kuiper H, Camoglio L et al. Does ursodeoxycholic acid mediate immunomodulatory and anti inflammatory effects in patients with primary sclerosing cholangitis? Eur J Gastroenterol Hepatol. 1999;11:129–36.
35. O'Brien CB, Senior JR, Arora-Mirchandani R, Batta AK, Salen G. Ursodeoxycholic acid for the treatment of primary sclerosing cholangitis: a 30-month pilot study. Hepatology. 1991;14:838.
36. Beuers U, Spengler U, Kruis W et al. Ursodeoxycholic acid for treatment of primary sclerosing cholangitis: a placebo-controlled trial. Hepatology. 1992;16:707–14.
37. Stiehl A, Walker S, Stiehl L et al. Effect of ursodeoxycholic acid on liver and bile duct disease in primary sclerosing cholangitis. A 3-year pilot study with a placebo-controlled study period. J Hepatol. 1994;20:57–64.
38. Lindor KD, The Mayo PSC/UDCA Study Group. Ursodiol for primary sclerosing cholangitis. N Engl J Med. 1997:336:691–5.
39. Olsson R, Hagerstrand I, Broome U et al. Sampling variability of percutaneous liver biopsy in primary sclerosing cholangitis. J Clin Pathol. 1995;48:933–5.
40 Hirano F, Tanaka H, Makino Y, OkamotoK, Makino I. Effects of ursodeoxycholic acid and chenodeoxycholic acid on major histocompatibility complex class I gene expression. J Gastroenterol. 1996;31:55–60.
41. Mitchell SA, Bansi DS, Hunt N, von Bergmann K, Fleming KA, Chapman RW. A preliminary trial of high dose ursodeoxycholic acid in primary sclerosing cholangitis. Gastroenterology. 2001;121:900–7.
42 Harnois DM, Angulo P, Jorgensen RA, La Russo NF, Lindor KD. High-dose ursodeoxycholic acid as a therapy for patients with primary sclerosing cholangitis. Am J Gastroenterol. 2001;96:1558–66.

43. Olsson R, Boberg KM, Scaffalitsky O et al. Five year treatment with high dose UDCA in PSC. Gastroenterology. 2005;129:1464–72.

44. Cullen SN, Rust C, Fleming K, Beuers U, Chapman RW. High dose UDCA for the treatment of primary sclerosing cholangitis is safe and effective. EASL 2006. J Hepatol. 2006;44:S234.

45. Broome U, Lofberg R, Veress B et al. Primary sclerosing cholangitis and ulcerative colitis: evidence for increased neoplastic potential. Hepatology. 1995;22:1404–8.

46. Tung BY, Emond MJ, Haggitt RC et al. Ursodiol use is associated with lower prevalence of colonic neoplasia in patients with ulcerative colitis and primary sclerosing cholangitis. Ann Intern Med. 2001:134:89–95.

47. Pardi DS, Loftus EV, Kremers WK, Leach J, Lindor KD. Ursodeoxycholic acid as a chemopreventive agent in patients with ulcerative colitis and primary sclerosing cholangitis. Gastroenterology. 2003;124:889–93.

48. Brandsaeter B, BroomeU, Isoniemi H et al. Liver transplantation for primary sclerosing cholangitis in the Nordic countries: outcome after acceptance to the waiting list. Liver Transplant. 2003;9:961–9.

49. Angulo P, Bharucha AE, Jorgensen RA et al. Oral nicotine in treatment of primary sclerosing cholangitis: a pilot study. Dig Dis Sci. 1999;44:602–5.

50. Schramm C, Schirmacher P, Helmreich-Becker I et al. Combined therapy with azathioprine and prednisolone and ursodiol in patients with primary sclerosing cholangitis. A case series. Ann Intern Med. 1999;131:943–6.

51. Stiehl A, Rudolph G, Sauer P et al. Efficacy of ursodeoxycholic acid treatment and endoscopic dilatation of major duct stenoses in primary sclerosing cholangitis. A 8 years prospective study. J Hepatol. 1997;26:56–61.

52. Gow PJ, Chapman RW. Liver transplantation for primary sclerosing cholangitis. Liver. 2000:20:97–103.

53. Van Hoogstraten HJ, Wolfhagen FJ, Van de Meeberg PC, vanBuuren HR, van Berge H, Schalm SW. Ursodeoxycholic acid therapy for primary sclerosing cholangitis: results of a 2 year randomized controlled trial to evaluate single vrsus multiple doses. J Hepatol. 1998;29: 417–23.

33
Primary sclerosing cholangitis: bile duct and colonic carcinomas after long-term ursodeoxycholic acid

A. STIEHL, D. ROST and H. KULAKSIZ

INTRODUCTION

Primary sclerosing cholangitis (PSC) is characterized by progressive fibrosing inflammation of the bile ducts leading to cholestasis and finally to cirrhosis of the liver[1-3]. The disease is frequently associated with ulcerative colitis[1-4]. A problem lies in the increased incidence of cholangiocarcinomas and colonic carcinomas and, according to a recent study, also pancreatic carcinomas[5].

URSODEOXYCHOLIC ACID

With the exception of one study[6], in all other studies with sufficient dosage, UDCA led to significant improvement of AP, GGT, -ALT, -AST and in part also of serum bilirubin[7-11]. Recent data indicate that high doses of UDCA (20 mg/kg) lead to significant improvement of liver histology, whereas lower doses are less effective[10]. The efficacy of high-dose UDCA has recently been confirmed[11]. Such high doses may be needed since in patients with cholestasis the absorption of UDCA may be reduced[12]. In the majority of patients the optimal dose is between 22 and 25 mg/kg[13].

A problem in the treatment of patients with PSC is the development of dominant stenoses which occlude the major bile ducts, which cannot be expected to be treated efficiently by medical treatment[14] and which need endoscopic intervention[14-16]. It seems very important that all endoscopic procedures are performed under antibiotic prophylaxis since bacterial cholangitis is a frequent complication of endoscopic procedures[17-19]. It is obvious that UDCA will have little or no effect on liver histology when dominant stenoses are present and are not treated by endoscopic means.

BILE DUCT CARCINOMA

An unresolved problem in the treatment of patients with PSC is the development of bile duct carcinomas[1-3,5]. At present it is very difficult to detect cholangiocarcinomas at an early stage. Brush-border cytology of dominant strictures is insufficiently sensitive[20]. Tumour markers CEA and CA19-9 are neither sensitive nor specific[21]. Imaging methods (CT, NMR) do not allow the detection of early carcinomas and the results with positron emission tomography need further confirmation in larger trials. When the carcinoma has developed the prognosis in general is very poor.

In a large multicentre study from Sweden, in which 305 PSC patients were followed over a median follow-up time of 63 months, a bile duct carcinoma was observed in 8% of patients, and 44% of these were asymptomatic at the time of diagnosis of PSC[3]. In 37% of the patients with bile duct carcinoma this diagnosis was made within 1 year after detection of PSC and, as a consequence, it seems possible that the patients already had a bile duct carcinoma when the PSC was recognized. The decrease of the incidence of bile duct carcinomas in the years following diagnosis of PSC has recently been confirmed in another study on the natural course of the disease[22]. No factors were found which would allow the identification of patients who will later develop a bile duct carcinoma.

A bile duct carcinoma rate of 8%[3] appears much lower than was suggested previously. Of interest is the fact that in the Swedish study overall only 8% of the patients developed a cholangiocarcinoma, and in patients with endstage disease who were considered for transplantation, 30% had bile duct carcinomas[3]. These data explain why the figures on the incidence emerging from transplantation centres are always much higher than the corresponding figures from prospective studies in gastroenterology units. Very high rates of bile duct carcinomas have repeatedly been reported in studies in transplantation centres[3], and it appears that they reflect very selected patient groups.

In a controlled study 0/52 of patients with PSC on UDCA developed a bile duct carcinoma, in comparison to 3/53 patients in the placebo group[9]. In a prospective long-term study on the effects of UDCA on outcome, the incidence of bile duct carcinomas in 150 patients was only 3%, and this decreased with time on UDCA treatment[23]. In a study of 225 patients listed for liver transplantation, hepatobiliary malignancies developed in 20%, and UDCA treatment was associated with a significantly decreased incidence of hepatobiliary cancer[24]. It seems possible that the reduced inflammation around the bile ducts observed after UDCA treatment[7,8,10] may reduce the incidence of bile duct carcinomas.

COLONIC CARCINOMA

Colorectal carcinoma occurs more frequently in patients with chronic inflammatory bowel disease than in the normal population. Risk factors are involvement of the whole colon and long duration of the disease. Recently it has been shown that PSC represents an independent risk factor for the development of colonic carcinoma[25]. In a study in which 40 patients with PSC and colitis were matched with 40 patients of the same age, and with comparable colitis and comparable duration of the disease, the absolute cumulative risk of developing colorectal dysplasia or carcinoma in patients with PSC was almost five times higher than in patients without PSC. The study also indicates that patients with PSC and colitis who develop colonic dysplasia or carcinoma are at a high risk of developing cholangiocarcinoma. It is evident that patients with PSC and colitis need colonoscopic surveillance at short intervals.

In animal experiments bile acids have cocarcinogenic effects in the development of colonic adenocarcinomas. UDCA has been shown to prevent this cocarcinogenic effect[26] and as a consequence the effect of UDCA on the incidence of colonic dysplasias, adenomatous polyps and carcinomas is of great interest. After oral administration of a single oral dose of 500 mg UDCA to patients with ileostomy at the end of the ileum, 59% were excreted from the ileostomy[27]. Thus, due to its poor absorption in the upper small intestine, substantial amounts of UDCA enter the colon, where it is bacterially degraded.

In two placebo-controlled trials on the effect of UDCA on liver disease in PSC the incidence of dysplasias and carcinomas has been evaluated. In a first study, in which 59 patients were included, the incidence of dysplasias and carcinomas in the UDCA group was 32% and in the control group it was also 72%[28], the difference being significant. In a second placebo-controlled study with 52 patients, of 29 patients in the UDCA group only 10% had dysplasias or carcinomas, whereas in the placebo group of 23 patients 35% developed dysplasias or carcinomas[29] ($p < 0.05$). Thus, in two controlled trials in patients with ulcerative colitis and PSC, UDCA significantly reduced the incidence of colonic dysplasias and carcinomas.

EFFECT OF TREATMENT ON SURVIVAL

PSC is a progressive disease, and survival of such patients is reduced. Survival is better in asymptomatic patients than in symptomatic patients. In patients treated with UDCA and, whenever necessary, by aditioal endosopic dilations, the actuarial Kaplan–Meier estimate of survival after treatment with UDCA and dilation of major duct stenoses was significantly improved compared to predicted survival[14,16]. The need for endoscopic treatment of dominant stenoses has been confirmed in a multicentre study in which 63 patients were included[15]. Actuarial survival compared with predicted survival was significantly improved after treatment[15]. In endstage disease liver transplantation represents the treatment of choice.

CONCLUSION

There is good evidence that the incidence of colonic dysplasias and carcinomas may be reduced by treatment with UDCA. The incidence of bile duct carcinomas in UDCA-treated patients is low, and decreases with time of treatment. It seems possible that UDCA treatment may lead to a reduction of dysplasias and carcinomas of the bile ducts. These findings await further confirmation. Dominant stenoses develop frequently and need endoscopic dilation. After UDCA treatment and endoscopic opening of dominant stenoses, survival may be improved in comparison to predicted survival.

References

1. Chapman RW, Arborgh BA, Rhodes JM et al. Primary sclerosing cholangitis – a review of its clinical features, cholangiography and hepatic histology. Gut. 1980;21:870–7.
2. Wiesner RH, Grambsch PM, Dickson ER et al. Natural history, prognostic factors, and survival analysis. Hepatology. 1989;10:430–6.
3. Broome U, Olson R, Lööf L et al. Natural history and prognostic factors in 305 Swedish patients with primary sclerosing cholangitis. Gut. 1996;38:610–15.
4. Olsson R, Danielsson A, Järnebrot G et al. Prevalence of primary sclerosing choanitis in patients with ulcerative colitis. Gastroenterology. 1991;100:1319–23.
5. Bergquist A, Ekbom A, Olsson R et al. Hepatic and extrahepatic malignancies in primary sclerosing cholangitis. J Hepatol. 2002;36:321–7.
6. Olsson R, Boberg KM, Schaffalisky de Muckadell O et al. High-dose ursodeoxycholic acid in primary sclerosing cholangitis. A five year multicenter randomised study. Gastroenterology. 2005;129:1464–72.
7. Stiehl A, Walker S, Stiehl L et al. Effects of ursodexcholic acid on liver and bile duct disease in primary sclerosing cholangitis. A 3 year pilot study with a placeo-controlled study period. J Hepatol. 1994;20:57–64.
8. Beuers U, Spengler U, Kruis W et al. Ursodeoxycholic acid for treatment of priay sclerosing cholangiis: a placebo-controlled trial. Hepatology. 1992;16:707–14
9. Lindor KD and the Mayo PSC/UDCA Study Group. Ursodiol for the treatment of primary sclerosing cholangitis. N Engl J Med. 1997;336:691–5.
10. Mitchell SA, Bansi D, Hunt N et al. A preliminary trial of high dose ursodeoxycholic acid in primary sclerosing cholangitis. Gastroenterology. 2001;121:900–7
11. Harnois DM, Angulo P, Jorgensen RA, LaRusso NF, Lindor KD. High-dose ursodeoxycholic acid as therapy for patients with primary sclerosing cholangitis. Am J Gastroenterol. 2001;96:1558–62
12. Sauer P, Benz C, Rudolph G et al. Influence of cholestasis on absorption of ursodeoxycholic acid. Dig Dis Sci. 1999;44:817–22.
13. Rost D, Rudolph G, Kloeters-Plachky P, Stiehl A. Effect of high-dose ursodeoxycholic acid on its biliary enrichment in primary sclerosing cholangitis. Hepatology. 2004;40:693–8.
14. Stiehl A, Rudolph G, Sauer P et al. Efficacy of ursodeoxycholic acid and endoscopic dilation of major duct stenoses in primary sclerosing cholangitis. An 8-year prospective study. J Hepatol. 1997;26:560–6.
15. Baluyut AR, Sherman S, Lehman GA, Hoen H, Chalasani N. Impact of endoscopic therapy on the survival of patients with primary sclerosing cholangitis. Gastrointest Endosc. 2001;53:308–12.
16. Stiehl A, Rudolph G, Klöters-Plachky P et al. Development of bile duct stenoses in patients with primary sclerosing cholangitis treated with ursodeoxycholic acid. Outcome after endoscopic treatment. J Hepatol. 2002;36:151–6.
17. Olsson R, Björnsson E, Bäckman L et al. Bile duct bacterial isolates in primary sclerosing cholangitis: a study of explanted livers. J Hepatol. 1998;28:426–32.
18. Pohl J, Ring A, Stremmel W, Stiehl A. The role of dominant stenoses in bacterial infections of bile ducts in primary sclerosing cholangitis. Eur J Gastroenterol Hepatol. 2006;18:69–74.
19. Kulaksiz H, Rudolph G, Kloeters-Plachky P et al. Biliary Candida infections in primary sclerosing cholangitis. J Hepatol. 2006;45:711–16.
20. Ponsionen C IJ, Vrouenraets SME, van Milligen AWM et al. Value of brush border cytology for dominant strictures in primary sclerosing cholangitis. Endoscopy. 1999;31:305–9.
21. Hultcrantz R, Olsson R, Danielsson A et al. A three year prospective study on serum tumor markers used for detecting cholangiocarcinoma in patients with primary sclerosing cholangitis. J Hepatol. 1999;30:669–73.

22. Burak K, Angulo P, Pasha TM, Egan K, Petz J, Lindor KD. Incidence and risk factors for cholangiocarcinoma in primary sclerosing cholangitis. Am J Gastroenterol. 2004;99:523–6.
23. Stiehl A, Kloeters-Plachky P, Rudolph G. The incidence of cholangiocarcinoma in primary sclerosing cholangitis during longtime treatment with ursodeoxycholic acid. Gastroenterology. 2006;130:A721.
24. Brandsaeter B, Isoniemi H, Broome U et al. Liver transplantation for primary sclerosing cholangitis; predictors and consequences of hepatobiliary malignancy. J Hepatol. 2004;40: 815–22.
25. Broome U, Löfberg R, Veress B, Erikson LS. Primary sclerosing cholangitis and ulcerative colitis: evidence for increased neoplastic potential. Hepatology. 1995;22:1404–8.
26. Earnest DL, Holubec H, Wali RK et al. Chemoprevention of azomethane-induced colonic carcinogenesis by supplemental dietary ursodeoxycholic acid. Cancer Res. 1994;54:5071–4.
27. Stiehl A, Raedsch R, Rudolph G. Ileal excretion of bile acids: comparison with biliary bile composition and effect of ursodeoxycholic acid treatment. Gastroenterology. 1988;94: 1201–6.
28. Tung BY, Emond MJ, Haggitt RC et al. Ursodiol use is associated with lower prevalence of colonic neoplasia in patients with ulcerative colitis and primary sclerosing cholangitis. Ann Intern Med. 2001;134:89–95.
29. Pardi DS, Loftus EV, Kremers WK et al. Ursodeoxycholic acid as a chemoprotective agent in patients with ulcerative colitis and primary sclerosing cholangitis. Gastroenterology. 2003;124: 889–93.

Index

Hat-Trick Hero

Celia Warren

One minute Josh had been fast asleep. The next he was wide awake. He didn't know what had woken him. By the faint light of his bedside lamp, his eyes struggled to focus on his alarm clock. It was one o'clock in the morning.

Out of the corner of his eye, Josh saw a movement. His football was rolling slowly but deliberately across the carpet towards him, just as if someone had given it a gentle kick. It came to a standstill beside his bed.

Josh switched on the main light. He reached down for the ball. It felt warm, as if it had been left lying in the grass on a summer's day. Of course, he had left it in the corner by the radiator as he did every night. But what had made the ball roll by itself like that? Josh shivered and snuggled down under his quilt away from the cold night air. He left the light on while he went back to sleep.

'Morning, Joshua,' said his mother, six hours later, as she opened his curtains.

Sunshine flooded into Josh's bedroom. Good. It was going to be fine for the match. It was the first time Josh had been chosen for the school team and he wanted the day to be perfect. Now all he had to do

1

was get through the grind of a morning's schoolwork and keep his excitement under control.

Josh rubbed his eyes and jumped out of bed. Automatically, he picked up his football and gave it a fond stroke, just like his sister, Alice, would give her guinea pig. It was not until he put the ball on his unmade bed that he remembered waking in the night. But surely he had just picked up the ball from beside the radiator, not from by the bed where it had rolled in the night? How odd!

'Mum must've put it back,' Josh said to himself, and thought no more about it.

As Josh's mother dropped him off at the school gate, she wished him luck.

'I'm sorry I shan't be able to watch you, Joshua,' she said. 'I'm afraid I just can't get away from work in time.'

Josh dodged out of the car before she could kiss him. Mum could be so embarrassing at times; like when she called him by his full name, Joshua.

'We're going to win tonight,' he told Alice, as they walked into the playground.

'I'm sure you will,' said Alice. 'I wish I could watch,' she added, 'but if I miss the auditions this afternoon I won't get a part in the panto.' Alice, like their mother, was keen on drama. Somehow Mum always managed to come and see Alice when she was acting. Josh wished he had a dad to come and cheer him on – but it was no good wishing.

'Your dad was never interested in football,' his mother had told him often enough, 'but *his* dad – your grandad – played all the time. He'd have been very proud of his grandson.'

Josh had never known his grandfather. Grandad Jim

had died before Josh was born, and Josh's dad had taken himself off to live and work in America when Josh was only a baby. He couldn't remember him at all.

The whistle blew. For a brief moment Josh thought he heard a crowd cheer and clap. It was as if someone had rapidly switched a radio on and then off again in the middle of a live broadcast of a football match. Josh shook his head. It was only a teacher, blowing the whistle in the playground. It was time to go into school.

The Head, Mr Henry, asked the team to stay behind after assembly. He reminded them of their responsibilities as hosts at that afternoon's home match. They must make the St Luke's team welcome. They must show good sportsmanship – it was the playing not the winning that counted . . .

Mr Henry's voice droned on. Josh's mind wandered. From the cloakroom the squeaky sound of a recorder drifted through to the hall. Someone was playing the theme tune to TV's *Match of the Day*.

Mr Henry's closing words jolted Josh back from his daydream.

'Now, some exciting news,' he said. 'There is to be a special feature about the school in the *Echo* this week. A photographer will be taking pictures of the match this afternoon, and I'm looking forward to seeing some exciting shots of you all in action. So now, heads down in the classroom and save your football thoughts for later. Off you go.'

As Josh turned to leave the hall, he felt a hand on his shoulder. It was Mr Henry.

'Your first inter-school match, isn't it?' he asked.

'Yes, sir,' nodded Josh.

'Good luck then, Jim,' smiled Mr Henry and marched off to his office before Josh could correct him.

'Oh well,' shrugged Josh. 'Jim's better than Joshua, I suppose.'

Time never goes so slowly as when you're waiting for something. The first half of the morning seemed endless. Break, when it finally came, was spent discussing tactics. Back in the classroom the morning dragged on and on.

Eventually lunchtime came. Josh was the first to get changed. Proudly, he ran with his friends on to the field to meet the St Luke's team. But even as they set off for a warm-up run around the field, the air was changing. It took on a sudden chill. Mist was beginning to rise from the nearby canal and drift across the school field. The games teacher from St Luke's and their own Mr Briggs had their heads together. Soon they blew the whistle and beckoned everyone over.

'This mist is already beginning to thicken,' said Mr Briggs. 'It's going to be difficult to see each other soon, never mind the goalposts.'

Josh and his mates grimaced. They knew how quickly these November mists turned to fog. Games often got cancelled at this time of year. Josh crossed his fingers.

'So we've agreed to shorten the game to thirty minutes each end, and we're starting now . . .'

St Luke's won the toss and chose the goal nearer the canal.

They're not stupid, thought Josh, as he looked at the clearly visible goal his team had to defend, compared with St Luke's goal, where the mist was already swirling around the net. On the other hand, they had the advantage of a slight slope.

The match began.

It was one of those games where the action is instant. Within seconds of St Luke's kick-off, Josh's team captain, Rob, had claimed control of the ball. Rob chipped it to Kev who headed it to Josh as they advanced down the field. Josh fed the ball through St Luke's line of defence but met stronger resistance from their goalkeeper. Back up the field went the ball. As Josh turned to pursue it, he realized just how quickly the mist was spreading. Already their own goal was almost hidden. St Luke's would have to work harder now.

Voices cut through the swirling fog, distorted in the damp air. Figures were growing harder to see as the mist spread patchily across the pitch. Josh could just make out that it was Kev who had succeeded in grabbing the ball back from St Luke's. As Josh shouted to Kev his voice sounded strange and detached, but Kev responded and the ball was Josh's.

He grabbed his chance. He plunged through the mist, weaving his way up the right wing, until he knew he had to pass the ball. Only one player was visible. Josh struck out and landed the ball in front of his team-mate's boot. A superb strike saw the ball fly home, past the goalkeeper's head, into the roof of the net.

As they ran back to the centre, Kev clapped Josh on the back. 'Brilliant shot,' he cried.

'That was some goal,' added Rob, their captain.

'It wasn't mine,' said Josh, breathlessly. 'I passed it to . . .'

Who was it? In the mist Josh hadn't been sure. It was a boy his own size. It might have been Andy. Josh gasped in the cold air and felt it as hard as glass in his lungs. He couldn't finish his sentence before everyone was in position and the ball was back in play.

St Luke's rallied and, having created an opening, they kept hold of the ball in a relentless attack. Twice Rob broke through their ranks only to have the ball taken back by a strong advance from St Luke's.

Now it was Josh's chance to tackle. He hurled himself forward. His boot connected with the ball but only briefly, and again the ball was disappearing towards its target. Now Andy tried to intervene, but the ball shot in the air off the end of a big St Luke's boot and slotted into their goal, scoring an equalizer.

'We're going to change ends now,' came Mr Briggs' voice. 'This mist is getting too thick too quickly.'

Josh glanced at his watch. They were only twenty minutes into the game. One–all, and only twenty minutes to go! He hated drawing. Josh's hands clutched his mud-encrusted knees. He tucked his head down. His boot lace was undone but he couldn't bend to tie it. He concentrated on his breath as it spread in a murky cloud to mix with the mist. In this half they would be playing upfield, but now both nets were lost in the mist. Josh took a painfully deep breath and watched Rob take the kick.

Motivated by their equalizer, St Luke's quickly took control. The ball switched from left to right, sometimes visible, sometimes obscured in the fog. All the players became an indistinguishable grey. Josh threw himself at the ball as a St Luke's striker flicked it right into his path. He shot it straight between the legs of the flailing opposition. Rob took it upfield and passed to Andy, who headed it straight back to Josh.

Josh kept moving, dragging the defence all over the place. He ran forward with the ball, skidded on the wet grass and recovered. His marker's boot shot towards the ball but, even as Josh swerved out of the tackle, the other boy lost his balance and landed with a squelch on the churned-up sludge.

A shout went up from the sidelines. *Yes, Yes, Yes!*

Josh felt the beads of sweat on his forehead. He could barely see the goal, but he fired. The goalkeeper was on it in an instant, palming it out of the goal mouth but, before he could follow up, Josh saw a boot, its lace flapping like his own, strike from a narrow angle. The ball flicked easily into the back of the St Luke's net.

'Goal!'

'Two–one!'

'Two scores, Josh!' cried Rob. 'Go for your hat-trick.'

'Well played, Josh.'

Even Mr Briggs was congratulating him now, as they ran back down the field.

'It wasn't me,' said Josh, but his voice was muffled in the mist and now the ball was back in play. He hadn't time to talk.

The second goal was a blow to St Luke's, but they were not dispirited for long. They quickly took the ball and kept hold of it. Their tallest, fastest striker pushed the ball towards the nearly invisible net. Emerging suddenly through the mist the shot took the lurking goalkeeper by surprise, but his quick reaction, a full-length dive, saved it. Brushing the hair from his eyes with the back of a muddy hand, he threw the ball

7

to Andy who dodged his marker with expertise, driving the ball over to Kev.

'Josh!' screamed Kev like a banshee in the fog, as he headed it over to his friend.

'This one's mine,' Josh responded and lashed out.

The ball spun through the air and bounced off the goalpost, momentarily disappearing in the mist, before it reappeared. Josh watched as, again, it was booted through the air and into the St Luke's goal. There was a flash from the sidelines, where the photographer from the *Echo* was trying to catch the scene despite the fog, and then the final whistle blew.

Only the cheer from his team confirmed to Josh that the ball had landed a third goal. Josh didn't see it. He kept his eye fixed on that one spot; the position of the player who had scored. He ran forward, searching for the invisible player. Who was it who was scoring all these goals?

Already Josh's friends were pressing round him with congratulations and cries of 'Hat-trick!' He shrugged them off, looking around him. Was it a St Luke's player who had a taste for scoring own-goals? he wondered, doubtfully.

'You mustn't be so modest,' Mr Briggs told him as they set off for the changing rooms. 'Visibility was poor to say the least, but nothing deterred you, Josh. You really were Man of the Match!'

'It was teamwork,' muttered poor Josh.

Nobody doubted Josh had scored all three goals. Nobody had seen anyone else near the ball each time it found its mark. Everyone was ecstatic and Josh was their hero. He got changed in bewilderment. His team had won. He was a hero. But all he could feel was disappointment and confusion.

As they shared biscuits and hot chocolate with the St Luke's players, Josh looked around. None of their team seemed anything but resigned to their defeat. None of them looked as if they had been playing any crafty games – only straight soccer. Josh had watched everyone's feet as they walked into the building at the close of the match. Nobody's boot lace was untied apart from his own. Whoever had kicked the ball must have found time to retie their lace.

'Here's our star striker,' Mr Briggs told Josh's mother when she arrived later.

He patted Josh's back as the boy climbed into his mother's car. It was dark now and the thick fog swirled in the glow of the car's headlights.

'And his sister's going to star in the panto,' Josh's mother beamed. 'I'm proud of the pair of them.'

Josh let Mr Briggs close the car door and they set off home. Josh felt his mother's sideways glances as she drove. He guessed he did not look like a hero. Most likely he looked as sad and lost as he felt.

'Tired?'

Josh nodded. He felt no pride in the victory that had been attributed to him. Why had nobody else seen the phantom scorer? Why did they all think it was him? He felt glad his mother and sister hadn't been there. They would have seen it wasn't him who had scored. Then Josh remembered the photographer.

'Mum, will you make sure you get the *Echo* tomorrow?'

'It's delivered, silly,' said his mother.

'Well, please don't chuck it out till I've looked at the sports page,' said Josh.

*

Thankfully the next day was Saturday. Josh did not have to go to school and face his friends' misplaced praise. When the paper came, he turned straight to the sports page. There was the photograph, under the caption, 'HAT-TRICK HERO!' Josh stared in disbelief. There was a picture of him, kicking the ball. Hazy in the background the goalposts were just visible, framing the shadowy figure of the startled St Luke's goalie as he dived in the wrong direction. Underneath was a description of the action, praising both teams for their tenacity and courage in difficult conditions.

'I thought this was a football match, not a war!' Josh's mother commented, as she looked over her son's shoulder.

Josh looked hard at the action photograph. It was him all right. There was his boot in the air, with its dangling lace. And there was the ball curving away to land smack between the goalposts.

He was still staring at the page when the doorbell rang. It was Mr Williamson, an elderly man who lived a few doors away. He had lived there for years and was a good friend of Josh's family. He was waving a copy of the *Echo*.

'Your son's a chip off the old block, isn't he?' the old man chuckled. 'Congratulations, Josh,' he added, seeing Josh appear behind his mother.

'Come in,' she said. 'I'm glad someone else is as excited as I am. Josh seems to be taking it all in his stride.'

'What's a "chip off the old block"?' Josh asked.

The old man laughed. 'You're like your grandad Jim,' he explained. 'I was at school with him, you know. We were best mates and forever kicking a ball around. We played in the streets then, when there

10

weren't so many cars about. I reckon you take after him, lad.'

'I never knew him,' said Josh.

'You look just like him at the same age. Funny thing is,' he went on, 'I remember playing in a game just like this one. It's almost like history repeating itself. It was Jim's first inter-school match – and down came the fog. November it was, too. We won the game, two–nil, and your grandad scored both goals. But old Jim, he never forgot that match. You want to know why?' Josh nodded. His eyes were fixed on his neighbour's face. 'Well, when Jim's second goal put us in the lead, the ref blew his whistle on us. Stopped the match there and then. We'd won, but Jim never felt satisfied. He always said the blooming fog stopped him getting his hat-trick.' The old man laughed. 'Seems you've done it for him.'

For a minute Josh didn't speak. He had forgotten that his grandad's name was Jim. That was what Mr Henry had called Josh by mistake yesterday. Then he remembered the football rolling across the carpet to his side in the night.

Josh's mother was looking at him.

'You're right,' she said. 'He does look a lot like his grandad at that age. Hang on a minute, I've got a photo somewhere.'

She pulled an old shoebox from the cupboard and began to rummage through its contents. It was full of old envelopes and postcards with old-fashioned postage stamps. Black and white photographs were scattered amongst them. At last she pulled out a rather dog-eared print.

'Here we are,' she said, showing the old man. 'He's even in his school football strip.'

'Eh, up – that makes me feel old,' he said. 'There's Jim. How old? Eleven, maybe? And look – his boot lace is undone as usual. Just like yours, Josh!'

He handed Josh the photo. Josh had only seen pictures of his grandad as an adult. In this picture there was a boy looking up at him. The photograph was black and white, just like his own picture in today's paper and, for a second, Josh felt as if he was looking at a picture of himself. Jim had the same slim build as Josh; the same straight blond hair and the same eyes, that smiled up at him. Josh smiled back.

'Hat-trick hero,' he said.

Fixer

Anthony Masters

Jack rolled over on the muddy ground in the goal mouth, hugging the ball tight as Clapham United's fans roared their applause.

'Brilliant save!' yelled Rob as Jack struggled to his feet. He'd done it again. How long was his luck going to last?

But surely it wasn't luck, was it? It was skill. Ted Gill, United's coach, had told him that over and over again.

'Remember you've got talent. Luck isn't in it.' Ted had been almost impatient, for Jack never thought much of himself. Now Ted was cheering hard.

But Jack's elation died away as Barney Dexter's big, confident smile swam into his mind. 'You'll fix next Saturday's final, Jack. You'll let Albion in.'

Today was a friendly. It didn't matter to Barney. But next week did. If Jack couldn't fix the match against Wimbledon Albion, Barney would fix *him*. And then what would Mum think when she found out he'd been shoplifting?

'What's the matter?' asked Rob as they ran to the changing rooms after the match. 'You look like you've let 'em all in, not kept 'em all out.'

'I'm knackered,' was all Jack could say, and Rob

stared after him in surprise as he grabbed his bike and began the long ride home.

Jack didn't want to hurt his mother. She had been hurt already – hurt so badly by the drunken driver that she had been in a wheelchair ever since. The man had driven off, leaving her unconscious, but the police had eventually tracked him down. He had got off with a heavy fine and two years' ban. That wasn't enough for Jack. He would like to have killed him.

So much had gone wrong for his mother. Dad had walked out long ago, and had never contacted either of them again. Then there had been the accident that had left her paralysed.

Now Jack was going to give her a final blow.

As he cycled down the hill he remembered the amazing news that Ted Gill had given him a few weeks ago.

'You're going to be picked for the training scheme. I reckon you should be proud of yourself, Jack. Of course there's the coaching fees and the travel expenses...' Ted had looked at him anxiously. 'What with your mum and all...' He had paused, wondering how to go on. 'Will you have any problem about the money?'

You bet I will, Jack had thought. Even with all Mum's allowances we're always flat broke. But aloud he'd said, 'I'll manage.'

Jack knew that Mum wouldn't be able to afford the fees. He already had an early morning paper round and had tried to get the evening one, but had lost out to Tim Hawkins. So Jack had decided to start shoplifting, reckoning that if he managed to steal food, Mum would have enough money left to pay for his football training.

Jack wasn't dishonest by nature. In fact, he had never even contemplated doing such a terrible thing in his life. But there seemed no alternative.

'I've got the evening newspaper round,' he had lied to his mother when he got home. 'I can get some of the shopping with that if you can afford to pay my coaching fees out of your allowance.'

His mother, delighted and proud, had only one worry. 'You'll be exhausted. Two newspaper rounds – and then all that shopping.'

But Jack had told her the cycling would keep him fit, and eventually she had been satisfied.

He had hated lying to her and he had hated shoplifting. But once Jack had stolen a pot of jam and a couple of tins of baked beans, the conscience that usually gave him a hard time seemed to get buried deep inside.

Jack took a shoulder bag to the supermarket, putting a few stolen items inside whilst the rest that he was actually going to pay for went straight into the trolley. It was too easy. What's more, he was well-known at the supermarket. After all, he'd been shopping here for the last two years and most of the checkout staff knew about his mother's accident. No one suspected him. Everyone thought he was a hero.

Jack had even begun to salve his conscience by convincing himself that he had every right to steal. The supermarket was a huge chain. They would never miss a few stolen goods. Mum was paralysed. They had no money. It was all he could do. There was no alternative.

'I can afford your training money,' Mum had reassured Jack as they had their tea. 'So when do you start?'

'After the final. The final we're going to win. We'll take Albion. No bother.'

Later, he had helped her out of her wheelchair and into bed as he did every night. Mum had got so thin that she was very easy to lift. He'd do the same in the morning. It always terrified him.

'Got you!' Barney Dexter had been holding a small camera.

Jack had gazed at him in horror. He'd forgotten that Barney was a shelf-filler in the evenings. A year older than Jack, he was one of the school's worst bullies.

'What are you talking about?'

'I saw you putting stuff in that bag last night so I decided to bring in the camera my granny gave me for Christmas.' His grin had widened. 'It's a Polaroid. Look at you then.'

He had held up the print, which showed Jack furtively snatching a tin of grapefruit segments from the shelf.

'So what?' Desperately he had tried to brazen it out.

'Where is it then? I don't see the tin in your trolley.'

'I must have made a mistake,' Jack had spluttered, his face reddening, the sweat standing out on his forehead, his heart hammering so much that it hurt.

'It's in your bag.'

'Keep your voice down.'

'Only if you show me.'

Jack had paused, panic blinding him, not knowing what to do.

Of course the tin was in his shoulder bag and so were several others, as well as half a pound of sausages.

'All right,' he had muttered, fighting back the

16

desperate tears, trying to keep control. 'What are you going to do?'

'It's more like what *you're* going to do, Jack.'

Barney had begun to replenish the stocks of canned fruit while Jack stood miserably beside him.

'You know my brother Warren?'

Jack had nodded. Warren was in his year. He was also the star striker for Wimbledon Albion, the team Clapham needed to beat at the final on Saturday. A dreadful flicker of understanding had raced across Jack's mind.

Barney had looked up, his grin malicious. 'I can see you're beginning to get the message.'

Jack had been determined he wasn't. 'I don't get you.'

'Try harder. You're going to let Warren in, aren't you?'

'He won't get near me.'

'Yes, he will. And you're going to let him in. Albion are going to win!'

'They're not!'

'Because you're going to fix the match. And if you don't, I'll take these prints to the manager here.'

'That doesn't prove a thing.'

'Didn't you hear what I said, thicko? I said – prints. In the plural, right?' Barney had reached into the pocket of his overall and held the second instant photograph close to Jack's eyes. This one all too clearly showed him putting a can of beans into his black shoulder bag.

'Get me?'

'Got you,' Jack had said, feeling sick.

'Of course, if you let Warren in I won't show them to anyone.'

Jack had tried to make a grab for the print, but Barney had been too quick for him, shoving it back into his pocket.

Without thinking of the consequences Jack had bunched his fists.

'Don't start anything,' Barney had said quietly. 'If you do, you'll give yourself away.'

Jack had walked home, his bag of stolen goods over his shoulder and the ones he hadn't stolen in two large plastic bags. What was he going to do, he had wondered. Barney Dexter had him completely in his power. If he was nicked for shoplifting what would Mum say? What would it do to her?

'Everything comes in threes,' she had once said bitterly. Jack had reminded her that it hadn't.

'Not yet,' she had replied gloomily.

Dad walking out. The drunk driver. And now her only son on a shoplifting charge. Who said everything didn't come in threes?

With two days to go to the match, Jack found that he couldn't sleep and was becoming increasingly irritable. He even took it out on Mum.

'It's the big one on Saturday,' she said enthusiastically over breakfast. 'Aren't you nervous?'

'Not really.' Jack's voice was flat as he pushed his cornflakes round his plate.

'You seem to have lost your appetite.'

No wonder, he thought. He was eating cornflakes from one of the miniature packets he'd nicked. He could hardly get them down without choking.

'I may be able to get to watch the match for once. Mrs Jennings said she'd bring me down.'

'I wouldn't bother.'

'Don't you want me there?' She was instantly hurt.

Jack stood up, knowing how badly he was upsetting her, yet knowing how much more deeply upset she would be if he was found out. He'd *have* to let the shots in. He'd *have* to fix the match. He didn't have any choice.

But suppose Barney Dexter didn't destroy those prints? Suppose he went on blackmailing him for ever?

'I've got to get to school.'

'But you're early.'

'Bye, Mum.' He gave her a peck on the cheek and was gone.

Looking back, Jack saw his mother gazing after him like a wounded animal.

Barney was waiting for him by the lockers.

'You're going to fix the match, aren't you?'

A dark red mist seemed to have drifted into Jack's eyes, and inside he felt tight as a drum – as if he could hardly breathe. 'Please,' he whispered. 'I *can't.*'

'Your mum's not going to like you being done for shoplifting, is she?' Barney grinned. 'Not after all she's been through.'

The red mist darkened until it was so dense that Jack could hardly see. 'You leave her out of it.'

'The police won't.'

Barney was taller than Jack and much stronger. Nevertheless, Jack threw himself at him, punching and kicking, yelling abuse.

As the blows connected, Barney was forced back against the lockers, head down, protecting his face with his hands, too afraid to fight back, as an interested crowd began to collect.

Then Rob arrived, broke through the spectators and grabbed Jack round the waist, pulling him away from

Barney, trying to defuse the violence. Jack struggled in his grasp.

Then the bell went and the crowd immediately dispersed.

'I'll get you for that,' Barney muttered as he limped away. 'You see if I don't.'

But Jack knew he already had.

'What on earth was that all about?' Rob asked.

'He said something about my mum.'

'What?'

'It doesn't matter.'

'You know what he's like.'

'You bet I do.'

'You don't want to start getting into fights. Not with the match a couple of days away.'

'Get off my back!' yelled Jack, all his frustrated rage and anxiety returning.

'I'm only trying to help.' Rob looked like Mum. Hurt and bewildered.

'Don't bother.' Jack ran off in the direction of his tutor group.

Jack stood in the goal mouth, poised and ready. The last couple of nights had been really bad and he had hardly slept at all for worrying about what he was going to have to do. He hadn't been near the supermarket, getting what they needed from the more expensive corner shop, and Mum had been surprised at how quickly her allowance had been used up again.

'I thought things would be easier with that extra money from your evening news round, but it doesn't seem to be making as much difference as I thought,' she had said last night, totting up her petty cash book.

Immediately Jack's lies had got more complicated. 'I've lost the round, Mum. I couldn't face telling you.'

'But how?' She had been bewildered again. 'Mr Dawson's always thought so highly of you.'

'I was a bit late the other night and he was in a bad mood. So he took the round off me and gave it to Will Rogers.'

'That's not fair.'

'It doesn't matter.'

'Anyway,' she had said. 'I'm glad.'

'Glad?' Now it had been Jack's turn to be bewildered.

'It was too much for you. Draining all your energy. It could even have wrecked the match.'

The match was wrecked already, thought Jack as Warren Dexter came pounding towards him.

'What's the matter, Jack?' Ted Gill was furious with him at half-time. So were the rest of the team as they gathered together for a briefing. But the briefing was more like an inquest.

Only Rob looked concerned. Everybody else was out for his blood.

'You've got to wake up!' snapped Ted Gill. 'You let two easy ones through. Why?'

'I don't know.'

'You looked like a performing seal,' commented Dean Harrison.

'More like a ballet dancer,' added Jake Thompson nastily.

'Who asked for *your* views?' Ted Gill turned on them angrily. 'We all have our off days. Jack's having one of his. But we're going to save the match, lads, and I'll tell you how.'

21

As Ted Gill talked tactics, Jack felt relieved that his mother hadn't turned up to watch him blow the game away. Not so far, anyway.

Ted had been right. The shots had been too easy to let through. Far too easy. What was he going to do? Everyone would soon realize he was fixing the match. If anyone was having an off day, it had to be Warren Dexter.

'Your mum's here,' said Rob as they walked back to the pitch.

Sure enough, she was on the sideline in her wheelchair, barely able to stop giving Jack a wave. Her appearance was the final blow.

Mrs Jennings was hovering behind his mother. Maybe she'd been late or her car had packed up.

'Show your mum what you can do,' said Rob. 'Don't let her down.'

Something clicked in Jack's mind. Of course he couldn't let Mum down. Not now. Not on the field. She was going to be properly let down later, he told himself. Even if he let the shots through he'd never get Barney off his back. He knew that now. How was she going to like having a thief for a son?

He glanced towards the sideline. Barney Dexter had been standing there all the way through the first half, a smile fixed on his big meaty face.

Now Jack was going to blow that stupid grin away.

Warren Dexter was on him again, running towards the goal mouth, manoeuvring the muddy ball with rather more skill while the Albion supporters went mad, cheering and shouting, chanting his name.

Jack gazed at him intently, trying to read his mind, watching his feet. Where was he going to put the ball?

Had his coach given him a talking-to? He seemed much more on form. For a moment Jack thought he knew what Warren's tactics were going to be. Then, just in time, he realized he was trying to fool him.

Jack dived as the ball shot towards the net.

Now it was the turn of the Clapham United supporters to go wild as Jack made his save, scrambled to his feet and kicked the ball out of the penalty area.

'Well saved, Jack!' shouted Ted Gill. He was standing next to Barney Dexter, whose grin was still firmly in place.

Jack knew that Barney thought the save was just part of his fixing strategy. Let in two, keep one out, let in the others, so they would look like mistakes. But now Barney had another think coming.

Jack turned to glance at his mother, who was clapping delightedly and shouting his name.

His love for her welled up inside him with such intensity that he could feel tears pricking at the backs of his eyes.

What was the best of the two options? Let her see him fail as United's goalie? Or see him branded as a thief?

Jack saved two more shots in spectacular style. His sudden return to form made Clapham United attack much more aggressively and soon there were two balls in Albion's net and it looked as if the game might end in a draw.

Then, just before the referee blew the whistle for full-time, Rob scored.

As the Clapham supporters cheered for all they were worth, Jack turned to face Barney Dexter. He was in exactly the same position on the sideline, the grin still on his face. But he was holding up a couple of prints and Jack knew exactly what they were, and what he was going to do with them.

Then he had a sudden and very risky idea.

'You did well, Jack. You really did well.' His mother looked younger, full of life – exhausted but also enormously excited. He had not seen her this way for a long, long time.

Her praise was worth more than Ted Gill's, more than his team-mates', more than Rob's.

But Jack realized that if his plan didn't work out – and it was a long shot – then his mother might be badly hurt once too often.

'I'll be home soon, Mum. I'm just going to . . .' he hesitated, 'cycle back with Rob. We want to talk over the game.'

'I bet you do, love,' she said. 'But don't be too self-critical. You were wonderful.'

Wonderful? he thought. I'm not wonderful. I'm a thief.

Jack found Rob in the changing room.

'I want to talk to you.'

'What about?' Rob looked at Jack curiously.

'My sudden return to form.'

'Warren seemed to have the same problem in the first half. But what went wrong with you?'

Slowly, hesitantly, Jack began to tell him.

When he had finished, there was a long silence.

'Come on then,' said Jack. 'Say you despise me.'

'I don't.'

'You should.'

'You were set up and you fought back. Now you've got me to help you.'

'We want to see the manager.' Rob was insistent.

'What about?' The supervisor looked put out.

24

'It's important.'

'Can't I help?'

'Not really.' Jack was trembling.

'Very well. Step this way – but I hope you're not going to waste Mr Johnson's time.'

'No,' said Rob. 'We're not going to waste a second of it.'

The office was small and functional with a few chairs, a couple of filing cabinets, a telephone and a nameplate on the desk: *Graham Johnson*.

The manager was young and friendly, unlike the supervisor, who snapped the door shut disapprovingly.

'Do sit down,' he told the boys.

They did as he said. A long silence developed. Jack's mouth was so dry that he could hardly bring the words out. Then he forced himself.

'I – I took some stuff,' he stuttered. 'Because my mum's ill. We don't have enough money. I've been picked for the football training scheme. I can't afford the fees. She's in a wheelchair. Mum can't afford the fees either. I told her I had a round. A newspaper round. But I didn't. I never had one – at least, I did in the mornings, but not in the evenings.' Jack came to a shuddering halt, knowing that he wasn't making any sense.

He glanced at Rob but he was looking away, red in the face with embarrassment.

Jack plunged on.

'Barney Dexter – he took these photographs. Like of me nicking stuff. He said if I didn't fix the match, he'd take them to you.'

As if on cue, there was a knock at the door and the supervisor reappeared, looking even more irritated.

25

'Yes. What is it now?' asked Graham Johnson briskly.

'There's someone else to see you.'

'Who is it?'

'Guy called Dexter. Works for us part time as a shelf-filler. Says he's got something you should see.'

'Tell him I'm busy right now.' The supervisor closed the door reluctantly.

'Now look,' said Graham Johnson. 'Why don't we begin all over again? I didn't really understand what you were on about.'

This time Jack spoke more slowly and clearly. But as he told his story, he could already imagine telling it again to a policeman.

When he had finished, all Graham Johnson could say was, 'I see.' The silence filled the room like cold lead. Then he spoke again. 'I think you've been punished enough, don't you?'

Jack gazed at him, unable to believe his ears.

'Our usual policy is to prosecute shoplifters, but I'm not going to this time. In fact, I'm going to ask you if you'd like a job. There's a vacancy going.'

'Is there?' Waves of shock filled him, and Jack could hardly grasp what was being said. Rob was looking incredulous.

'It's just come up. A shelf-filler.'

'But I'd be working with—'

'Dexter's leaving.'

'Is he?'

Graham Johnson got to his feet. 'So how did the match go then?' he asked.

As Rob and Jack left the manager's office, feeling not only bewildered but amazingly relieved, they saw

Barney Dexter standing outside, the prints clasped in his hand, his grin unusually strained.

'Mr Dexter?' Graham Johnson's voice was cold. 'Would you like to come in?'

'Thanks for coming with me, Rob,' said Jack as they walked over to their bikes.

'That's all right.'

'I can hardly believe what's happened.'

'Neither can I. But what are you going to tell your mum?'

'The truth.'

'Is that a good idea?'

'If I don't, Barney might get to her first. If I can tell you and the manager, I can tell Mum.'

'Want me to come?'

'Not this time.'

Rob nodded, and Jack knew that he understood.

When Jack got back home, Mum was in the kitchen, doing all she could to make tea on her own. She was still full of excitement.

'You were great, Jack,' she said.

'I wasn't till you turned up.'

'I'm sorry. Mrs Jennings' car broke down and—'

'You saved me. And then I stopped the shots. But I've got something to tell you – something I'm ashamed of.'

She looked up at him calmly. 'What is it, Jack?'

Slowly, and then more confidently, he began to tell his mother what had happened.

A Dog Called Lineker

Eric Johns

'We're going to have a knock-out competition,' Claire announced.

'Which teams are playing?' Speed wanted to know.

'Mine and Russo's.'

'What d'you mean, *your* team?' Speed asked indignantly.

'It's my idea, so I'm the captain,' Claire told him.

'But you're the goalkeeper,' Speed objected. 'Goalies can't be captain.'

'Peter Schmeichel is sometimes,' Claire said.

'We've never had a captain before,' Danny put in. 'We've all just *played*.'

'Well, this time we're playing Russo's mob, so we need a captain and that's me. Does anyone not want to play?'

The five players who suddenly found themselves in Claire's team looked at her. She was short and broad with bristling fair hair which was about one centimetre long all over. She had scabby knees, torn shorts and trainers with splits in them.

Dave, Nicky and Sam glanced at each other and shrugged. They didn't really care who was captain or whether there was one at all. Claire glared at Speed and Danny.

'Even if we let you be captain,' Speed said, 'it won't

make any difference because you'll be too far away in goal to tell us what to do.'

'I'll be thinking up tactics so we win,' Claire said firmly.

It was the summer holidays. The weather was hot and Claire and her friends had nothing much to do. They met each morning on the recreation ground and messed about on the swings and other apparatus, or kicked a football about.

It was while the others were taking shots at her in goal, that Claire came up with the idea of a knock-out competition. What she wanted was something more exciting than just stopping endless shots she could see coming a mile off.

'So who's in this competition besides us and Russo?' Danny asked.

'That's all. There aren't any other teams round here.'

'You can't have a competition with only two teams,' Speed told her.

'Why not?'

'It's not a competition, just a game.'

'Well, it's the final,' Claire decided. 'The Summer Cup Final.'

Speed looked doubtful. 'You know what Russo's lot are like,' he told the others. 'If it looks like we might win, they'll start to cheat.'

'We'll just have to watch them all the time,' Claire said.

'Have you asked Russo whether he even wants to play?' Danny asked.

'Not yet. I was just going to ask him now.'

The six of them set off to see Russo's team. They played at the other end of the recreation ground – the end with the goalposts. No one knew why the recreation ground only had one set of goalposts, but everyone knew why Russo and his team had to have that end. They thought they were better than anyone else. Claire's team made do with bags or coats for goalposts.

As they approached Russo's team, Claire looked with envy at the kit they wore. All six of them were dressed in the latest strip for Manchester United. Not that she wanted that strip for herself. She supported Southampton (just to be different), but it would have been nice to have a proper strip. Her team looked like tramps.

'Look at them!' Speed snorted. 'As soon as they see us they start acting big.'

It was true. Mel, Russo's best striker, took a shot at goal, missed and threw up his arms in despair as if he'd been cheated out of the goal of the season by an unexpected earthquake.

'What d'you want?' Russo wanted to know, sounding as if he thought they'd come to steal his goalposts.

'We thought you might like a game,' Claire told him.

'Unless you don't want to risk getting your kit dirty,' Speed added, just to encourage them to accept the challenge.

'We might,' Russo said, and turned to his team. 'What d'you say? D'you fancy teaching them how to play?'

'All right by me,' Tone, their goalkeeper, said. 'So long as they agree to stop when it gets to twenty–nil. It'd get boring after that.'

'Yeah,' Mel put in. 'We'd better decide on the rules before we start, so they can't change them after.'

The teams spent some time sorting out the rules and

agreed to play the next morning. That would give them enough time to work out tactics.

'Right,' Claire said when they'd returned to their end of the recreation ground. 'Speed and Danny, you're strikers. Nicky and Sam, you'll mark Russo and Mel, and Dave, you'll be sweeper. OK?' she asked.

No one argued about the positions because those were the positions they always played in.

'We'll have a practice,' Claire said. 'Speed, you be Russo, and Danny be Mel.'

Speed and Danny took the ball up the field, then started passing to each other as they returned to attack. Speed ran easily round Nicky, and Danny avoided Sam without difficulty. That only left Dave. They switched the ball between them to get past him, and Danny shot. It was only a brilliant save by Claire that prevented a goal.

Claire could see that her team's defence was its weak point. Nicky and Sam were doing what she told them, but somehow it didn't look right. It wasn't the way they usually played. Perhaps, she thought, proper tactics, like marking, only worked with real teams where everyone was used to doing what they were supposed to. She sighed. 'All right. Forget about marking. Play the way you usually do,' she told her defence.

The three defenders smiled happily. Claire threw the ball to Dave to clear. Nicky and Sam closed in on him, and the three of them raced past Speed and Danny with the ball hidden somewhere in the middle of them. They kicked the ball away and ran back to take up defensive positions while Speed went to fetch it.

Speed and Danny attacked. Nicky deflected the ball, and the three defenders closed in on it. Claire frowned.

The three of them were like three different bits of one player instead of three different players. They always raced in the same direction like lemmings. That was what her defence reminded her of – lemmings.

'We'll call ourselves the Lemmings,' Claire shouted down the field.

'Why?' Danny asked.

'It just seems right.'

'I agree,' Speed said glumly.

Just then Claire heard her mum's voice echo across the recreation ground. 'Claire! Dinner.'

'Are we going to practise this afternoon?' Claire asked her team.

No one seemed very enthusiastic.

'All right. We'll meet tomorrow, half an hour before the game for a warm-up.'

She trotted off to her mum. Lineker, her black and white collie dog, was standing on his back legs straining against his lead as he tried to get to her. Her mum let him go and he charged at Claire. She dived sideways and grabbed the lead as it whipped past. She was pulled along until Lineker decided she was too heavy and came back to lick her instead.

'Look at the state of you,' Claire's mum said. That was what she usually said instead of hello.

Claire was a mess because she was a fearless goalie. She never hesitated to take the ball away from a striker. Even in summer, when the ground was as hard as the flapjacks they cooked at school, she still threw herself in the path of anyone who jinked past her defence.

After lunch, Claire practised goalkeeping. The garage wall was the goal and Lineker was striker. Claire threw the ball into the air and let Lineker hit it with his nose. He never missed, but Claire never knew which way the ball was going to go. Lineker definitely tried to punt it back to her. He understood the game all right, but accuracy wasn't his strong point. Claire didn't mind. It was good practice not knowing which angle the ball was going to come from.

'You must have a nose like an old boot,' Claire told Lineker, after twenty minutes. She always worried that he'd hurt his nose, but he never seemed to. 'I don't think the Lemmings have got much chance tomorrow,' she admitted to him. 'I wish you could play.'

Next morning, the Lemmings met as arranged. Speed and Danny did muscle-stretching exercises, Claire bounced up and down in the space between the two piles of jackets and bags, and Dave, Nicky and Sam ran round in circles like lemmings looking for a cliff to jump off.

At the other end of the pitch, Russo's team fired balls at Tone who was in goal. Claire looked at them enviously. They had four proper leather footballs to practise with, while all her team had was a plastic one which was starting to go down since Lineker had tried to bite it.

Claire sighed. The Lemmings' chances seemed to be about zero. Things weren't going to turn out anything like she'd imagined. There were no roaring crowds, no floodlights, no scouts from famous clubs who'd been tipped off about the unknown goalie everyone was talking about.

Russo jogged down the pitch. 'You ready, then?'

'Yeah. We're warmed up,' Claire said, trying to sound professional.

'We'll use one of our balls,' Russo decided, glancing away from Claire's ball as if it hurt his eyes.

The two teams spread out. The ground was far too big for teams of six players. If anyone got away with the ball he'd have so much space he'd never be caught. It would be striker against goalie.

'OK,' Russo said. 'You call.' He tossed a coin.

'Heads,' Claire said.

'It's tails,' Mel yelled.

'We kick off,' Russo decided.

Claire looked at his team. They all seemed bigger than her players.

Russo kicked the ball forward, and Mel ran deep into the Lemmings' half. He and Russo swung the ball from wing to wing, and Claire winced as Dave, Nicky and Sam charged from one side of the pitch to the other. She knew what was going to happen. Any second now, Russo or Mel was going to make a run at goal and her defence would be on the other side of the field.

It was Mel who did it. Claire came out of her goal to narrow the angle of his shot. Dave, Nicky and Sam came charging back but were far too late. She was lucky, though. Mel's shot was just to her left and at an easy height. Claire dived and pushed it wide.

Russo's team all yelled, 'Corner!'

Two of his defence came up to help the attack, and Speed dropped back. Mel took the kick. Claire had to admit that it was a good ball. It came over high and dropped in the centre of the goal mouth. Dave, Nicky and Sam closed round it so that Claire couldn't see where it was. They all lashed wildly at the ball and got in each other's way. Suddenly, the ball rocketed out of the scrimmage and shot towards Danny who was standing near the halfway line. Claire yelled at him.

Danny pounced on the ball and sprinted away. It ran easily, always a pace in front of him. There was plenty of space. The over-confident Russo's team had left him unmarked. By the time the one defender still in their half had woken up to what was happening, Danny was too far ahead to catch. He ran right up to the goalie, dribbled past him and put the ball between the posts.

The Lemmings whooped in triumph. Dave, Nicky and Sam ran round in circles chanting, 'One–nil. One–nil!' Claire tried to look as though this was what she had planned. What she was really thinking was that they couldn't be that lucky again.

Russo didn't look pleased. 'What d'you think you're playing at?' he shouted at his defender.

'He was asleep,' Mel said scornfully.

As soon as they started again, Russo sprinted straight down the pitch. Mel lobbed a long ball to him. He held onto it until Dave, Nicky and Sam, in their usual tight group, were almost on top of him, then he ran round them contemptuously. Claire groaned to herself. Russo charged towards her. She ran forward, but knew that this time she would not be as lucky as before.

Russo checked his pace and swung his foot at the ball. It was going slightly quicker than he thought, and when he hit it he was at full stretch. The ball rose in the air and soared over Claire's head.

'Goal!' Mel roared.

'That wasn't a goal,' Claire objected. 'It was too high. It would have gone over the bar.'

'There isn't any bar,' Russo said calmly.

Speed came jogging back to support his captain. 'You've still got to keep the ball low enough so's it would go under the bar, if there was one.'

'You didn't say that when we agreed the rules,' Mel said.

'We didn't need to,' Claire objected. 'It's obvious.'

'Oh, yeah. It's obvious now we've scored a goal,' Russo said mockingly, 'but you should have thought of it before.'

'Either that's a goal or we don't play any more,' Mel told them.

'You can't change the rules after the game's started,' Russo added, smirking.

Russo's team jogged back to their positions.

'I told you they wouldn't play fair,' Speed said glumly.

From then on, Russo's team were all over the Lemmings. Claire made several heroic saves, but it was only going to be a matter of time before a ball came out of a goal area scrimmage and got past her.

It happened when, not for the first time, Dave, Nicky and Sam were between her and the ball. Mel came charging at the ball, obviously intending to blast it straight at the three defenders. Acting like true lemmings they fled out of the path of the shot, and the ball hurtled through the space they'd left and past Claire before she even saw it.

'That was typical Lemming defence,' Claire muttered as she jogged to fetch the ball which did not stop until it hit the wire fence at the edge of the recreation ground. 'As good as an own goal,' she added.

She felt fed up. This was not what she'd hoped for. She'd known her team were unlikely to win, but she'd hoped they would look a bit more like a proper team.

In the distance Russo's team were laughing and jumping on each other in triumph.

They kicked off again. Speed tapped the ball to Danny and he passed back to Dave who was supposed to pass forward again to whoever of them wasn't marked.

Claire stood in her goal and watched Speed and Danny run up the field on either wing. Two defenders ran out to mark them, while the third stayed in front of the penalty area. Russo and Mel ran towards her, ready to be fed a ball once the defence had stopped the attack. Claire nodded approvingly. Russo's team looked as though they knew what football was all about, even though they did cheat.

She waited for Dave to pass to Speed or Danny. He didn't. Instead, the three Lemming defenders closed round the ball and headed down the centre of the field towards the defender on the edge of the penalty area. Even at that distance Claire could see the puzzled expression on his face. Standing in goal with no defence, she knew how he felt. Her team's tactics made her feel like switching to tiddly-winks.

Dave, Nicky and Sam looked like three lemmings who had suddenly spotted the edge of a cliff and did not intend to stop until they'd thrown themselves over it. They swerved round the defender, who seemed unable to decide which of them had the ball or which way it was going to go. The goalkeeper seemed just as puzzled. The ball bounced around between the three Lemmings like a ball stuck between three posts in a pinball machine.

The goalkeeper threw himself in their path, but the three of them curved round him as if each of them

38

knew exactly which way the other two were going to go.

Somehow, the three of them dribbled the ball over the goal line.

'Goal!' the Lemmings screamed. Claire, Speed and Danny rushed to congratulate the three defenders. They leapt up and down in the centre of the pitch.

'Two–all! Two–all!' they chanted.

'Come on!' Russo shouted. 'Let's get on with the game.'

'Or you'll be penalized for time-wasting,' Mel added.

Claire jogged back to her goal mouth. Her team might not look much like real footballers but they were holding their own against a team with proper kit and four leather footballs between them.

When Russo's team kicked off, Mel made a bad pass and Danny won the ball. He ran round a defender and crossed to Speed.

'Pass back. Quick!' Claire shouted. Then she saw a movement by the gate to the recreation ground. It was her mum with Lineker on his lead.

'Oh, no,' she moaned. 'Don't call me to go in. Not now we've got a chance to score.'

They'd agreed at the start that if either captain had to go home, that would be the final whistle.

It would be just her luck to be called now.

Speed and Danny were in front of the goal. There was only one defender and the goalkeeper. Danny struck the ball. It was a beautiful shot, heading towards the top corner of the goal. The keeper ran off his line and jumped. He just got a fist to the ball. It was a brilliant save. Claire wished she'd made it.

The ball arced up high and dropped towards the

edge of the penalty area. At that moment Claire glimpsed a black shape streaking across the pitch.

'Lineker!' she exclaimed.

The dog was going so fast that his lead was flying straight out behind him. He hit the ball with his leather-hard nose. It was the finest shot of his career.

The ball cannoned into the bottom corner of the goal.

'Goal!' Dave, Nicky and Sam yelled, laughing. They were joking, but suddenly an idea came to Claire – an idea that would teach Russo to play fair.

'Goal!' she shouted. 'Goal! We're leading three–two!'

'Don't be stupid,' Russo said crossly. 'Dogs can't score goals.'

'Why not?' Claire demanded.

'It's against the rules.'

'You didn't say that when we agreed them,' Claire argued.

'Everyone *knows* dogs can't score,' Mel objected.

'Well, you should have said so before,' Speed told him. 'You can't change the rules after the game's started.'

'We'll abandon the game if you're going to be stupid,' Mel threatened.

'What's the matter?' Danny wanted to know. 'You scared you won't score another?'

'Right, let's show them,' Russo cried. 'You can have that goal and we'll still beat you.'

Just then a voice from the edge of the recreation ground called out, 'Coo-eee! Russell!'

Russo seemed to shrink.

Both teams turned to see where the voice had come from. Standing by the fence was a tall lady in a big, purple sunhat, a tight, green shirt, pink shorts and silver shoes with stiletto heels. She was waving at Russo.

'Russell, darling,' she called. 'It's time for lunch and your vitamin pills.'

'We'll finish this game another time,' Russo grunted, his ears turning as red as his shirt.

'If you go,' Claire said, 'the game ends – and we've won. That's what we agreed.'

Russo tried to shrug to show he didn't care, but his shoulders drooped defeatedly.

The Lemmings sportingly clapped the losing team off the pitch. They heard Russo say to the woman, 'I *told* you never to come up here!'

'D'you think that's his mum?' Speed asked, giggling.

'Poor old Russo,' Danny said. 'I've never felt sorry for him before.'

Claire ran over to her mum to tell her the result.

'I'm sorry about letting Lineker go,' her mum said apologetically. 'When he saw the ball he jerked the lead right out of my hand.'

'That's OK,' Claire said laughing. 'He was definitely Dog of the Match!'

Jessica's Brother

Gus Grenfell

'Keep your eye on the ball!' How many times had people yelled that at him? Well, they wouldn't need to this time.

The midfielder's hurried clearance was still high in the air, and Owen Foley fixed all his concentration on it. It was going to overshoot him so he backpedalled quickly, positioning himself for the header. He rose as the ball fell. His timing was perfect.

Crunch! The charge from the left caught him in mid-air. The opposing striker didn't look big enough to have such an impact on Owen, but he was knocked sideways like a skittle. He turned as he fell and landed front first, knocking the wind from his lungs. The striker gathered the ball, sidestepped the keeper and calmly side-footed into an empty net.

Owen lay there for a moment, then slowly hauled his lanky frame upright. He scraped the mud off his arms and pushed his sandy fair hair out of his eyes.

'Are you blind, Owen? Didn't you see him coming?' Chris, the goalkeeper, hands on hips, was staring at him angrily under the bill of his green baseball cap.

Owen said nothing. How could you keep your eye on the ball *and* on your opponent at the same time? He dragged himself dispiritedly to the edge of the D for the restart.

The whistle went a minute later, before Owen had really got his breath back. He turned and headed for the changing rooms, disappointed with the way he had performed. He had tried to play a sensible game, not be drawn out of position, but he seemed to have been stuck in the same spot most of the game.

He hadn't missed all his headers, and he'd made a few decent tackles, but he hadn't been very adventurous. He had tried to be solid and dependable in central defence, but he was afraid he'd ended up being dull.

Chris ran up and clapped him on the shoulder, his usual grin back in place, his baseball cap under one arm. Owen grinned back and punched his arm. No hard feelings; they were mates. After all, this was the pre-season trials, not a cup final.

It was all right for Chris, he had been a regular in the Under-12 team and there was no one to touch him, so his place in the Under-13s was assured. Owen had been convinced he was going to make it this time. Until now. The grin went. He felt like crying with frustration. It would be 'We'll let you know', and then the phone call saying, 'Sorry, I'm afraid we haven't got a place for you in the squad at present.' Again. Just like the other times.

There were other games still underway on nearby pitches. Some involved boys younger than him, some older, and, to judge from the shrill cries coming from a pitch over to the right, the girls – about to get their own team for the first time – were going through their paces.

Owen could see a familiar red head bobbing up in the middle of a bunch of players. Jessica, his sister, had insisted that if he could have a trial, so could she, and Mum had taken her part, of course. So Dad had driven them all down. Embarrassing or what!

When he was changed, Owen walked over to the car park. Dad was in the car alone.

'Where's Mum?' he asked, sliding into the back seat.

'Still waiting for Jessica, I expect. How did you get on?'

'Not very well. I don't think I'll get in.' Owen couldn't trust himself to say anything else. He could feel his throat tightening.

'Never mind. I expect you did your best. We can't all be footballers.'

That was Dad all over. He was so easy going. He never seemed to get upset. Owen sometimes wished his father would shout at him, say what did he mean by not getting in the team, and if that was his best then it wasn't good enough. Then Owen could let go and shout back and get it all out of his system. Instead he had to bottle it all up and pretend it didn't matter.

Owen had read halfway through his copy of *Shoot* before Mum and Jessica appeared. Jessica was jumping up and down, and they were both grinning like Cheshire cats. A terrible thought occurred to him. Surely she couldn't have; he'd never considered it remotely possible. But a cold certainty was forming in the pit of his stomach. He didn't need to hear Jessica's jubilant announcement as they came within shouting distance.

'I'm in the squad, I'm in the squad!'

She rushed to the car, wrenched open the door, bounced onto the seat and flung her arms round him. 'Owen, I'm going to play for the Under-11s! They said I was ever so good, didn't they, Mum? They said I've got good ball skills and a solid left-foot shot, didn't they?'

Mum was pink-cheeked and breathless, almost as though she'd been playing herself. She was talking to Dad.

'Sorry we were so long,' she said. 'I've been talking to the manager and the other mums. Isn't it exciting? They want her to go for training twice a week. I said we could manage it.'

She paused and turned to the back seat.

'What do you think, Owen?'

Owen was busy trying to fight Jessica off.

'I'm sorry, I ought to have asked how you . . .'

The thundercloud on his face must have made it obvious.

'Oh, Owen, I'm so sorry, really I am.' She put her hand through the gap between the front seats and rested it on his knee. He tried to squirm away, but there was nowhere to go.

'Well, at least,' she said, 'you'll be able to be happy for Jessica.'

Happy for Jessica? That was the last thing he felt. At this moment he wished a great hole would open in the upholstery and swallow him.

School. Monday morning. At least it was a relief to be out of the house, away from all the excitement and Jessica-centred conversation.

What kind of boots should she have? 'Knee-length patent leather with high heels,' he'd said. Frowns all round. Not funny.

How would she look in the new yellow strip with red shorts? 'Blood and pus,' he'd said, deliberately

46

jolting the table as Jessica had a spoonful of cornflakes almost in her mouth.

And a mouth guard. She'd need a mouth guard. 'A mouth guard?' He was scornful. 'Nobody suggested I should have a mouth guard. I suppose it doesn't matter if I get my teeth knocked right down my throat.'

Oh, and they were having a competition to find a name for the team. 'Barbies!' he'd said, leaving the room and slamming the door.

It was morning break, and Chris was coming towards him, holding a slightly out-of-shape football with most of its surface scuffed off, and gaps where the stitching had gone, like gaping underwear.

'Fancy a kick-around?' he said.

'Why not?' They ran out into the yard, gathering others as they went.

The yard at the front of the school had once been tennis courts and was surrounded at the back and sides by high, chain-link fencing. The wall of the school itself formed the other side.

Owen found himself attacking the school end, the goal between a drainpipe and a litter bin. Good. In his present mood he could just fancy belting the ball against a wall, and not having to bother about the finer points of the game.

Chris threw the ball in the air and there was a rush as it came to land, mainly from the few year seven boys who were allowed to play and were keen to impress. They'd only been at the school a week.

Owen stood back as the melee sorted itself out and the ball trickled loose. He hacked it towards the wall where Pete, the largest and laziest of his team-mates, was lounging. Pete didn't even need to lever himself off the wall or take his hands out of his pockets. He simply stuck out a leg and guided the ball into the goal area.

'One–nil!' Owen shouted. 'I bet we get twenty before the bell goes.'

'Bet you don't,' said Chris, kicking the ball from his hands. Nobody intercepted it. The chain link rattled and bulged.

'One–all!' It wasn't a game for midfielders.

Owen set off with the ball at his feet, taking advantage of the lack of touchlines, and did a mazy run round two other games going on in different parts of the yard, pursued by a gaggle of year sevens.

'Show-off!' Chris shouted.

Owen paused, taking stock, seeing if there was anyone to pass to. One of the year sevens nipped in front of him and took the ball off his toe. The cheek of it! Everybody laughed, which didn't improve Owen's mood at all. He ran after the kid, grabbed his arm and pulled him back.

'Hey, foul, ref!' the boy called.

Owen ignored him. That was another advantage of school yard soccer; no officials.

'Are you Jessica Foley's brother?' said the cheeky little year seven kid. 'My dad says she's the best lass he's ever seen play.'

Owen was seething. He eyed up the ball, bobbling unevenly on the pitted asphalt, and whacked it. The ball hit the bin with a clang and knocked it over, scattering crisp packets and coke cans in the goal mouth. The ball rebounded, still in play.

'Leave it!' Owen shouted, determined to quieten the laughter, and charged forward. He let fly with an uncontrolled swing. His foot went under the ball and sent it ballooning over the heads of his mates. And right through the library window.

It wasn't Owen's day.

And it got worse. Owen had a letter from the Deputy Head to hand over when he got home, which included a bill for the broken window. He'd thought of chucking it on the way back, except that the Deputy Head said he would ring to make sure it arrived and 'talk about the issue'. The ball had been confiscated as well, and they were banned from playing football in the yard. And he was on lunchtime litter duty for the rest of the week.

Dad was on the phone when he opened the door, talking in that smarmy voice he used for people like deputy heads. Yes, of course. He would take it out of Owen's pocket money. Yes, boys did need to learn how to act responsibly around the school. Traitor. Why didn't he tell the Deputy Head to stuff it and pay for the window himself? Some boys had dads like that.

Owen walked into the sitting room and wished he hadn't. Mum and Jessica were all in a tizz about football practice; they had to go in ten minutes. He slammed out and went upstairs to his room. He would get something to eat while they were out, then stay in his room all evening. Even if it did mean watching Monday evening football on the miserable little black and white telly they let him have.

He hadn't bargained on the invasion later. They came rushing upstairs and burst into his room as soon as they got back, ignoring the *Area 51 – Keep Out* sign he had on the door; ignoring the fact that he was watching the match.

Jessica was full of herself.

'I'm in the team!' she said, bouncing around as if she were on a pogo stick. 'I'm going to play for the Beacons.'

'The *what*?' Owen asked.

'The Beacons. Beamsley Beacons. That's our name. Yellow shirts, see? And there used to be a beacon on top of the hill outside the town. It sounds right. Don't you think it's good?'

'No, it's rubbish,' he said, scowling.

'Well, everybody else likes it. We're going to play Stanbury Sparx on Saturday. They've just formed as well. I can't wait.'

Dad was standing in the doorway now. 'What position do you play?' he asked.

'Oh, everywhere!' she replied, whirling round with her arms stretched out. 'I just watch what's going on and run to the best place.'

And after ten minutes you fall flat on your back, exhausted, Owen thought. Somehow he didn't think his sister was ready for total football. He moved his head to the left to see round her to the television, but she moved and blocked the screen again. He moved his head back.

'And I scored lots of goals in the game at the end, didn't I, Mum?' she said. 'How many was it?'

Mum laughed. 'I can't remember. Seven or eight?'

'The last one was the best. I ran all the way down the pitch.'

The increased tempo and pitch of the commentator's voice told Owen he had missed a goal.

'Do you mind?' he said, jumping up off the bed and pushing Jessica aside. 'I'm trying to watch the match.' He swore as he was just too late to catch the action replay.

There was a tense silence.

'Well! Sorry, I'm sure,' Mum said. 'We thought you'd be interested, that's all.'

'Well I'm not. OK?'

They withdrew, deflated.

He knew he hadn't heard the last of it. Mum would come up and talk to him 'when he'd calmed down a bit.'

He flopped down on the bed again, drew his knees up under his chin and fixed his gaze on the screen. The tall, fair-haired central defender was rising majestically to meet a long clearance from the opposition penalty area. A striker was there too, but there was never any doubt about who was going to get the ball. With a powerful flick of his head the defender directed the ball into the path of a wing back already racing up the touchline.

That's how it should be done.

Next day Owen arrived home to find a pair of new football boots on the kitchen table. Not quite top of the range, but far better than any pair he'd ever had.

He felt himself go hot as a wave of resentment swept over him. One measly trial and she gets a pair of new boots. It wasn't fair. He felt an urge to pick them up when no one was looking and chuck them in the bin. Except it wouldn't stop her playing; they'd just buy some more.

Then Jessica came clattering in wearing another pair; a pair he recognized. They were the first new ones he'd ever had; they were a tenth birthday present. He'd been so proud of them he'd worn them around the house all day.

'They're mine!' he said.

Mum laughed. 'Not much use to you now. They're far too small. They're just right for Jessica to play about in.'

Mum didn't understand, did she? And there was no point in trying to explain. He had to get out of the house.

'I'm off on a bike ride,' he said, heading for the door.

'Oh, would you take Jessica? She's been dying to go, and I don't like her going out on her own. Don't go out of the estate, will you?'

Owen said nothing, but stormed out to the garage to fetch his bike. As he wheeled it down the path, Jessica was sitting on the step pulling on her trainers.

'Wait for me!' she said.

He had no intention of waiting for anybody. He mounted his bike and rode it out of the gate, down the avenue and round the circle at the end, skidding his back wheel round. As he came back past his house, Jessica was emerging from the gate but he ignored her. He wasn't going to let her cramp his style.

He pedalled furiously up and down the streets as fast as he could go. Jessica kept appearing out of little passageways that linked the streets between some of the houses, yelling, 'Wait for me!' It would have been quite funny if he'd been in the mood.

And then, suddenly, she shot out in front of him. He tried to swerve round her, but his arms seemed locked to the handlebars. It was like somebody else was steering and he was just a helpless passenger.

It seemed like minutes as the distance between his bike and Jessica's grew less and less. He watched his front wheel hit Jessica's bike side on. He watched her fall off and the bike come down on top of her. He jumped as his own bike toppled and joined the heap in the road.

He was vaguely aware of Chris running up and pulling the bikes off Jessica's still form. No sound. Then she started whimpering and a wave of relief swept over him.

Other people arrived; eventually Mum, who took charge. She checked Jessica over.

'I don't think there's anything broken, but that ankle doesn't look too good. We'd better get you down to casualty,' she said.

Jessica's crying had turned to shuddering sobs 'I . . . I'm sorry, Mum. It was my fault. I wasn't watching where I was going.'

Was that true? Owen wasn't sure. If he hadn't been rushing around and ignoring her . . .

'You and Chris can take the bikes back home.' Mum was talking to him. 'And the Beamsley manager rang. He wants to see you play again tomorrow. It's a practice match against Hightown.'

Chris grinned. 'That's what I was coming to tell you.'

By kick-off time Owen had got over the surprise of being called back. He was feeling nervous, but excited as well. The manager had talked to him and told him to try to do more with the ball once he'd won it – little layoffs to midfield, more deliberate passes upfield rather than a hurried blast to no one in particular.

'You're good in the air,' he said. 'You win a lot more than you lose. And not many get past you once you're committed to the tackle.'

Did he mean it? The trouble was, Owen remembered the ones he missed, especially when he was punished for them. At least he now had another chance to prove himself.

Chris came over. 'You feeling OK?'

'Sort of.'

'Just don't let any weedy little striker come and knock you over, right?'

'If you don't let them sidestep you!'

Chris threw his baseball cap at him. 'How's Jessica?'

'Fed up. Her ankle's strapped and she'll be out of action for a couple of weeks or so. Could have been worse.'

Funny how things worked out. Now that she couldn't play, Owen felt quite sorry for her. He'd even promised to play with her when she got better. After all, ever since he could remember he'd wished he had a younger brother to play football with.

Meanwhile, he was going to go out there and play out of his skin. So, when Jessica did eventually don the yellow shirt of the Beamsley Beacons, people would say, 'Hey – isn't that Owen Foley's sister?'

The Boffin Bounces Back

David Harmer

When Brian Butterworth walked in through the door of Atko's classroom that first day of term, I can honestly say I had never seen anything like him. I was used to brainy kids – there was Charlotte Adams, there was Joe Stubbins – but Brian Butterworth was in a different league. When it came to brains, we were all in Division One and he was champion of the Premiership.

He even looked brainy. Big glasses, skinny legs, skinny arms, red hair all over the place, old-fashioned clothes, shoes with laces, proper grey trousers, even a tie. A tie! There hadn't been a lad in a tie at Thorpe Lane Primary for twenty-five years – not since my dad went there, and Basher Briggs was the headmaster with the longest, twitchiest cane in South Yorkshire. But Brian wore a tie, and you know what? It suited him!

That first morning, on the yard during break, we all talked about our holidays. Sean Davies went on and on about Florida, and I told my mate Dekko about Whitby. Brian came over to us.

'Look,' he said, 'let's get it sorted out right away.'

'What?' I asked.

'My nickname.'

'How about Softie Cedric?' sneered Billy Stones. We all grinned.

55

'Ridiculous!' snapped Brian. 'You have two choices. I'm either called Brain, a simple anagram of my name, or the Boffin. I don't mind which – you choose.'

Billy closed his open mouth. Then opened it again. 'I still think Softie Cedric's best,' he said.

Brian looked at him coolly through his enormous glasses. 'You, I take it, are the Tough Kid. Very well, here's the deal. No rough stuff and I help you with that maths Mr Atkinson set us before break, which,' and here he gazed at all of us with a smile, 'I am afraid to say was so pathetically easy that I wondered if I was in Year Six or Reception.'

'The Boffin,' said Billy firmly. 'My pal the Boffin.' And they walked off, heads together, whispering numbers.

The next day, Brian was wearing a home-made badge with *It's Cool To Be a Boffin* written on it, and he delighted us all by correcting Atko's maths.

Atko is a great teacher, really friendly and really firm. No messing with Mr Atkinson. He also runs the school football team and that makes him a bit special. I play in goal, and most games I let in just one or two less than our team scores. Some games I don't.

I think Atko was as surprised by Brian as we were.

'I'm sorry, young Butterworth,' he said, smiling, the piece of chalk rolling in his hands, 'I've done *what*?'

'Well, Mr Atkinson, you've multiplied 57 by 73 and got 4,217 when in fact the answer is 4,161.'

'Brian, did you work that out in your head just now?'

'Yes. I can do that sort of thing. My last teacher, Mr Baines, used to shout at me for doing it.'

who stank of the curing ponds – no one would want to get into a close ruck with them. And there were a couple of young butchers, who were built almost as solidly as the great sides of beef they could haul around and chop up as easily as if they were bundles of kindling.

The field of battle had also been agreed. The game was to be played between the Clopton Bridge and Holy Trinity Church, along Waterside, the road which ran beside the river and marked the northern edge of the town. It was ideal. Waterside was so close to the Avon that there were few houses, so little chance of an outraged shopkeeper or an interfering nosy parker calling out the Watch.

The rules of the game were simple, like those of the Asherton match Will had once seen. Each team had a goal to aim for: the apprentices had to try to carry the pig's bladder ball to the bridge, and the schoolboys had to ground it at the churchyard gate. There was no limit on the number of players on each side, and the ball could be kicked, punched, thrown or carried; so could the players.

There was the muffled creak of a floorboard outside the bedroom. Will tensed. There was a soft scratch at the door. Barely breathing, Will inched open the door. The dim, lanky figure on the landing beckoned to him, and began tiptoeing down the narrow wooden stairs. Will followed. Every step was heart-stopping. If his father discovered them creeping out, there would certainly be a sound beating for both boys. Will sighed. They would face a beating anyway, whether they woke Will's father or not. There was work to be done, and Will's father stood no slackness from either his apprentice or his son – especially since the money troubles had begun.

Tom and Will slipped out of the back door and ran past the stinking pools in which the skins, which Will's father and Tom made into gloves, soaked until they were as soft as the finest velvet.

They walked quickly along Henley Street.

'Well?' hissed Tom. 'Are you with me or against me, Will? It's one or the other.'

It was the question Will had been dreading. All week they had been asking him – first Tom, then Dickon:

'*My team or his . . .*'

'Me or him . . .'

'*Friend or foe . . .*'

'Which is it to be?'

'*Which is it to be?*'

It was the day of the game, and Will *still* didn't know.

'Well . . .?' repeated Tom.

'Hurry or we'll be late,' said Will, ignoring the question.

He jogged round the corner in the High Street, with Tom close behind. They sped past the darkened shops and silent houses into Chapel Street. With every second, the weak morning light was getting stronger, and the moment when Will would be forced to take sides was getting ever closer. Which team *would* he be on?

'I want neither,' he muttered to himself. 'Don't they understand?'

Will and Tom turned right up Chapel Lane. Up ahead, at the agreed spot, midway between the church and the bridge, two gangs of about twenty boys stood facing each other, glowering.

At the head of one gang stood Dickon, a blown-up pig's bladder in his hand.

'Come on, you grammar school milksop! Or are you too much of a molly-coddle to see this through?' shouted one of the apprentices.

Dickon bunched his fists together. Tom took his place at the front of his team.

'We're ready!' called Tom. 'Ready to crack your skulls until you plead *Mercy! Mercy! Mercy!* Like the mewling little maids you are!'

'Begin!' shouted one of Tom's team. 'Begin!' echoed another. 'Begin! Begin! Begin!'

Tom turned to Will. 'It was Will's suggestion,' he bellowed over the apprentices' chanting. 'Let him start us off!'

There were cries of 'Yes!' from the apprentices. From the schoolboys' side a voice shouted, 'Who cares for the ball – let's just give them the thrashing they deserve!' followed by a cheer from a handful of the other boys.

With a curt nod, Dickon flung the pig's bladder to Will. Will fumbled the catch and dropped the bladder. Blushing, Will picked up the bladder. It was round and greyish-yellow: it felt slightly spongy beneath his fingers, as if it could do with a couple more hearty puffs. But it was too late to worry about that now.

Squinting with concentration, Will threw the ball as hard as he could at a spot in the dirt road between Dickon and Tom. With a great roar both gangs of boys rushed at each other. They locked together in a single struggling, grunting mass of flailing fists and bellowing voices.

'Where's the ball?' shouted a voice that sounded to Will like Tom's.

'At the bottom!' shouted back a heavily built red-haired boy, who was digging like a huge mole at the mass of struggling bodies. He lifted the ball high with a shout, cut short by the fist of an opponent crunching into his jaw. He disappeared down into the struggling mayhem still clutching the ball.

Will had been trying to avoid the struggling kicking mass and work his way round the scrum to the far side, by the river, where he thought he'd be safe. He'd just reached the far side of the road when the ball squirted out of the bottom of the scrum and rolled to a stop at his feet. For an endless fraction of a second Will gazed at the ball in horror before being engulfed in the howling mob. As the wall of bodies swallowed him, a fist hit Will in the throat and made him gag, his legs were knocked from under him and he was rolling helplessly backwards. He felt a kick in his back and then the awful stifling weight of someone falling across his back.

'Get off me!' he screamed. 'You're crushing me!'

The mass of bodies swayed, then pushed back the way it had come. Will frantically burrowed his way on all fours to the outside of the pack. He didn't care who he was gouging and clawing and scratching on his way out, nor did he care where he was clawing and gouging them. Tears of pure fear were running down his cheeks. He knew his life was in danger in that awful, heaving, suffocating mass of bodies. He knew that the enormous beast – the many-headed, many-limbed howling monster that the schoolboys and apprentices had become – could crush and tear and kill without a second thought.

Will fought his way out onto the green mossy bank beside the river. He hauled himself to his feet, sobbing and gasping for air just as the mob swayed back in his direction.

'No!' screamed Will. '*No!*'

An elbow smashed into his chest. Someone's knee knocked him behind the legs. As Will turned round to protect his front, someone else gave him a shove in the back. Will felt his feet start to slide down the bank. He whirled his arms desperately in the air to try and keep his balance. He teetered on the brink, frantically trying to clutch onto a handhold in the empty air. Then with a final, despairing, yodelling cry, Will fell into the filthy river with an enormous splash.

The coldness of the water drove the breath out of Will's lungs. He struggled to get his footing on the slimy, shelving river bottom.

'Help!' he shouted. 'I've—'

His feet slipped and his knees buckled again. He splashed face down in the water, taking in another foul-tasting mouthful of brown water.

'Splouff! Arcch!'

He spat out the water and began thrashing his way along the bank towards a small clump of willow trees where the muddy slope was less steep.

'*I command you to stop!*'

Will heard a familiar voice boom above the shouting and cursing of the football players.

'Stop!' it bellowed again. 'As Alderman of this town, I command you: *Stop at once!*'

All through Will's childhood, the stern voice of his father had stopped even the most harmless of childish pranks as swiftly as the stinging cut of the birch rods which his father kept hanging on the kitchen wall. That same voice now stopped the game of football.

There was a sudden, shocked silence. Will cowered beneath the overhanging willow branches.

'Captain of the Watch – *arrest them!*'

There was a sound of shuffling feet, and a few muffled snuffles and whimpers. Will pressed himself against the cold, slimy banks of the river.

'And where is my son?' demanded the voice. 'Where is the one who has brought disgrace upon my household!' he bellowed.

Will closed his eyes and held his breath.

'*Well?*'

There was no reply.

'Let him hear this,' boomed the voice. 'He has brought shame upon his family, and let him be sure that he will be sorely punished when he returns. And the longer he hides, the harsher will be his punishment!'

There was another long pause.

'Take them back!' he snapped to the constables of the Watch. Will listened to the shuffle of feet, gradually fading as the schoolboys and apprentices were marched away from the river side. He stood, shivering in the icy water, for one minute . . . two . . . three . . . four . . . five.

Then there was a crack of a twig and the sound of someone slithering down the bank.

Will shut his eyes and tried to press himself into the bank.

'What have we here?'

It was light, musical voice. Will turned round. Peering down at him was a short, plump young man dressed in a bright scarlet doublet, with a bundle of linen under his arm.

'Is it an eel? Or maybe a particularly slimy newt? Eh?'

The young man laughed and held out a hand. He helped Will out of the water and onto the bank.

'So, you were in the riot and got clean away, eh?' asked the man.

'It wasn't a riot,' said Will, horrified. 'It was a football match.'

'Is that so?' asked the fat man, with mock solemnity. 'And, pray, whose idea was it to play this football match?'

Will sighed. 'Mine,' he admitted in a soft voice.

'Speak up!' said the man. 'No use speaking if you can't be heard. I'll ask you again: whose idea was it?'

'Mine,' admitted Will again, in a louder voice.

'Better,' said the man thoughtfully. 'A good voice – a little reedy, perhaps. No good for singing, but adequate for an attendant lord, or perhaps a messenger of no great consequence.'

Will stared at the young man in the garish clothes. What was he talking about?

'So you were the playmaster of this little shenanigans,' said the man. 'I was just come down to wash our costumes here in the stream, when I see a full-scale riot going on and the Watch pelting along the lane to crack a few heads. So I say to myself: time to hide, Will Kemp, until matters are settled. So I hid behind this clump of trees, and merry amusement it was to be sure, especially your dive into the River Avon!' And he laughed heartily.

'Costumes?' asked Will.

'Yes, lad,' replied Will Kemp, patting the pile. 'Tonight we play the comedy of *Damon and Pithias* at the Swan Inn.' He pointed to one of the two squat

99

thatched buildings standing beside the bridge. 'And if I don't get these washed and dried before this afternoon I'll be capering with a toe up my backside!'

'Players?' asked Will. 'Are you travelling players?'

'Aye, lad,' said Kemp. 'Or, as some call us, stout beggars and vagabonds. This evening we play here at Stratford, then we're away before midnight, and tomorrow we play at . . .'

'You leave tonight?' Will interrupted.

'We surely do.'

One of Will's lightning ideas came to him.

'Take me with you,' he begged. 'I must leave the town tonight, or . . . or . . . or . . .'

'Or you'll get the beating you so richly deserve?' suggested Will Kemp and guffawed again. 'So you'd rather go for a player than face the music – is that it?'

Will nodded.

Kemp laughed again. Then he shook his head. 'It would do you no good and it would do no good for us, either. I'm sorry, lad, if we were to take a rich man's son – a grammar school boy too, I would guess – the Watch would be on us before we left the parish boundaries. We'd all be getting a thrashing – you, me and all the rest of my company. No, lad. It's not worth it. Besides, the life of a player's not the life for the likes of you, I can promise you that.'

'But *please* . . .' implored Will.

Kemp shook his head again. 'No, my fine young gentleman. You stay here and take the beating that's coming to you. And when you're grown, then you may come to the Swan Inn one fine evening and watch old Will Kemp caper his way through some fine entertainment for your pleasure. And you can clap, and cheer, and spare a silver penny to give to old Will

Kemp, and in the morning think no more about it than a pleasant dream that gave pleasure and hurt no one – unlike your game of football!'

Kemp squatted down by the river and began to soak the soiled costumes.

Will got to his feet, shivering, river water running off his clothes. He clambered up the bank. Then he turned and looked down at the tubby figure, sluicing the clothes in the grimy water. Then he looked over the meadows towards the Swan Inn, and the bridge, and the road that led out of Stratford.

'One day . . .' he muttered to himself. 'One day I will run and run and run and never come back.'

He looked down at the scarlet back bent over its laundry. 'One day, Will Kemp, we will meet again,' he declared in his grandest voice, 'and then you'll be sorry you didn't take me with you today!'

Will turned and began limping towards the road.

Kemp gave a roar of laughter and clapped his wet hands together.

'Bravo!' he called out to Will's retreating back. 'A splendid exit line, young sir! *Bravo!* Maybe you *do* have the makings of a player after all. But one thing I can promise you – you'll never make a *football* player!'

And Will Kemp roared with laughter once again.

Strikers and Keepers

John Goodwin

The huge crowd were up on their feet. 'Penalty! Penalty!' they shouted. The referee blew his whistle and pointed to the spot. The crowd cheered and held their arms aloft. Now surely the winning goal would be scored and for their team it would be triumph yet again. Still their cheering echoed round the stadium and mingled with chants of 'Paggio . . . Paggio . . .'

Carlo Paggio, the team's captain, stepped forward and placed the ball on the spot. The crowd were quiet now. All the players stood quite still. Paggio too stood still. He looked at the ball, then at the goal, and then back at the ball again. He shook his hands by his sides and then took three very deliberate steps back. All eyes were on the ball.

He ran forward swiftly and hit the ball hard and true as only a great player can. It was right on target and zoomed towards the bottom right corner of the net. Perfection. Yet a blurred shape in green was hurling itself towards the ball. The goalkeeper! Arms were flung forward and in a rolling mass of ball and gloves and goalkeeper's body the penalty was . . .

I switched off the video and dressed for school. Tuesday is can't wait day. It's straight downstairs. Sneak past Mum and Amber's bedrooms and don't make a sound on the creaking floorboard to wake the dog. Pull the magazine out of the letter box and stuff your fingers in the letter box flap to stop it shutting with a crash. Then fly upstairs as fast and quietly as you can, clutching the magazine tight in your fist. Close your bedroom door without a sound and then breathe more easily. Get ready for your fist full of football fantasy and magic. For Tuesday is the day of *Score* and its free football stickers.

Only it wasn't. Not this Tuesday. The letter box was closed, its mouth shut tight. No football magazine stuck out of its jaws. No stickers to add to the collection.

I stared hard at the letter box, half expecting the flap to open at any second and the roll of the magazine to be pushed through. I waited for ages. I waited until my toes were blue with cold and my teeth started to chatter.

No magazine.

I levered open the flap of the letter box to look through it and see if the magazine was lying outside on the pavement. It wasn't. My fingers slipped on the letter box flap and it shut with a crash. There was only one thing for it.

I opened the door as quietly as I could and set off along the pavement faster than the players come out of the tunnel at the start of a match. I had one target in my view: Goodall's Paper Shop. There was just enough time before school, but I'd have to run all the way.

The trees in Lime Grove were the players of the other team. I passed three and they didn't move a centimetre. I was just too quick for their lumbering branches to catch me. The goal was in sight. I went round a fourth – I was flying.

Then the defence showed their dirty play. A huge root of a tree burst viciously through a crack in the pavement. It was a brute of a root, deep from the black earth. Then it was round my ankle and pulling me crashing to the ground.

'Penalty! Penalty!' screamed the crowd. First I was Carlo Paggio, the striker, and then I was in the goal-keeper's green strip, hurling myself sideways along the High Street and straight into Goodall's Paper Shop. My gloved goalkeeper hands were ready to grab that fistful of football stickers. Behind the counter stood Mrs Goodall in her referee's black uniform.

'Steady on, lad,' she said, taking a pencil from behind her ear and licking the end of it.

'I want . . .'

'I know what you want,' she said, licking the pencil for a second time. 'You came in here last week, didn't you?' she asked as her thick black pencil scrawled the numbers of houses onto a huge bundle of newspapers.

'Yes,' I said.

'Then you'll know the paper boy delivers your papers.'

'Yes,' I repeated.

'So why have you come here?' she asked, lifting an even bigger bundle of newspapers onto the shop counter. 'Actually, I know why,' she said, without looking at me. 'It's those football stickers, isn't it?'

I nodded a silent nod.

'And your stickers are in the magazine which the paper boy has with him.'

'Oh,' I said and took a step back towards the shop door.

'Here, I've got a spare packet of them,' said Mrs Goodall as she pulled a set of stickers out of her pocket and threw them towards me. I dived forward and caught them with the best goalkeeper grip I could manage.

'For me?' I asked her.

'Well, they're not for Gary Lineker, are they? Now take them out of my way. I need to get on with these papers.'

I was out of the shop in a stride. Once outside I ripped open the packet of stickers with my teeth. Ben Buck. I'd got him. Vinny Capstick. Everybody's got him ten times over. Two to go. Please, *please*! I'll do anything if it could be him. Not be rude to Amber for a whole week. I'll promise anything, if only . . . Giorgio Fabrizi. Oh no. He's the worst player ever. And now for the last one. The big one. I can't look. It won't be him. I know it won't.

I don't believe it!

Look again. Pinch yourself. It is.

Mika Tailer

The sticker everybody wants and nobody, but nobody, has got so far. Except me. And I'm going to keep him. You bet I am. Mika, the only goalkeeper to save three penalties in a World Cup final. Mika, my hero.

I just stood and stared at his face. I had been trying to collect his sticker ever since the magazine had first come out. I put my finger on the sticker and let it go right round the shape of his face. My finger was coming up to the top of his head for a second time when the expression on Mika's face seemed to change. It was smiling. You might think I was dreaming, but I tell you it's true.

Then my eyes started to go blurry and I couldn't see straight. I put the sticker carefully into my trouser pocket and ran all the way to school without stopping.

I knew that sticker would bring me luck. It had to. Now the kid they all called 'wimp head' would show them a thing or two. They were in for a few surprises.

When it was time for our football lesson, I hid the sticker in my sock, ran out of the changing room and sprinted up and down the pitch. Knocker and his mates started to giggle and call out, 'Wimp head . . . wimp head . . .'

But I didn't listen, because it was time for the wimp to triumph. No more miskicking for me. No more feeble attempts at heading the ball. This time I was a striker – a striker with a red hot sticker in his sock.

Mr Brailsford, our PE teacher, gathered us round and picked two teams like he always did in the football lesson.

'Charlton, Wayne, Woody, Dannie, Josh, Edward and Ben . . .' Mr Brailsford's picking was just about complete. 'Oh, and James, Ryan and . . . Jack.'

There were only two players left without a team. One was Knocker, a giant of a boy with size ten boots. The other was me – a skinny little lad they called wimp head.

'Would you believe it, I almost forgot you two,' he said with a grin. I'd thought perhaps we were going to get the red card before we'd even started.

'There's an odd number today. You can play in the same team. We can swap someone over at half-time.'

Knocker glared at me and said, 'Oh sir, can't he play in the other team?'

'No,' said Mr Brailsford firmly.

'But he's useless. A wet wimpy spider with . . .'

But Mr Brailsford didn't let Knocker finish his sentence and blew his whistle for the start of the match.

We kicked off. I positioned myself as striker and ran up towards the other team's penalty area. I ran fast and hard and found myself with a bit of open space around me. I eyed up their goalie, Josh. He wasn't that good. He only went in goal because nobody else in their team wanted to. Surely I could put a shot past him and find the back of the net. All I needed was one good chance. One neat pass from midfield, a quick dart up the pitch, and the shot was on. We could be one–nil up, no sweat.

I waited for ages in that open space by myself. Nothing happened. No neat pass came from midfield. No pass came at all. I might as well have been on a different planet for all the part I played in the match. Most of the play happened in the other half of the field, and we were soon two–nil down.

When we did get the ball, Knocker had it. It was as if it was glued to the end of his size tens and there was nobody else in the team but him. He was the biggest kid in the class. Big boots and big mouth. He ran all over the pitch. He barged and pushed, then ran some more, lost control of the ball or shot miles wide of the goal.

Out of nowhere we got a free kick. Mr Brailsford blew his whistle hard.

'Free kick,' he said to me. 'You take it, Sam. Give it a big kick upfield.'

He placed the ball on the ground.

'Not him!' shouted Knocker. 'He couldn't kick his way out of a bag of chips!'

Some of the kids began to giggle, and I could hear Josh far away in the goal with his loud, stupid laugh. The more he laughed, the worse it was.

'Don't take any notice of the rest, Sam,' said Mr Brailsford. 'Just give it one big kick.'

I looked at the ball and tried not to think about being a wimp. I tried really hard, but somehow I just couldn't block them out. My foot hit the ground in front of the ball and instead of it flying high into the air, it just trickled forward a few centimetres and then stopped. I could hear loud booing coming from Josh in goal.

Mr Brailsford blew his whistle.

'Half-time. Change ends... and cut out that booing.'

The second half started. Mr Brailsford put Knocker into the other team. I ran upfield just like before, and just like before nobody passed the ball to me. The other team scored and we were three–nil down. It was a complete waste of time. I was so busy feeling sorry for myself that I hadn't noticed the ball roll towards me. A perfect pass from midfield. I just stood and stared at the ball. Behind me, the others were shouting and yelling. Their cries were getting closer.

'*Kickit, kickitup. Goforgoal. Samkickitup.*'

If I didn't do something soon it would be too late.

I ran forward three steps and looked at the goal. It seemed miles away. Surely I couldn't shoot for goal from this far back! Behind me, the rest of the players were so close. The ground was shaking as two size-ten boots pounded the turf a few metres away.

It was now or never. The sticker in my sock was

burning hot. Then my whole leg was burning, and pulling itself slowly back.

I could see the studs of Knocker's size tens out of the corner of my eye. My leg went forward at galactic speed. It struck the ball at seventy miles an hour. Off zoomed the ball goalwards – right on target.

Josh saw it coming. He wasn't booing now. That volley had shut him up for sure. He placed himself in the centre of the goal and watched the ball like a hawk. His hands and body were ready to block its movement when the right moment came. Yet the ball was swerving and gathering speed as it travelled through the air.

Faster and faster it went. I wanted to shout out and tell everybody that it was impossible to stop a shot like this one. That Josh had better move out of the way before he was killed. But before I could say a word, the ball was near the goal and heading for the top corner of the net.

Yet it missed the net and crashed into the goalpost. Crunch went the post and down fell the net as the goalpost was broken into two pieces.

All the players stood on the pitch and looked at the broken mess. Mr Brailsford was leading Josh away from the tangled web of net and post, and Josh was scratching his head in a daze. I just stared at it all silently. Had *I* done this? I should have been dancing round the pitch with my shirt pulled over my head like they do on the telly. Instead I just felt numb. It was like a hurricane had struck.

'What a strike!' said Mr Brailsford, excitedly. 'The strike of the century. I've never seen a kick like it. We shall all have to wear crash helmets next. How on earth did you kick the ball like that, Sam?'

For some questions it's best not to try and find an answer.

The flu came. Loads of kids were off school with it. Josh even fainted in assembly and had to be taken home in one of the teacher's cars. It meant the school football team were short of players. Things were so desperate I was picked for the eleven for the match on Wednesday afternoon.

Mr Brailsford gave us a pep talk in the changing room before the match.

'This is the big one,' he said. 'You know the Under-12s haven't won a match all season. Some of the other school teams have had victory after victory, but all we've done is crash from defeat to defeat. We're going to win today, aren't we?'

All our voices spoke as one. 'Yes, sir!'

It was a tight match. Nil–nil and well into the second half. But the opposition were spending more and more time in our goal mouth. We managed to clear attack after attack, but it could only be a matter of time before they would find the back of our net. Somebody had to do something. Somebody with a sticker in his sock. Mr Brailsford's words at half-time were pounding in my head.

'Wear your shirts with pride.'

It was up to me. It was time for me to show some pride. To stop playing like a scared wimp. The next time the ball came anywhere near me, I'd do it. Mika wouldn't let me down. I could crack the ball all the length of the pitch just like last time and smack it right into their goal. If I kicked from near our goal it would be safe enough not to break the goalposts. Then we'd be one–nil up with the game in the bag.

They won another corner. This was it. The moment I'd waited for all match. I positioned myself on the goal line, waiting for the sticker to burn hot in my sock and for my leg to get strong and powerful. Only it didn't seem to be working. The ball was almost on me when I began to jump. Up in the air I went, propelled by Mika power. Higher and higher I climbed. I had a sudden panic. Maybe I was going into orbit. Look out, Jupiter, here I come!

Out shot my arms like a spring uncoiled as I caught the ball just before it hit the back of the net.

'Penalty! Penalty!' screamed the opposition.

I fell to the ground clutching the ball.

'You caught the ball . . . but you're not the goalie,' said a quiet voice. 'You've given away a penalty, and now we'll lose the game.'

I heard what they were saying, but my legs were out of control. The sticker power had taken over. I was up on my feet, clutching the ball to my chest. The ref's whistle was blowing, but I took no notice.

'Penalty, Sam!' shouted Mr Brailsford. 'Put the ball down.' But I didn't. I ran two steps with it.

Now everybody was shouting, 'Put the ball down!'

Still I ignored them. I pulled my arm back and hurled the ball high in the air. Miles high. And now I was shouting. The words just said themselves.

'Go on . . . Go for it . . . Chase that ball. Let's have a goal. Go for it, Knocker . . . Go for goal.'

Only Knocker didn't chase out. Instead he ran to me and shouted, 'You stupid wimp. You've lost us the game!'

Then he pulled back his fist and punched me in the mouth.

I ripped the sticker into tiny pieces and watched them fall all over my bedroom floor. This was the end of football for me. I'd let everybody down so badly. Mr Brailsford, the team, everybody. I'd made such a fool of myself. To think I could score a winning goal like that. It was pathetic. Mr Brailsford's record of defeats was getting worse. I'd made a promise that he could rely on me, and this was how I paid him back.

I looked at the bits of sticker strewn over the floor. Mika wasn't to blame. He was a world-class goalie. What would he do if the ball zoomed towards him, heading for the net? Of course he'd jump up and catch it with both hands. That was his job. It was why he was famous.

My mother's voice called out from downstairs.

'Sam . . . Sam.'

I didn't answer.

'Sam . . . somebody to see you.'

'I'm not in!' I shouted back.

A few minutes later there was a knock on my bedroom door. 'Go away,' I said.

It went quiet and then a small voice said, 'It's me, Sam . . . Charlton. I've come with some good news.'

'Go away, Charlton.'

'Knocker has been banned from the team and you've been picked for the next match . . . only this time you're the goalie.'

I ran along the pavement. I ran past the trees in Lime Grove and their lumbering branches, their outstretched arms ready to trip me up. But I needed to run faster

113

or Goodall's Paper Shop would be closed for the day and then it would be too late. I needed another Mika sticker. If I was going to play again in the school team I had to have zap power. I couldn't do without it.

Into the High Street I sprinted, just as Mrs Goodall was turning the notice in the window from *Open* to *Closed.*

'You've cut it fine,' she said, moving off towards the shop counter.

'I ran all the way,' I said, trying to get my breath back.

'I can see that,' she said. 'You're all of a lather.'

I didn't know what a lather was, but I knew what I had to ask for.

'I was wondering if . . .'

'No,' she said, turning off the light above a display cabinet. 'Sold out.'

She took off her referee's black uniform and hung it on a nail in the wall.

'I need some stickers . . .'

'I said we've sold out. Last lot went ages ago.' Then she peered closer at me. 'What do you want them for anyway?'

'I want the luck,' I said.

'There's no luck in them,' she said gently. 'The only real luck you need is in that head of yours.'

'Oh,' I said, not making any sense of what she was saying. Her hand moved towards the light switches. The shop went dark and I found myself outside, feeling numb.

It seemed a long way back home. Mrs Goodall's words were pounding over and over in my head. How could I manage without the sticker in my sock?

How could I make my own luck? How could I become a great goalie for the school team?

By now a bit of a wind was blowing down Lime Grove. It made a strange noise in the branches of the trees. Not a scary sort of noise, but a noise like people talking. And the talking was growing louder and now the sound filled the air. People were clapping and chanting and waving. They were up on their feet.

'Penalty! Penalty!' they screamed.

The imaginary ref looked very much like Mrs Goodall in her black uniform. She blew her whistle and pointed to the spot. It went very quiet now. I pushed my fingers to the very tips of my goalie gloves and took a deep breath. Somehow I had to save the penalty. If I did that, we would win our first game.

'To the right . . . he's going to kick it low to the right,' said a voice inside my head. I took another very deep breath, stood quite still and waited for my moment. Then the whistle went and the ball was struck cleanly, bang on target. It seemed a certain goal. I dived for the ball, just like Mika would. My arms were flung forward, and in a rolling mass of ball and gloves and goalkeeper's body . . .

The penalty was saved!

Lyon Heart

Ann Ruffell

There had been a student demonstration on the streets, a police chase round the city, a multiple crash on the Boulevard (Lyon's ring road) and a bin-men's strike. And that was just for starters.

But here, in the flat on the outskirts of Lyon, one of France's biggest cities, I was so bored that I wanted to push somebody into one of the overflowing dustbins just to see what they'd do about it.

It had seemed such a good idea at first. Dad had to go to a conference, and our friends who lived in Lyon invited the whole family to come too. Mum wanted to go, and they couldn't just abandon me, so I got a whole week off school when everyone else was still glumly slogging through projects that they'd long ago lost interest in.

'*South of France?*' they said. 'You lucky thing, Jane.'
'Well, it's only sort of middle-to-south,' I told them.
'Can you get me in your suitcase?'
'Send us a postcard!'
But all the time we'd been here, Mum and Dad had spent their time talking to their friends in bad French which I couldn't understand, eating strange food (including terrifyingly stinky cheese), drinking wine that made Mum go all giggly, and going out in the

golden light of Lyon to look at museums and boring churches.

Michel, who was the only son, was at school all day. Like I should have been if I'd had any sense and said I'd stay with Laura for the week. It makes you glad to be English when you see them going off to school at crack of dawn. They start at *eight o'clock* and don't finish till half past five! And then they've got loads of homework to do.

I wrote that on my postcard to Laura to cheer her up.

Michel was all right, I suppose, but like I said, I didn't see a lot of him.

Until Saturday.

They were talking about the bomb on the Paris Métro. And talking half French and half English, because Dad was feeling a bit fierce about it and couldn't find the words in French.

'It's terrible that you have to throw a bomb and risk killing people to make yourself heard,' he said.

Michel's father made French noises like a kind of puffing spit. 'A bomb is meant to kill, and to kill – that is never reasonable.'

'Nobody was hurt, which was lucky, but if nobody listens to reason about important issues . . .' my mother began.

And Michel's mother stood up for her. The argument went on well into the afternoon, and you could see they were all enjoying themselves immensely. And practising their French and English like mad.

We were to go home next day. *Thank goodness,* I thought to myself. I've never had such a yawning holiday in my life. But instead of making my last evening something wonderful to be remembered, my parents announced they were going out to dinner. Without me.

Out. To dinner.

As if they hadn't spent all the rest of their time *eating!*

Michel, they said, would look after me.

Big deal.

Michel wanted to go to a football match. 'It's a match between Lyon and our deadly rivals, St Etienne,' he explained to Dad. 'Every Lyon supporter will be there!'

Football! I ask you! I could just hear my friends when we got back: 'So – what did you do in France?' They would be expecting me to say we did things like hunting in the forests for wild boar, like Asterix and Obelix. Or picking grapes in the fields. Or going clubbing. Not going to a boring football match! It was about the last thing I would have chosen to do on my last day.

I said no.

'Come on, Janey, you'll enjoy it,' said my father.

I said no.

'But Jane,' said my mother, 'it's only polite . . .'

'It would be more polite of him to take me somewhere *I'd* like to go,' I sulked. 'Why can't I stay here by myself if he wants to go?'

'You're too young! You certainly can't stay here by yourself. And anyway, where *would* you like to go?'

But that was the trouble. I didn't know where, and I'd used up all the French I knew a hundred times over and was definitely running out of conversation. I suppose I was lucky that Michel knew a bit more English than I knew French, though he had a nasty habit of laughing at me when I did try.

So I just shrugged my shoulders in what I hoped was a proper French way. 'I suppose I'll have to go,' I said.

Mum sighed, and Dad looked angry, but I'd *said* I would, hadn't I, so what were they moaning about?

'Enjoy yourselves!' said Mum brightly as I followed Michel to the door, carrying my small back-pack with a spare sweater, sandwiches and a plastic bottle of mineral water in it. Sandwiches because we weren't getting any dinner, and water because Michel said they wouldn't let us in with drinks cans because of the bomb in Paris last week.

It was just the same as home on match days. As the bus got nearer to the stadium more and more people got on, and more and more people could be seen, all walking in the same direction, towards a blaze of floodlights.

'Don't people queue?' I asked Michel as he joined a crowd round the first of a row of ticket booths.

'Queue? In France?' He laughed, and pushed evilly at the group in front of us. I grabbed onto his coat. There were far too many people here. The road was packed with people, walking, pushing, laughing.

Just as Michel got to the booth, the woman behind the counter slapped a large book in front of the window to show she was closed, and the crowd surged to the next one.

'Well, she might have said!' I muttered indignantly, but Michel simply laughed and began to elbow his way to the front again.

You won't believe this, but *each* time we got near a booth they decided to run out of tickets and we had to move on to the next one. I began to feel quite cheerful. Perhaps we'd never get a ticket, then we'd have to go home, and I could go to my room and read a book or something.

But from the fifth one Michel emerged, triumphantly waving a pair of tickets.

And we joined another crush.

This was definitely the worst night of my life. If this was what football was about – standing in huge crowds of people, absolutely all of whom were taller than me so that the only view of anything I could get was the small of someone's back – then I'd rather not, thank you.

'La police,' Michel bawled into my ear.

'What?'

'Searching. I think because of the bomber. They do not find him yet.'

'He's in Paris anyway, isn't he?' I couldn't see why they were searching us here, in Lyon, when the bloke was five hundred kilometres away in the capital of France.

But they were certainly searching for something. As the shove of people swayed, centimetre by centimetre, nearer the stadium gates, I saw them on top of the stand. With guns. You could see them quite clearly, silhouetted against the orange and pink evening light.

Mum and Dad would definitely *not* have wanted me to go if they'd known. But there was no way I could get home now – it was clear Michel wasn't bothered. Perhaps it happens all the time at French football matches.

We reached the gate. The ticket collectors ripped tickets. We joined another crush. Security men searched our bags and took away our bottles of water. Michel protested, but it happened to everyone: there were heaps of leaking bottles of Vittel muddying the ground. 'In case we make a bomb with one,' explained Michel, and we laughed at the thought of water bombs crashing down on the teams.

Another crush. And policemen and women doing body searches.

'I hope we get in for the kick-off,' Michel was saying anxiously as we milled up the steps to the back of the stand.

Who cared about kick-offs? I thought. *There* was something to tell my friends! Guns *and* body-searches! Better than a pop concert!

As we fought our way to a sort of plastic cushion on a concrete step, men were striding up the steps with sheets of blue paper, thrusting them into our hands.

'What's that for?' I asked Michel suspiciously. I had a horrible memory of school trips. You go out for a fun day, and they spoil it by giving you sheets of paper to write about it.

'To wave,' explained Michel.

So we waved, and great flowers of colour – blue from our stand, red from the next – flashed over the crowd.

And at last the match began.

I settled down for a couple of hours of boredom, and wondered what the toilets would be like. (I found out. I won't describe them. You'll be sick.)

Half my mind watched the pattern of red-and-blue and green figures on the emerald pitch, while I thought about our early start tomorrow to catch the plane back home. It would be cold in England. Grey skies, grey buildings, grey school uniform.

For goodness' *sake* – is that all you do at a football

match? Run up and down after that stupid ball, trying to kick it into a net?

Michel began to explain that there was more to it than that. He pointed to a red-and-blue-clad player, who even I could see had deliberately kicked the ball off the pitch, and told me that this was the right strategy for this moment. I couldn't see it myself, but the whole of the red-and-blues surged up to our end, and suddenly one in black, who had been sort of loafing about by the goalposts, sprang into action but didn't quite make it.

The crowd went mad.

Michel leapt to his feet, clapping and shouting.

There were two people sitting by me, the only people apart from me in the whole of the stadium who didn't jump up and down. We looked at each other sympathetically. *These mad football fiends!* we said with our shrugs. I wondered who'd dragged them along.

But somehow, now that our team had got a goal, I began to be interested. The patterns of players started to make some kind of sense.

'Why did he do that?' I said indignantly as a green-clad Stéphanois (what they called the St Etienners) shoved one of our side to the ground to get to the ball.

Michel stopped his insulting chant to answer me. 'They try to win by cheating, because they are not as good as us,' he said contemptuously.

But as I watched, there was a sort of motorway pile-up somewhere in the middle of the pitch, where a heap of players fell on top of one another and a medical team rushed out with a stretcher and took one of our red-and-blue ones off.

And suddenly, across the pitch, there was a great movement of people from the corner to the centre.

'What's going on?'

Michel dragged his eyes away from the game. 'Oh dear. I think trouble.'

Following the shifting mass was a wave of black-clad people. Police.

Then Michel laughed. 'They move the Stéphanois away from the Lyonnais. They start to fight at the corner.'

There was a different feel about the stadium now, a tense excitement. The match went on, and I began to understand what was going on.

A St Etienne player fell dramatically and lay on his face for several seconds on the bright grass. The referee came over, walked away, and a derisive chant filled the place.

Michel grinned. 'He try to get sympathy, but the referee will not blow his whistle, so they do not gain any time.'

I watched. The green man lay for a few more seconds, then got up. He limped away with the whole of the Lyonnais fans laughing and chanting.

'Suppose he's really hurt!' I said.

But he'd made his point, and when he thought no one was looking, melted back into the game with no sign of injury.

Now I was getting really interested, and when the Lyonnais team came up our end again I rose with the rest, trying to see better, cheering them on.

Another goal for us! I jumped and yelled and waved the shreds of my blue paper.

Then it was half-time and the terrible toilets and a sandwich. I put on my spare sweater, but when the match started again I didn't need it. I was sweaty with shouting and jumping up and down and laughing at our goalkeeper, at our end now. He was dressed in mustard yellow and, when the play was at the other end, he danced about and played up to the crowd. Michel told me he was a Corsican. 'He is famous for doing mad things!' We cheered his contemptuous catch when St Etienne dared to kick the ball towards our goal. We roared with disappointment when, in spite of his springing efforts, a sneaky ball got past him into the net.

Two–one. The atmosphere was electric.

Somewhere over the other side of the stadium the police moved like black beetles.

Another Stéphanois desperately tried to fake another injury. A Lyonnais had a real one, and was carried off on the sinister stretcher. An ambulance slowly drove round the running track at the edge of the pitch and disappeared somewhere in the corner.

A knot of faraway people shifted uneasily. More police beetled in, and a police car followed the path of the ambulance.

There was tension on the pitch. There was tension in the stands. The joyful waves of spectators, like a great sea surge, were no more.

Over in the covered stand to the left of us, a sudden stream of people ran uphill.

Michel looked sharply over.

'More trouble with St Etienne?' I asked. Then I looked back onto the pitch where a desperate struggle for the ball was going on.

'I think no,' said Michel. He narrowed his eyes. 'These are all our supporters. I do not know why . . .' Then the police started running uphill too, and people seemed to fall into the sides, onto other people, until they were flattened in swathes like a combine harvester cutting through standing wheat.

'Some kind of real trouble!' said Michel in a fascinated, nervous whisper.

I felt a sudden curl of terror creep up my stomach. The bomber! It made sense. He hadn't been found. He could easily have travelled down from Paris to strike somewhere else. Lyon was France's second city, after all . . .

He couldn't be carrying a bomb. Not possibly. Not after all that searching. Though there had been so many people to search. Michel had told me the stadium held forty thousand people and it looked packed full to me. Forty thousand! Wouldn't it be really easy to slip past the net of *agents de sécurité* and police?

They were spoiling the match. If St Etienne got another goal . . . I really couldn't bear it. Not unless we got another one in first.

I tried to watch the match as well as the swirls of agitation over on the covered stand. Were they coming near us?

Our goalkeeper, the Corsican in mustard yellow, rushed forward to meet a challenge that I didn't even know was coming, left his goal in what looked to me a very dangerous way, and kicked the ball practically to the other side of the pitch.

'Wow! He's fantastic!' I cried and joined the crowd round us in a standing ovation.

And then there was a sudden rush through the standing people. Someone pounded the plastic seats behind me. I looked back – as did everyone else. Some people put their arms out to stop him. Others pushed them away, trying to save him.

I saw his face suddenly right next to mine, gasping for breath, sweating as much as any footballer, but with his eyes wide with fear. I recognized his face. It had been in the papers. Mum and Dad were talking about him only this morning. Just a person. Like me. Like Michel. A person who minded so much about something unfair that he had planted a bomb to make his point.

One person, with all those police after him. It didn't seem fair, even if he might kill people with his bombs. If people listened to him instead . . .

He had reached the gangway – not much room there. It was full of people sitting on the steps. They'd never allow that in England, I found myself thinking crazily. And the police came running along our seats, running, running.

I sat down.

Michel, with a startled look round, sat too.

Most of the people in our row sat, then the people behind, following each other just as they had when they rose to clap a goal.

And the police had to get off the seats to push their way past our knees, trampling on bags, kicking shins.

I sort of saw him, fighting his way to the top, with the police wading through people after him.

But then there was a roar from the crowd, and I had to look towards the pitch.

All was quiet behind us, nothing more happened to disturb the match.

I forgot the bomber, and gripped Michel's arm as we went into injury time. People kept turning their heads to look at the great clock behind us.

I nearly screamed when the ball came close to our goal; really screamed when it went the other end.

And at last, the relief. It was the end, and we had won!

I had forgotten the bomber, as I said, until we tried to get out. The message came down from the top: the police weren't letting anyone out just yet.

But the singing had started already. Voices, already hoarse, roared songs of victory and insult. And at last we could go, though the St Etienne supporters would have to wait a bit longer.

From the top of the stand, waiting to get out of the gates, it was like a volcanic eruption – people moving in the slow heat of victory like a lava flow down the street.

'I wonder if he got away,' said Michel.

'I don't know,' I said. 'I suppose he should be punished, really. Do you think someone might listen to what he has to say, though?'

'Who knows?' said Michel, but his shrug suggested that he didn't think it was very likely.

We had to walk all the way home: there weren't any more buses going in our direction. Cheerfully we marched with the cars, singing the victory song, klaxons hooting the victory rhythm, windows open in the apartments we passed and people looking out, knowing that Lyon had won.

The lights were still on in the flat when we reached home.

'We've just seen it on the news!' said Dad. He gave me a surprisingly fierce hug.

'Yeah! We won!' I cried with satisfaction.

'That man who did the bombing. They showed us

128

the struggle outside the stadium. Are you all right?'
Mum was pale with anxiety.

'Of course I'm all right,' I said, emerging from her suffocating embrace. 'It didn't spoil the match, at least only for a little bit.'

Michel's French was far too fast for us to follow. His father would translate for Mum and Dad later. The police had had a tip-off that the bomber might be at the match, Michel's father said. Mum wasn't really reassured that the security had been very good, and that if he had been carrying a gun or a bomb they would have found it. She kept on looking at me as if to make sure I was still around.

I had to remember to buy a paper at the airport tomorrow. There'd be some really good pictures, with any luck, to show my friends.

Of the bomber? Well, I supposed there'd be that, too. But what I wanted was a picture of my favourite goalkeeper, doing a flying save!

Will I ever go to a football match again?

Try and stop me!

Jennings Uses His Head

Anthony Buckeridge

(From *Jennings Goes to School*)

Jennings spent most of Saturday morning with his fingers crossed. So many obstacles had arisen to block his path to the Second Eleven, that he could hardly believe that they had been successfully overcome. Now, however, with bilious attacks and detentions safely behind him, there was nothing to stop him from realizing his ambition. All the same, he was on his guard lest fate should intervene with another cruel blow.

His usual method of going down to breakfast was to take the stairs two at a time, and the last three in one enormous leap, but today he walked sedately, grasping the banisters firmly in case a chance slip should result in a sprained ankle. Carefully he scanned the faces at the breakfast table, in case some wretched creature had come out in spots during the night and it would be Linbury's turn to telephone messages of cancellation. However, everyone's complexion seemed as flawless as could be expected, and Jennings breathed again.

At two-thirty, two taxis turned into the school drive, and the Bracebridge team arrived, accompanied by an apologetic Mr Parkinson.

'I'm most terribly sorry for that stupid mistake about the quarantine,' he said, as Mr Carter greeted him. 'It must have put you to considerable inconvenience.'

'That's quite all right,' Mr Carter assured him. 'It didn't cause us any trouble, did it, Wilkins?' He turned to his colleague for confirmation.

'Eh? Oh, no, no, no, not at all,' Mr Wilkins replied hastily, avoiding Mr Carter's eye.

The home team was already on the pitch, wearing quartered shirts of magenta and white. In honour of the occasion, Jennings had washed the back of his knees as well as the front, and had obtained some new white laces which he had twisted under and over and round his boots in a cat's cradle of complex design. He then tied two knots on top of the bow for safety, and a third one for luck. The youngest member of the team was ready for the fray!

As soon as the visitors had changed, they streamed out on the field and Mr Carter, in shorts and blazer, blew his whistle and the game began.

It was soon obvious that the teams were evenly matched, but to start with both sides were keyed up, with their nerves sharpened by the importance of the occasion. As a result, the standard of play suffered, for an excited atmosphere breeds wasteful energy rather than careful play. During the first ten minutes both goals were bombarded with shots, some lucky, some wildly impossible. Gradually, however, their nerves were steadied and their play improved: tactics and skill replaced brute force and ignorance. In fifteen minutes, they had settled down to concentrate on control of the ball, and combination of movement.

The teams played in silence, while the spectators on the touchline shouted encouragement.

'Linbury!' they yelled, in rolling waves of sound, and held on to the last note of their cry until their breath gave out. 'Linbury! Come on, Linbury!'

Loudest of all the school supporters was Mr Wilkins. It was as though he kept an amplifier in his throat for these important occasions, and as he swept up and down the touchline, his tremendous encouragement surged out across the pitch so that the players had difficulty in hearing the referee's whistle.

In contrast to this, Bracebridge had only the thin and reedy tones of Mr Parkinson to urge them on, and his voice was as the soft sighing of the west wind compared with Mr Wilkins' stentorian north-easterly gale.

The only other supporter for Bracebridge was their linesman who, owing to his role, should really have been impartial, but he was an opportunist, and carefully waited for the lulls between the shouts for Linbury to squeak, 'Play up, Bracebridge!' at the top of his voice.

The play swept from one goal mouth to the other. Now, the Bracebridge forwards had the ball and were attacking strongly. A long, low, swerving shot came in from the left wing and Parslow, in goal for Linbury, dived to make a brilliant save. The school clapped and cheered and smacked each other on the back, and Mr Wilkins switched on his loud-hailer at full volume.

'Good save,' he boomed. 'Jolly well done!'

The ball was cleared and away went the Linbury forwards, Temple, at outside-left, streaking down the field with the ball at his toes. A moment later he, too, had made a long, low, swerving shot and it was the Bracebridge goalkeeper's turn to dive and gather the ball safely to his chest before kicking it clear.

Linbury clapped the goalkeeper dutifully while their faces registered disappointment, and Mr Wilkins reduced the volume-control to halfway for his congratulations to the opposing goalkeeper.

The headmaster, perched on his shooting-stick, looked down the line of spectators to make sure that none had committed the fault of failing to applaud his opponents.

All through the first half the battle raged evenly and neither side scored. Jennings was playing a hard game, but he knew that he was not playing his best. As it was his first match and he was so much younger than the rest of the side, his sense of nervousness would not wear off. Desperately he sought to make up in energy what he felt was lacking in control.

His first chance came in the second half – and he missed it!

Linbury were attacking, and a pass came to him from the left wing. The goalkeeper was out of position and Jennings, with the ball coming straight towards him, was unmarked, less than ten yards from the goal. Even Darbishire could not have missed such an easy shot, and had Jennings been content to direct the ball gently into the net he would have scored.

But the sight of the open goal filled him with a desire to drive the ball with net-severing force. He drew back his right foot, swung it forward with all his might – and missed the ball completely!

Johnson was just behind him, cool-headed and capable, and avoiding the floundering Jennings, he trapped the ball dead and casually propelled it into the net.

The whistle blew: one–nil.

The crowd on the touchline went wild with delight

even. Sometimes, just sometimes, he wasn't sure whether his mum was talking about Matt or him.

'Here you are,' said his mum, placing a steaming bowl of chicken casserole in front of him. 'Food for the troops. How did the practice go?'

'Fine,' Chris replied, tearing apart a bread roll and stuffing some in his mouth. Couldn't talk with his mouth full, could he?

'Do well, did you?'

He spooned in some casserole and nodded. Not that she waited for an answer anyway.

'Great. Tell Mr Mackenzie not to forget to let me have the strips for the final well in time. Have to make a special effort with them, won't I!'

That was another thing. She didn't only turn up at all the matches. She washed the match strips, helped with refreshments – there was no escape. He was just thankful she didn't trot on as team mascot as well! Luckily, his dad came in with his tea at that point and started talking to him about some wildlife film or other he'd seen.

Give me wildlife over Mum any day of the week, Chris thought to himself.

His luck didn't last, though. The back door opened and his two uncles breezed into the kitchen.

'Getting psyched up for the big match then, Chris? Not long to go now,' said his Uncle Eddie, giving him a thump between the shoulder blades.

'Of course he is! One of us, isn't he? Thinks positive,' his Uncle Pete laughed. 'Just turn it on for those scouts, mate. Got an old contact of mine from United coming over to have a look, too. Do your best and you'll be in, no sweat.'

'He always does his best, just like Matt always did,'

his mother chimed up, 'and he'll get just as far, you mark my words.'

Chris couldn't stand it any more. He pushed his chair away from the table and made for the door.

'Where are you going?' his mum asked, surprised.

'Over to Alec's. Said I'd help him with his bike. Be about an hour.'

Out in the hallway he grabbed his anorak. As he tugged at the zip, he heard his dad's voice.

'Why don't you lot leave the poor lad alone?' he said mildly.

'Oh, *y-o-o-u* . . .' he heard his mum reply, in that voice she always used when she thought his dad was probably right but she wasn't going to admit it.

At least he could get everything off his chest down at Alec's. *He* wasn't football mad – and he listened. The two of them had been going round with each other for most of this school year, ever since they'd landed up in the same class.

Alec was into bikes; properly into them, belonged to a racing club and everything. Chris had never liked mountain bikes much; he had a pretty good road bike himself. Alec had helped him sort out some upgrades that he was going to ask for next birthday. He'd even been out on a couple of rides with the club and had a great time. They'd said he could go any time, and he would, too, when the football season was over. Same old story!

Once he had started helping to clean up Alec's stripped-down bike and had told him everything, Chris cooled down. Alec did his best to help.

'How do you know you'll make the grade with the scouts anyway? Sounds as if this Jason would be the first choice.'

'You can't make a team out of eleven strikers, or geniuses like Jason Gilmore. They'll be looking for good all-rounders, too,' said Chris.

That was him to a T.

'I just don't want it, Alec,' he said. 'Do you know how many cubs actually make it to senior level?'

Alec grunted between the screw he had clasped in his teeth and shook his head.

'Not many, I can tell you,' Chris went on. 'Imagine it, all those months – years even – the hours of playing before they tell you, *Sorry, lad, but . . .*'

Something else was niggling him, something he didn't even want to tell Alec. How many ears had 'the uncles' bent about him? Were they trying to pull strings? He hoped not, but it was one more reason to stick to his plan now that he had made up his mind.

'I don't reckon you can do it,' Alec said.

'What do you mean?'

'It's OK in a practice,' said Alec, 'but can you really see yourself backing off in the actual match, not wanting to win, letting your mates down?'

'I won't be letting them down! I'm not the whole ruddy team, you know!'

'Why not just take a sicky, then? Come up with some mysterious bug? Or play your usual game and say "no thank you" when the scouts recognize your outstanding talents?' Alec said, half-jokingly.

Chris shot him a sarcastic look. 'You have *met* my mum – and the uncles?'

Alec pulled a face. 'More than once. It was just a thought. Best of luck, that's all I can say. Want me to come along and watch?'

'So you can pick up the pieces? No thanks.'

*

It was here. The day of the final. The inside of the Town Boys' changing room buzzed as if it was wired with high-voltage electricity. Chris looked around. Jack Briggs, who ran midfield with him, gave him his 'I am an alien' impression as he pushed his head through his crisp, royal-blue match shirt. Timmo was high as a kite and already plucking imaginary balls out the air. Jason was as cool as ever, a quiet smile on his face but his eyes sparkling, ready for anything. Real winner's eyes.

The door opened. A smell of outside and the hum of voices came in with Mac, and went as he shut the door behind him. They weren't at any of their usual venues. It was a tradition for the county non-pro club to offer their ground for the District Final, so it was like the real thing: terraces, a small stand, loud-speakers, the lot, even the county ref and linesmen.

'OK,' said Mac, 'this is it. You know you can do it, so just go out there and give it all you've got. *And enjoy it!*'

They all groaned at the old clichés.

'I mean it,' said Mac. 'Now come on, let's show Delingham what for.'

They clattered out after him. Chris hung back and walked out with Timmo.

'How are you feeling, Chris?' his friend asked, tossing a ball from hand to hand.

'Nervous!' Well, that was true enough.

'Me too,' said Timmo, his grin coming back. He rolled his eyes heavenwards. 'Please, God, help me to keep 'em out.' And he was off down the field, heading for a pair of goalposts.

Chris sprinted into midfield and began a kick-around with Jack. Whistle, toss, ends, positions; he went through the familiar routine as if he was only half there. He looked round. The ground wasn't exactly crowded out, but it might as well have been for all the noise the families and friends of the two sides were making.

He could see his lot, too, behind the barriers, bang on the centre line. His mum waved. His Uncle Pete nodded towards a row of stand seats, pointed with his raised arm. The scouts, Chris supposed. His uncle gave him the thumbs-up sign. The ref raised the whistle to his mouth and blew. The game was on.

Everything was fine for the first ten minutes. The Delingham players were as nervous as the Town Boys and Chris got by, playing a steady but unspectacular game – nothing to bring him to any scout's attention, one way or the other. Then a Delingham winger broke.

Now, thought Chris. He left his run a fraction late and his leading foot met fresh air as the winger sailed past him. Trouble was, he sailed past Liam, one of their backs, too, and sent a corker screaming across to the big Delingham striker everybody knew all too well. Wham! Timmo caught it, safe as houses. Chris breathed a sigh of relief and ran back upfield. He told himself Timmo would be glad to have got into the game, to have the ball between his gloves. He tried not to think how he'd have felt if Timmo had missed – and Delingham had scored.

They did, five minutes later, but the play was well away from Chris. There was nothing he could have done about it.

After that, Delingham piled on the pressure but the Town Boys fought back. Chris could feel his team-mates' determination so strongly he could almost touch it. Liam blocked another Delingham charge and smartly sent the ball up to Chris. It was an obvious chance for a quick break but Chris held back, dribbled right a bit, left a bit.

'Chris!' screamed Jack. He moved in, took the ball and flicked it forward to Jason. Jason was off across the pitch, slicing through the defence like butter. He turned and sent such a good ball across the goal mouth that all Wilkie, their other striker, had to do was stick out his foot. One–all. The crowd erupted and the ecstatic Town forwards raced back to the centre, grabbing every blue shirt they could on the way back. Jack didn't join in. He was on his way over to Chris.

'Thumping heck, Chris, what was all that about?' he asked, half puzzled, half angry.

Chris could feel himself going red. 'Nothing, sorry,' he mumbled and ran back to position, waiting for the whistle. His head was in a whirl. The look on Jack's face! Then he gritted his teeth. He hadn't done anything drastic, put them in any real trouble. He couldn't give in now.

He didn't, but the rest of the half was like hell. No way was he going to mess up something vital, but whenever he thought the team was in a pretty safe position he stuck to his plan: a corner even Gascoigne couldn't have converted, a few kicks into touch, tackles that stopped short of being real tackles.

Then, just before the half-time whistle, the Town made a break. The ball was with Chris and Jason was right where he knew he'd be, running into a space on the right ready to take it. So was the green shirt of a Delingham centre-back. He sent the ball just slightly towards the Delingham player, his heart pounding with more than the effort of the game. If Jason was really quick he'd get it anyway, he thought. He didn't. The green shirt got there first and the Delingham player charged up the pitch. The whistle went.

Before he could get anywhere near the half-time team talk, Chris's arm was clenched in a tight grip and Jason swung him round to face him.

'I don't know what you're playing at, Davenport,' he spat out, narrowing his eyes, 'but a few more dumb moves like that and you'll have lost us the match. Pull yourself together.'

He didn't even wait for a reply. Chris swallowed hard. He felt rotten. He felt even worse when he joined the rest of the team and saw the down-beaten looks on their faces.

'Come on, you lot! It's one–all, not ten–nil. You're doing great!' Mac enthused. And by the time he'd finished ten more minutes of the same build-up they were all looking a lot happier. 'That's more like it,' he said. 'Now get out there and finish them off.'

But as they broke up, he caught Chris by the arm.

'Don't let it get to you, Chris,' he said quietly. 'Just play your normal game. We'd never have got this far without you in midfield. Remember that.'

Chris went back onto the pitch with his mind in turmoil. He hadn't been as clever as he thought. Mac had noticed – except Mac thought he was letting the big match get to him. He could see the others, high on adrenalin, raring to go. Would they think that, too? That he'd bottled out? Then he saw Jack and Jason talking, heads together, and looking over at him. Timmo joined them. Chris could see him waving his arms about, shaking his head. No guesses what they were saying. What should he do?

With the first touch of the ball, clear as a bell, he knew. It was nothing to do with Matt, his mum or anyone else; it was his decision. He'd do what Mac said, play his normal solid game. He'd probably done enough to put the scouts off in the first half, anyway!

He made mistakes. It wasn't that easy, switching his head round from playing for himself to being part of the team, and at first he had a sneaking feeling that Jack wasn't sending all the passes he usually would. But gradually he got back into the swing of things and his game began to flow. With the team in this mood, he could hardly help it anyway. He'd never seen them like this – playing with everything they'd got and then some. And he was in on it, one of them again. It felt brilliant. Alec was right, he'd been an idiot. Now he'd do his best to make up for it.

But Delingham weren't favourites for nothing. They were pushing like mad and it was taking every ounce of effort and determination for the Town Boys to hold them. Twice Jason broke through, twice a horde of green shirts blocked him. There was not much time left and both teams knew it. Chris had the ball, Jack was with him. They took it upfield between them. Jason feinted, left his marker and ran across in front for a forward pass. The mid-centres ran on as he flew like a rocket down the wing and swept in towards goal. The keeper came out, Jason flicked back. It was on Chris's right foot before he knew it – the perfect ball, an open goal.

He hesitated for a split second, something he would never have done normally. This was his chance to put things right, he mustn't make a mistake. Even as he thought it, he felt the charge and his feet went from under him as a burly Delingham back smashed the ball off his boot. A sickening wrench went through his ankle and a fierce pain shot up his leg as he hit the turf.

Mac took no chances. Chris was on the bench and stringy Darryl Wright, their sub, was haring off across the pitch as if he couldn't believe his luck. Chris didn't know whether to laugh or cry. How about that for showing the scouts what he could do? It was almost as if he'd asked for it! He buried his head in his hands, wincing as Mac propped up his foot.

Then he heard a roar and Mac was on his feet, jumping around like a demented kangaroo. Chris looked up in time to see Darryl go sprawling in the box. Somehow he'd got his foot to the ball and sent it skying towards Jason. The tall striker rose, his head met it like a dream and he cracked it into the top left-hand corner of the net. The crowd erupted, Mac was yelling and pumping the air with both fists, blue shirts swamped the Delingham area and went mad. They were ahead! All they had to do now was hold on.

Chris forgot everything else for those last few minutes. He went as wild as the rest of them when the final whistle blew and he knew that the team had won. There was pandemonium – they even had him on his good foot and dancing around until Mac rescued him. He saw the scouts coming over to congratulate Mac, saw one of them strolling over in Jason's direction.

Suddenly his dad was there. Behind him Chris could see the rest of the family and the excitement drained out of him.

'Well done, lad,' said his dad. 'Great match, you lot. Thanks for everything, Mac. I'll get that foot to the hospital for a check-up, just to make sure. You go back home in Eddie's car, Helen. I'll give you a ring from casualty.' There was no mistaking the firmness in his voice. He helped Chris over to the car park and had him in the car before his mum had even moved.

'Thanks, Dad,' Chris said weakly. The pain was getting to him now and he felt a bit sick.

'Don't mention it, son,' said his dad, giving Chris a big wink as he opened the passenger window to let in some fresh air.

Chris took in a few deep breaths and closed his eyes. He finally had it sorted. He wouldn't stop playing with Town Boys – he enjoyed it too much – but that was as far as it was going. He'd give the cycling a proper go, do some real training, and if that meant missing the odd football practice, so what? It wasn't the end of the world. There was still his mum and the uncles to handle but he'd manage it somehow. What he needed was to get somebody onside with him. He glanced across at his dad and grinned. He'd do! He couldn't think why he hadn't thought of it before. He'd have a good talk with him later.

He relaxed into the seat and let the wind fan his face. 'Move over, life. Make way for Christopher Davenport,' he said silently.

He was on his way.

He's the Man!

David Clayton

One Saturday morning in March, the entire St Mary's Juniors football team were feeling fed up. Most people who have just won six–nil are happy – but they weren't.

After the game they went to the burger bar as usual. They were saying goodbye to Mighty Mark Mullen. Soon he would be far away in America and they would have no goalkeeper.

'You'll be OK. You've got the Professor!' Mark said and they groaned.

The Professor, Paul Parker, was tall enough and keen enough. Nobody knew more than him about the game. He had everything – except talent. If he put his head in his hands, he'd drop it!

The lads couldn't bear to talk about it. They knew that putting the Prof in goal would never work, but they didn't want to make Mark feel bad.

'Do you *have* to go?' Tom Smith, the captain, wasn't a softie but even he had a lump in his throat. Mark was brilliant. If he wasn't diving at people's feet, he was catching high crosses. If he wasn't catching high crosses, he was hurling the ball to the half-way. With him, St Mary's were great; without him they were ordinary.

Once, Mark had been away on holiday and the

Professor couldn't play either. Steven 'Stick-'em-up' Stanley had been brought in and it had been a disaster.

They called him 'Stick-'em-up' because he held his hands wide apart above his head like the victim of a robbery. Anything right over his head was in. They drew five–all against a terrible team. It was a sad memory. Now they'd have the same problem every game.

Monday came and Miss Murray met the team.

'It's St Joseph's on Saturday. What shall we do about a keeper?' she asked.

There was no reply.

'Ann Bowers is very good,' she said. 'She can catch anything.'

The striker, Adam Roberts pulled a face. 'That's true, miss, but she's got a netball tournament.'

'What about Paul?'

'No. Drops it too often.'

'Steven Stanley?'

'No way!' they roared.

Miss Murray's face went pink.

'Well then, lads,' she said. 'If none of my ideas are any good, *you* sort it out.'

And she turned and walked off.

Chalky looked at Tubby. Adam looked at Butch. Charlie looked at Des.

Finally, Tom said, 'You know something. It *might* have to be the Prof or nobody!'

The team were *not* happy.

It was a miserable day. The game in the yard was duller than usual. Tom sighed as he went over to talk to the Prof. Suddenly there was a shout. Tom turned to see the ball hurtling towards him. There was no time to move.

Whap! A great long arm with a big hand on the end of it appeared in front of Tom's face. He turned and looked up at the body that went with it. The towering boy held the ball *in one hand!*

'Hey!' said the boy in an American accent. 'A guy could get hurt round here!'

The giant beamed down at Tom and shook his dreadlocked head. Then he gave the ball a little flick and spun it on one finger without even looking at it.

'Wow!' gasped Tom. 'Who are *you?*'

'Harrison T. Eccles,' said the lad. 'I'm in England for a year. Mark Mullen's dad and my dad exchanged jobs.'

Now he let the ball roll down his arm on to his neck. He ducked forward and it rolled on down his back and into his other hand behind him.

'Dead easy!' said Stick-'em-up Stanley, looking green with envy.

'OK, man, be my guest!' Harrison flicked the ball to Stanley who dropped it on the floor. Everyone burst out laughing.

'Give him a dustbin. Then he'll be able to catch it!' someone shouted.

Steven Stanley booted the ball away and stomped into school, looking furious. How could he compete with *that?*

Meanwhile the mob had closed round the new boy.

'Hey, how would you like to play football for our team?' asked Adam.

'Soccer? I don't know anything about that!' said Harrison. 'It looked pretty rough out there when you were playing.'

He looked at the scuffed knees of their trousers. Tom had blood coming through his where Adam had tripped him up. Tom hadn't noticed and didn't feel it in the heat of battle.

'No, you'll be OK,' said Tom. 'We just need someone who could teach you.'

Just then the Prof came strolling by playing a computer game.

'And I know just the right person to do it. Paul! Paul! Come here!'

Tom explained the situation to the Prof. The lads watched Tom waving his arms and the Prof shaking his head.

'You have *got* to be joking! By *Saturday*?' The Prof was horrified.

'We need him, really need him, otherwise . . .' Tom stopped – even he could see what he had been going to say. He never did think much.

'Otherwise you're stuck with me or Stanley?' the Prof said sadly.

'Hmm . . . er . . . well . . .' Tom was turning pink.

'OK,' agreed the Prof. 'But it won't be easy.'

'You're brilliant!' muttered Tom. 'I know you can do it!'

Just then the ball came flying across the yard towards Harrison. This time it was ankle high. The big boy craned over but missed it. It was less than a metre from his feet. Harrison was good in the air, but low balls seemed to be a problem!

Why did I agree? thought the Prof. 'I'll get a roasting if we lose now!'

Harrison and the Prof were strolling in the yard together.

'Haven't you *ever* played soccer, not even once?'

'Well, the Hispanic guys played all that stuff. Me, being black *and* a beanpole, I played basketball.'

'You mean, "No, I haven't played".'

'No.'

Down at the other end of the yard, Tom and his mates were all laughing and joking. They thought they'd solved their problem. It was a good job they didn't know what the Prof was thinking.

'Do you know the rules?' the Prof asked, but not hopefully.

'Sort of.'

'Do you know what a goalkeeper is?'

Harrison grinned.

'Yep, got that one. He's like a goalminder in ice hockey, isn't he?'

'Let's go out on the field.'

It was easier to *show* him. Steve Stanley tagged along.

'Man, this is messy!' Harrison looked out on the sea of mud, then down at his trendy trainers. 'No way! These cost me a hundred and fifty dollars!' He perched on a little bank behind the goal. 'Now *this* is OK,' he said.

'He can't keep goal from five metres behind the nets!' Steve chipped in.

'I know! I *know!*' snarled the Prof. It wasn't like him to be ratty but the whole thing was getting to him.

'Stay there!' he snapped. 'We'll show you what you can do if you're a keeper.'

The Prof trudged out on to the swamp. Steve Stanley stood with Harrison.

The Prof pointed downfield. 'Goalkeepers can handle the ball in this area.'

'Wow! That's kinda small. I mean, can't be more than six paces out.'

The Prof could feel his head caving in.

'Not *that* area,' he explained, pointing to the six-yard box. 'The area out to *that* line!' And off he went, stomping round the line like an angry gnome.

'OK, man, but you just didn't say. You said . . .'

'I know! I know!' groaned the Prof.

'But you didn't say, did you?' Steve added.

Ten minutes later, the Prof was walking gloomily back towards the school. It was going to be a hard week.

'Well, I guess I know about goalminding now,' smiled Harrison. 'How about me teaching you basketball?'

The Prof sighed. Saturday stood like a dark cloud before him.

The next day, the Prof brought a big box to school. At break, he opened it in his form-room. Inside the box was a table football game.

'Great!' said Tom.

'Yeah!' chortled Adam. 'We'll all play.'

'Oh, no, you *won't*!' growled Harrison's coach. 'This is to teach Harrison how to play football.'

Just then Miss Murray came along.

'Out, all you boys!'

'But, miss, I need to teach Harrison to be a goalminder . . . I mean goalkeeper.'

Miss Murray gave the tall American lad a long stare. He looked like a bit of a joker to her.

'OK, but no messing!'

Then they were alone. Harrison watched as the other boy set out the game on the classroom table.

'Hey! This is cool but where are the controls?'

'There *are* no controls. It's not a computer game. We're not going to *play* it. I'm just going to show you where to stand.'

'My feet are kind of big for standing on that diddy little field.'

The Prof turned to see Harrison grinning from ear to ear.

'It isn't funny. The guys in the team will be all over us if we lose.'

Harrison turned to see Tom and his mates with their noses pressed against the window. 'Cool!' he said.

Later, a shivering Harrison was bribed by Tom and the lads to have a game in the yard. The Prof watched from a distance and couldn't believe his eyes. Harrison was saving everything. Then Paul worked it out. Tom had the American on his team. Tom, as captain, always picked the best team so almost everything was blocked before it reached Harrison – *and* the ball was so bouncy that it hardly ever stayed on the ground for long. Harrison's long arms gobbled up all the high, wide shots. He looked like a star, but it was too easy. He needed a stronger opposition if he was to show just how good he was.

After a while, Steve Stanley came up alongside the Prof.

'It won't be like that on Saturday.'

'I know!'

'I was watching you before. You can't show him how to play on a table footy board. He'll have to play a proper game. And someone will have to tell him what to do as he goes along!'

203

The idea hit the Prof like a flash of lightning. Steven Stanley had said something good for once. In American Football they have a coach shouting orders. That's what he had to do. And make sure that the ball was really light and bouncy so that it wouldn't just dribble along the ground.

Suddenly a shot skidded through Tom's defence and clean through Harrison's giraffe legs. Ice ran through the Prof's heart. Basketball players weren't used to picking up the ball from around their knees!

Tom just laughed and said, 'He was unsighted. That's all. You were in his way.'

Harrison smiled gratefully. The Prof walked away sadly. Steven Stanley came up and muttered, 'He's great with the high balls, but he's rubbish with the low ones! Worse than me!'

The Prof had nothing to say. On Thursday, all years 5 and 6 played football. On Thursday, Harrison would play on a real pitch. It was crunch time for them both. Steven Stanley was smiling.

All day Wednesday, the Prof tried to teach Harrison the basic skills. Harrison was quite clever. He understood the rules when the Prof tested him but it would be a bit different when he was actually out there playing.

When Thursday came, the lads noticed that the American boy had a guitar case with him.

'Are you a rocker, then?' asked Adam.

'No, I play the blues like my dad.'

He took out the guitar and was soon picking out a great rhythm. Just then, Miss Conway came by.

'That's really good. Today's our day for the music teacher. You'll have to play for her.'

'Yes, ma'am.'

The Prof felt his brain frying again. The music tutor came in the afternoon. That was when they were supposed to be playing football.

But he needn't have worried. Just before lunch, rain started to pour down. The field was flooded. There was no chance of playing footy now anyway.

On the Friday, the weather was better and the hall was free. The Prof decided that he would teach Harrison one or two commands.

'When someone runs at you like this, I'll shout *Out!* You come out and block them. I'll also shout *Catch! Punch!* and *Kick!*'

They did a few dummy runs. Harrison was still all arms and legs, but he did get in the way of the ball and he was very quick.

At the end of the session, the American gave the Prof a little dig in the shoulder. 'We'll be OK, bro! You call the shots. I'm the man!'

But the Prof wasn't so sure. All afternoon he watched the others. All afternoon he saw how happy they were, even Steven Stanley who was named as sub after the Prof dropped out, saying he had to help Harrison.

That night the Prof played the match a hundred times in his dreams – or rather, nightmares. All the shots were low, and tall, gangly Harrison was letting in goals by the bucketful. Short-tempered Tom was glaring at the Prof and muttering terrible threats.

Next morning the sky was gloomy, but the bad weather held off. The bumpy St Mary's pitch was in good shape, with just a muddy diamond in the middle of the field.

The changing room was buzzing, especially at the St Joseph's end. All their eyes were on Harrison in his jazzy jersey. From the other end a little ginger tough with a pug nose came over to him.

'You aren't playing, are you?'

'Sure thing, son!' said the giant keeper, giving the kid a little pat on the head. 'Stay tuned!'

The boy slunk back to his team-mates. They were not happy.

Meanwhile the Prof was giving Tom some advice.

'You've got to keep it tight at the back, Tom. You've got to keep them shooting from way out. If you do that he'll catch everything.'

'Yeah, yeah, yeah!' You couldn't teach Tom anything. The teachers at the school had the same problem. 'I know what I'm doing,' he added. 'I wasn't born yesterday!'

Tom always did things his way. At the start of games, he would stay back. He was a good central defender but then Adam would get a goal or two and away Tom would go, glory-hunting down at the other end. Then the other team would break away and there'd be a hole as big as the Channel Tunnel in the middle of their defence.

'Think about it!' shouted the Prof as Tom walked away. Tom got on his nerves sometimes. He never thought anything through properly.

'I'm not thick, you know!' the captain snarled, running outside.

The Prof pumped up the ball like mad.

The ref took it off him. 'It's a bit hard, son!' he said.

'It's muddy out there, sir,' explained the Prof. 'It'll help if the ball's a bit lighter.'

When they kicked off, Tom kept to his word and defended. They had a flat back four. The Prof stood behind the goal, calling the moves for Harrison.

'Go out towards the ball a bit . . . Go left . . . More in line with the ball.'

The Prof's plan was working. It was hard to break through the back four and Tom's tough tackling. When they ran past they were offside. When they shot from way out, Harrison caught the ball easily.

The Prof was happy. Harrison was grinning. However, Tom was *not* happy. The score remained nil–nil. Tom *had* to win. Adam, the flying striker, drifted further and further back. Tom moved up until they met in the middle.

'What're you doing up here? Why aren't you down there?' snapped Adam.

'Because you're down here when you should be up there!' yelled Tom, pointing to where the striker should have been.

Meanwhile, a gap had appeared in the St Mary's defence. The ball was at David James's feet; he was St Joseph's best striker. He was in full stride and Harrison was in big trouble.

'C'mon, you guys, cover me!' he called.

'Out!' roared the Prof and off stormed Harrison.

James saw the fearsome sight coming, took a big swing and almost chopped down the corner flag with his shot.

'You duffer!' yelled one of his team-mates.

He turned in anger.

'All right then! Let him run *you* over!'

'Well played, Harrison!' Steven Stanley shouted from the subs area.

'Didn't do nothin'!' smiled Harrison calmly.

Tom trudged back with a red face to take the goal kick.

'I told you . . .' the Prof started.

Tom turned, giving him the evil eye. 'Don't say anything! I know . . .'

All the rest of the half, Tom was itching to storm upfield again. But every time he thought about it, he could imagine the Prof saying, 'You'll be sorry!'

Then St Mary's won a corner after some tricky footwork by Adam. Their opponents had all eleven back. Tom, Joe, Mark and Jim, all the back four, charged up in spite of the Prof's warnings. The other players were packed like sardines in the other penalty area. Harrison stood alone. There was a huge gap in the middle of the pitch.

'Go out! Go way out!' called the Prof.

'But there's nobody coming and it's kinda muddy out there.' Harrison was happier with dry feet in the sandy goal mouth.

'Just do it, OK?'

Harrison advanced to the penalty spot. 'Here?'

'Further.'

Harrison stopped on the edge of the penalty area. 'Here?'

'Further out,' the Prof pointed.

'But, man, if I go further, I can't handle the ball.' Harrison wasn't happy.

'Further,' nodded the Prof. 'Halfway to the centre.'

Harrison looked round when he got there. 'Hey, this is stupid!'

He stood with his arms folded. He was ankle-deep

in mud like porridge. He was not smiling as he turned towards the Prof.

'Watch the game!' came the cry.

Then the corner came over. It was a bad one. A big defender gave the ball a hefty hoof towards the halfway and the race was on.

'Go get it! Boot it!' yelled the Prof.

Harrison was on his way, teeth gritted, knees flying as if he was riding a bike. He was running one way; twenty others were running the other. *Now* he saw why he was out there.

Whap! He gave the ball an almighty crack. It cleared the St Mary's defence, the St Mary's attack, the ref, the St Joseph's attack and all their defence but one spindly red-haired boy. Just as it was sailing wide, the boy decided to poke his head at it. This was a bad idea. The goalie was in front of him. The ball squiggled, squirmed and spun, slipped and stopped just over the line. Terrible words were spoken. St Mary's jumped for joy.

Harrison T. Eccles smiled.

'I'm the man!' he said.

When half-time came, Harrison was a hero and St Joseph's slunk like ghosts from the field.

'Will you stop jumping out of their goalie's way?' their manager moaned. 'He isn't Arnold Schwarzenegger!'

'But, sir!' protested James. 'He's just so big!'

'He hasn't done anything yet!' snapped the teacher. 'Try to get round the outside. Test him a bit on the ground.'

The second half started. St Mary's were still glowing.

St Joseph's were still steaming. Right away, nippy James switched to wide on the right and sprinted clear.

'Out!' yelled the Prof, and off raced Harrison towards the penalty spot.

'No! No!' screamed the Prof. 'Not out there. Out towards him!'

'You didn't *say,* man!' gasped Harrison as he started to leg it back.

Nearly everyone was laughing. It was obvious now that Harrison had never played before.

James saw his chance and smashed the ball hard and low towards the open goal. Harrison got a leg to it but only succeeded in kneeing the ball violently into the net.

'I don't believe it,' groaned Tom.

As the ball bounced back onto the pitch, Tom lashed out at it. Unfortunately, the ball flew off his boot past the post and smashed the Prof right between the eyes.

'*Aaaaaagh!* I've got mud in my eyes!' he yelled.

'Yeah,' said Harrison, 'and your nose is bleeding.'

The Prof wobbled away towards the school. St Joseph's were looking at Harrison as if he was a turkey at Christmas.

'What do I do now?' said the keeper.

Tom coughed. 'Dunno!' he said.

Sam Carter, St Joseph's captain, was full of glee.

'C'mon. Their keeper's rubbish! We'll hammer them!' he shouted to his team.

And, right away, they were swarming like ants all over St Mary's. Tom went charging at Sam in midfield. The other lad slipped past him and James was on his way towards Harrison again.

This time, he kept his eye on the ball. This time he steadied himself.

I

THE PAOLOTTI TOWERS and the bell towers of the Cathedral and San Giovanni were gradually disappearing under a blanket of mist, their outlines dissolving. It was like an evening from times gone by, before the seasons blended into one another, an evening when the city wrapped itself in a misty shell, when it seemed suddenly familiar again and the noise, bustle and frenzy died down. In the enveloping mist, Parma had stopped yelling and had taken instead to whispering, like an old lady in church.

Soneri was strolling through the streets, in the grip of a not displeasing nostalgia. Each step summoned up a litany of memories: the university, rushing along Via Saffi, and Ada, lost too soon. He stopped in Piazzale della Pace when he could no longer make out the austere lines of the Pilotta or the houses in Via Garibaldi. There was now nothing to be seen but mist, ahead, behind, beside, above. The only sure thing, and a fleeting one, was the pavement on which he walked. Then his telephone rang. Life, illusory and deceptive life, was reaching out to him.

"Am I interrupting something, sir?" Juvara said nervously.

"Not at all. Just imagine that you've grabbed me by the hair of my head a split-second before I fell down a well."

The words were so gnomic that Juvara had no idea how to respond. "So what is it?" Soneri added.

"There's one hell of a pile-up on the autostrada, a near catastrophe . . ."

"You get catastrophes in other places apart from autostradas. And you tell me it's only a *near* catastrophe . . ."

"Alright, an accident. A really nasty one. More than a hundred cars, lorries, some on fire . . ."

"O.K., so you've alerted the traffic police, no doubt?"

"No need . . . they're already on the case."

"Good. So everything's in order?"

"No, not entirely . . ." the inspector stuttered.

"What then?"

"The questore has asked if one of us could go along. Somebody's been on the telephone to say that some gypsies are wandering about among the cars, stealing things." Juvara was struggling to get the words out.

"Why doesn't he send in the flying squad?" Soneri said with some feeling, but at the same time he was aware of a need to escape from loneliness and the trap of nostalgia.

"He already has, but with the mist the way it is . . . well, the fact is, they can't find the place. There's no-one on duty who knows his way around the Lower Po Valley."

Soneri felt a threat taking form somewhere above his head, like a coiled spring about to snap. Instead, it was he who snapped as he turned in the direction of the Steccata.

"Where is this place?"

"Near the service area at Cortile San Martino. There's a road running alongside the Autostrada del Sole."

"I know the one. What about the flying squad?"

"They're driving around in circles. The questore says you're the only man who knows the roads well enough . . . the only one in Parma."

"Fetch the car and pick me up in the piazza in five minutes."

Juvara was unable to find him. The commissario had to wave his arms and jump over the chain between the columns to attract his attention.

"I'll drive," he said the moment the inspector rolled down the window. "With you at the wheel, the best we can hope for is to end up in a ditch."

Juvara did as he was told, with some relief. "I had a problem getting out of the gate at the police station," he mumbled, as he got into the passenger seat.

"That's why you never land a girlfriend. You're hopeless."

Juvara smiled awkwardly and said nothing, relaxing only when Soneri gave him an affectionate poke in the ribs as he settled behind the wheel.

The mist rose over the bonnet of the car. As they left behind the creamy light of the street lamps and moved into the narrow country roads they were plunged into a near impenetrable darkness.

"You can see why they couldn't find the place," Juvara said.

"On a night like this, everybody should stay at home, preferably in front of a roaring fire, better still with a cat on their lap. Think of all the great opportunities we miss. But, maybe it's just as well," Soneri said, thinking back to his earlier nostalgia trap.

Juvara looked at him uncomfortably, making no reply and staring tensely at the road, or at the little he could see of it, which was hardly more than two metres ahead. "Even if we do manage to find the place, with all this mist about, how are we going to catch the people we're after?"

"O.K., one thing at a time. Let's concentrate on finding the right road," the commissario said curtly. Whenever more serious subjects came up, the inspector was quickly out of his depth. It was impossible to know if it was due to indifference or shyness. Or maybe it was on account of his youth. When Soneri had been thirty, what did he care about weighing up choices or roaring fires at home?

They drew up at a fork in the road where there were no signs. Soneri was not sure which was the right way, but some instinct made him turn to the left.

"Might be this one. Who knows?" he muttered to himself.

They carried on for a few hundred metres until they heard a menacing roar in the darkness, like the despairing bellow of an animal in the slaughterhouse.

"Did you hear that?" Juvara said, sitting bolt upright as the figure of a bull came into view in the fog lights.

"Yes, and we're on the right road," Soneri said.

The animal must have weighed several hundred kilos but seemed more apprehensive than aggressive. The commissario noticed Juvara take hold of his door handle and stiffen up.

"I'm wearing red," he said.

"Relax. He's vegetarian. Even if there's a lot of good eating on you, it's of no interest to him. Be careful not to upset him, though." Soneri laughed as he flashed the lights at the bull. The beast turned lazily to face them, before lumbering off with his great scrotum swinging between his legs.

"He's well hung," the inspector said, plainly relieved.

"What did you expect? He's not like our dear Chief, Capuozzo."

They drove on in the mist from which emerged bellows and cries like the pleas of orphans at night. They caught a second bull in the headlights, its tail raised as it trotted across the road.

"A limousin. Good beef cattle."

"I thought they were less dangerous," Juvara said.

"You're thinking of limousines, and even there I'm not so

sure. Think of what happened to J.F.K., not to mention all the Cosa Nostra men who've met their end in one of them."

They came across an enormous cow, which began to moo as they drew up close. "She's going to have a memorable night of passion, with all those bulls on the loose," Soneri chuckled.

"So long as they find each other."

"They're not shy and retiring like you."

They continued on their way until the mist took on a yellowish tint.

"It's either a motorway café or a hypermarket," Soneri said.

They stopped at another fork in the road. Everything around them was the colour of moscato wine. The engine was just turning over, allowing them to hear the rhythmic strains of a primitive, metallic music, heightened by the mooing and pawing of the bulls running free in the mist. When the commissario rolled down his window to look out, the interior filled with the acrid stench of burning. "Roasted tyres on the menu," he said, swerving to the right in the direction the smell seemed to be coming from.

"We're near the accident," Juvara said.

"Smart deduction."

"What about those bulls? Where did they come from?" the inspector said, apprehensive once more.

"Am I right in thinking that you suspect that they were on a lorry which crashed into another vehicle?" Soneri said in the same ironic tone as before. "Disasters can sometimes give rise to liberation."

There were now black streaks in the mist, and the smell of burning was even more pungent. The commissario leaned forward and looked upwards through the windscreen. The sky had the appearance of a huge peroxide wig with darker patches. He turned to Juvara, who looked as amazed as a child in a fairground. Ahead of them a herd of pigs was clustered together, as though homesick for their sty. Meanwhile a horse, bringing its own aura of mystery, galloped past through the darkness which was now filled with plaintive animal cries.

"What's this? *Animal Farm*?" Juvara said.

He was answered by a neighing sound somewhere in the surrounding darkness, but almost at the same time they became aware of a flickering brightness on their left which had the colour of a good Lambrusco. The sight disconcerted the commissario, who stopped the car.

"That's carcasses burning," Juvara said.

"That's impossible. The autostrada should be on the far side." It was the only thing he seemed sure of. He remained silent for a few moments, trying to get his bearings. He was lost and floundering, overwhelmed by memories of the days when he had walked those remote roads on the plain searching for isolated spots. The past was yet again taking hold of him and this time the memories were the names of girls with whom he had long since lost all contact.

He inched forward, and rolled down his window a little. He decided to follow the smell, as do animals on heat, as the bulls were doing at that moment in pursuit of the invisible. Shortly afterwards, over to his right, patches of more intense brightness appeared. The autostrada was indeed there, a long stretch of road indifferent to its burden of tragedies.

Soneri turned onto a track running alongside it and drove towards the fires. There was a little space on the footpath and he parked there among piles of rubble, broken tiles, waste paper and used handkerchiefs. Juvara too got out, but he stayed close to the car and kept the door open.

"Now what?" Soneri asked himself as he looked at the

slope strewn with rubbish on the other side of the barrier. The inspector, continuing to look cautiously about him, made no reply.

The commissario walked a little further along the path. The flickering light of the fires, the dome of mist tinted with yellow, the bellowing of the stricken animals and music in the distance made the whole scene somewhat surreal. The countryside behind him was swarming with life not native to it, and he knew that ahead of him lay rows of crashed cars, and hanging over them was the pall of death, disturbed only by the coming and going of breakdown trucks and the sirens and flashing lights of the emergency services.

He turned back. "Call headquarters and tell them we're on the spot. Ask them what we should do next."

The inspector was only too pleased to get back to the car. "Sir, that fire . . ." he asked, leaning out the window and pointing to a bonfire on the far side.

"The gypsies, obviously," Soneri said.

"They're telling us to be patient and stay put until the police cars turn up," the inspector told him. "Can you hear the fairground?"

"What fairground?"

"The one they've put up at the shopping mall behind the service station."

"Ah, so that's where the music's coming from."

"That's right. A lot of people are going there."

At that point, the barking of a dog could be heard above the animal chorus. The mist made it difficult to tell if the sound was coming from the slope or from ditches on the far side of the barrier.

"Another lost soul," Soneri said.

"It must have been in one of the cars caught up in the crash," Juvara said.

There was a call on the radio. Pasquariello, the head of the flying squad, wanted directions to find the commissario. A sudden gust of wind made the column of smoke change direction and the stench of burning tyres came through the open window. Juvara started coughing and threw open the car door to get a breath of fresh air.

"That's how they flush out foxes," Soneri said. He saw the inspector leap back into the car with unexpected agility. He turned and became aware of a bull's head a couple of metres away. The beast's snorts made it seem like a cartoon caricature, but this effect vanished when it opened its mouth, let its tongue hang out, arched its back and gave a roar that made the mist vibrate. The commissario was unsure if it was looking for food or wanted to mark off territory of its own, but Soneri remained there rooted to the spot, while Juvara, already inside the car, shouted to him to get in.

It all seemed to him unreal, a fairground scene like the one in the distance with the blaring musical background. There he was, confronting his own Minotaur, enveloped in a mist which had taken on the improbable colours of a showground. He heard Juvara's imploring voice, but he stayed where he was, staring at the motionless beast, watching his own reflection in its large, resigned eyes. It lasted no more than a second; the bull lumbered away and vanished into the mist.

"Your shouting nearly got me gored, Juvara."

"You take too many risks. It was about to charge you for real."

"Always remember that animals are much less dangerous than human beings. A policeman is always more likely to be killed than a vet."

Meanwhile the dog went on barking, the sound growing more shrill and irritating. "He's really scared," Juvara said.

"He's afraid of the bulls, just like you." As he spoke, head-lights shone out ahead of them.

"Here come the police cars," Juvara announced.

"We turned into a half dozen farmyards," one of the officers said, getting out of his car.

"You've seen nothing yet. Your real troubles will start when you try to find your way back," Soneri said, intending to be facetious but succeeding only in unsettling them.

"Where's that dog?" snapped the man who seemed to be in charge of the detachment.

The commissario made a vague gesture, raising his hand and waving it about. "There's no sign of gypsies," the officer said.

In reply, Soneri pointed to the fire on the opposite side of the road. The officer in charge mumbled something before putting a cigarette in his mouth and lighting it. The com-missario did the same with his cigar. They stood facing each other in silence until a loud moo came from very close by and another stray animal appeared, this time little more than a calf, as the commissario understood from the short horns.

"Fuck me!!" The commanding officer leapt to one side, pulling his Beretta from its holster.

"No need for that. It'll do you no harm. Anyway, with this mist, there's no knowing where the bullets will end up."

The officer moved back towards the safety of his car. The bullock pawed the ground as though it was considering charging, but then changed its mind.

"If it sees you're afraid, it might be tempted to rough you up a bit."

The officer lowered his pistol only when he saw the beast trot off, but his hand was trembling as he replaced the weapon in its holster.

"Will I take the M12?" one of the policemen said,

referring to the semi-automatic they had been issued with. His superior officer said no, but he appeared badly shaken. Soneri stared at him. "First time you've seen a bull?"

The officer shook his head. He was young, one of a generation who had received all its training in a police academy. Soneri was conscious of belonging to a different age, when a peasant world still existed and a bull did not seem such an alarming, extraordinary rarity. Before he had time to feel superannuated, the headlights of the second car shone on them.

"Will someone tell me why the fuck we've been sent to this godforsaken place?" shouted the new arrival.

"Because of the gypsies, Esposito," his colleague reminded him.

"This is a jungle. We've got pigs, bulls, cows . . ."

"The world is full of pigs and cows," a policeman said.

"But not of bulls," Soneri said, cutting short the conversation.

"Commissario, can you tell me what we're supposed to do even if the gypsies *are* looting things? I can't even see the tips of my shoes," Esposito said.

"You'd better ask Capuozzo," the commissario said, plainly annoyed. "Drive up and down this road with the headlights full on, just so they know you're here."

The officer in charge was struggling to make out what was being said, because the dog was barking wildly.

"Fuck that bloody dog," Esposito cursed. A new chorus of moos struck up, muffled by the mist.

"We should continue patrolling until fresh orders come through," Soneri said.

The officers got back into their cars. In the yellow-streaked darkness, the disco music continued to blare out while the firefighters were in all probability dragging the dead and injured from the twisted metal. Soneri watched the flickering blue lamps of the police cars until they were swallowed up by the darkness. He was left on his own, a cigar in his mouth. From the direction of the autostrada he could hear a constant racket occasionally interrupted by the sound of a car accelerating away. From time to time the plain around him would come alive with some sudden agitation, animals running, chasing and perhaps facing blindly up to each other.

"Commissario!" He heard Juvara call out.

"What is it?" Soneri moved back to the car.

"I thought I heard someone running from the autostrada into the fields."

Soneri stretched out his arms. "What are we supposed to do? Unless they run into us . . ." He stopped when he saw one of the squad cars coming towards them too quickly for a routine patrol. Esposito jumped out and ran towards the commissario, waving his arms in the air. "We've found a body, a badly burned body. I think it was one of those involved in the pile-up."

Without saying a word, Soneri got into his car and followed them along the road. When he got out, the dog was barking nearby. Esposito switched on his torch and turned it onto a body, disfigured and mutilated by the flames, lying on the other side of the metal fence. There was a little Pomeranian of an indefinable colour two steps away, yelping loudly.

"Do you think he was its master?" Juvara said.

The commissario shook his head. "Normally they keep watch in silence. This one is trying to tell us something."

"The accident happened right here. He must have been thrown from the car," said one of the officers.

Soneri looked up towards the autostrada. He struggled to make out the wrecked cars, still in a long line, each one concertinaed into the one in front. A little further on, a burning tyre was giving out black smoke. "Maybe," he said, but he did not sound convinced. He took the torch from Esposito's hand and went over to the barrier, staring at that dead body whose features were now only vaguely recognisable as human.

"I don't believe he was one of the motorists. We'd better call in the forensic squad. Be careful not to trample on anything. Cordon off the area around the body."

Juvara trotted at his side as he made his way back to the car. "Do you really think . . . ?"

Soneri nodded. "That body was dumped there, but was burned somewhere else."

He took out his mobile and dialled Nanetti's number, leaving the inspector consumed with curiosity. "At the toll booth, go in the direction of the Asolana . . . you know, where Guido's *osteria* used to be. No, before you get to the grain store," he explained to his colleague, listing places which were no longer there.

When he hung up, Juvara tried to question him, but Esposito butted in. "We've taped the site off. Pasquariello is in the office and he says one car is enough if the situation is under control, but he said to check with you first."

"One will do. Apart from anything else, if there was anything to steal, they'd have gone off with it before we turned up. Besides, it's a secondary matter now," he said gravely.

Juvara remained silent, reflecting on those last words. "Are you saying we were called out on a routine matter and discovered a murder?"

"Most things are a matter of chance," Soneri said. "You ought to know that by now, seeing the number of years you've been with the force."

They went back to where the corpse was and at that

precise moment they heard a high-pitched cry, something between a scream and a groan, from a field nearby – enough to unnerve Esposito and his colleague. "Good God, what's that?" Juvara exclaimed. "Not even in the wilderness . . ."

Soneri alone remained calm. The cry caused him no anxiety but reawoke in him old experiences of farmyards, frost and horseback rides at Christmas. It was a sound he recognised from his childhood and which at that moment resurfaced from the depths of his memory as a recognition. "It's nothing to be alarmed about. There's another death, but this time it's only a pig."

Esposito and Juvara looked incredulously at each other. "So who did it?" they said, almost in chorus and in the stern tones of an interrogating policeman.

"By a process of simple deduction, I'd say it must have been the gypsies. There's no-one else in the vicinity."

"I thought they were all Muslims," Esposito said.

"The majority are one hundred per cent Italian," Soneri said in a tone of reproof. The ignorance of fellow officers on issues on which they should have been properly briefed always astonished him, but just then a car drew up to take their minds off pigs and gypsies. The forensic squad had arrived.

"One day you're going to get in touch with some good news," were Nanetti's first words as he got out his car. "You're lucky I know this zone, otherwise we'd have been looking at this corpse tomorrow morning."

"We're the only ones who know this territory," the commissario said, as though confiding in an old comrade.

"I know what you mean. We're ready to be put out to grass."

"The correct term is care home," Soneri laughed. "That's what Capuozzo calls it, and he means care of the mind."

"His," Nanetti shot back, giving him the V sign. "Anyway,

are you sure this isn't somebody who got battered about in the crash?" he asked, pointing to the autostrada.

"First a car crashes, then it catches fire. If someone is thrown onto the road, he escapes the fire, doesn't he?"

Nanetti nodded, but he could not hide a certain exasperation at the commissario's ostentatious display of logic.

"Perhaps the car went up in flames, and perhaps this poor soul tried to escape from the fire which was already engulfing him and ended up here. But in that case, he would have rolled about on the grass and there would have been some traces. Those paper hankies and those bottles, for instance, they would have been blackened or at least there would be some mark on them, no? And the grass would have been scorched, wouldn't it?"

Nanetti ran his torch up and down the slope and had to agree that there was no trace of all the things the commissario had listed. He let out a groan and said, "I'm afraid you're right. O.K., let's cut the fence and search the ground, then we can carry off the body when we get authorisation from the magistrate. The autopsy will be the real test."

"By the way, who's the on-duty magistrate?" Soneri asked.

"We're in luck: it's Dottoressa Marcotti. You know how good she is."

"Excellent. We'll not have to waste time spelling out the totally obvious." Soneri went towards his car, signalling to Juvara to follow him. The two men were walking along the autostrada barrier when they heard a deep groan, sounding as though it were produced by bronchial tubes clogged up with catarrh. The sound was accompanied by something frantically pawing the ground, and they found themselves face to face with an enormous, rotating mass topped by a majestic pair of horns. A bull and a cow were coupling on the road, almost knocking down the iron railing of a little bridge.

Juvara looked on, in part troubled and in part excited by the sight. The commissario was amused to see that Juvara was so engrossed that there was no trace of fear on his face.

"Cheers!" Soneri said to the inspector, who seemed hypnotised. He could not tear himself away even when the bull got down from the cow's back, quivering, his head lowered, his great detumescent penis dangling and almost touching the surface of the road.

"Is that the same one we saw before?" Juvara wanted to know, finally getting a grip of himself.

"Of course it is. Can't you tell from its balls?"

"Seriously?"

The commissario gave him a nudge. "How the hell should I know? It certainly doesn't look like a limousin. It lacks class."

At that moment, the cow arched its back and peed loudly on the road.

"Usually it's the male who does that afterwards." The inspector had a beatific smile on his face, as though it was he himself who had just been making love.

"So, I hope you picked up something there. Anyway, it's time to go."

The two beasts had disappeared. The mist was still all around them and Juvara seemed hopeful that another miraculous vision would emerge. On Soneri, however, that unexpected juxtaposition of past and present created in him a kind of alienation. He was in the Lower Po valley and in a familiar mist, but somehow it all seemed unreal to him, a caricature of what was imprinted on his memory.

He started up the engine and inched forward into the dense wall of mist. "And they called this road the Autostrada del Sole," muttered Juvara at his side.

2

FOR ABOUT A quarter of an hour they circled round the bonfire which was blazing in the distance like an unattainable sun.

"Where is this road?" Soneri said, growing impatient.

"You're not really planning to go to the gypsy place, are you?" Juvara said in alarm.

"Why not? Calm down, they're not as bad as the bulls."

"But there's only the two of us . . ."

"Nothing's going to happen. These are not aggressive people."

"If you say so."

"How come you're so prejudiced? You're scared of animals, but bodies burned by the roadside have no effect on you. You're afraid of gypsies and yet you hang out in discos filled with thugs with knives in their pockets, drugged to the eye-balls."

The inspector gazed at him as though the thought had never occurred to him. "I suppose it's a matter of habit . . ."

"No, it's simply that people are fearful of the unknown. Anyway, let me introduce you to them."

He drove on for a few minutes but the camp and the fire seemed to keep changing position. After a bit, he turned the car round and went back the way he had come. Thirty seconds later, the headlights lit up a white, rusting sign on which it was just possible to make out the word: DUMP.

"This has to be it," the commissario said, turning into the site.

Juvara remained silent and impassive as he watched Soneri manoeuvre the car and drive up towards some huge metal dustbins filled with rubbish. A group of children emerged and ran off in all directions. The two men drove on towards the fire, around which at least twenty people were seated, feasting. A side of pork with some meat still on the bones was hanging from a kind of trestle.

"You see now who is more dangerous?" Soneri asked ironically, pointing to the slaughtered animal.

Their appearance among the caravans had brought the barbecue to a halt. All eyes were trained on the commissario and inspector. An age-old distrust was evident on the faces of all those present, giving a chill to the scene. For a few seconds the only sound to be heard was the crackling of the fire, but then a middle-aged man with a floppy Borsalino cap and a tight-fitting jacket came over to them, stopping a few feet in front of Soneri and making a enquiring gesture with his chin.

"Police," Soneri said, with every appearance of calm. Juvara took up a position one step behind, watchful and wary.

"If you're here about the pig . . ." the gypsy began, but stopped as he saw the policeman shake his head.

"I couldn't care less about the pig," Soneri said. "God rest his soul," he added, smiling over at the remains attached to the hook.

"Well then?" The gypsy stretched out his arms.

"How long have you been here?"

The man turned towards the others to seek help. "Must be a couple of months now. Look, we've got nothing to do with any thefts. We killed this pig because it was already injured.

It was losing blood and would have died in any case. It was trying to force its way in everywhere, even into our caravans."

"Served it right, then," Soneri said sarcastically. "Anyway, I'm not accusing you of having stolen . . ."

"You always do. Every time something goes missing, it's always our fault."

Soneri turned and saw that a group of boys had gathered round his car. The man shouted out something in an incomprehensible dialect and they all scarpered.

"Someone was burned to death by the autostrada . . ." he began again, approaching the topic warily.

"Two people. That's what we heard. We went along to take a look, but the traffic police told us to go away. We only wanted to see if we could give a hand, but we got the usual stuff – only there to rob and steal, and all that. So they can get on with it themselves. There were other people doing the stealing," he said with a snigger.

"I wasn't talking about those who died when their cars went up in flames after the accident. There was a burned body at the side of the road, but that one had nothing to do with the pile-up."

The man turned back to the group with an expression of bewilderment. "And what does that have to do with us?"

"I don't think it has anything to do with you, but you might have seen something."

"In this mist?"

"It was light during the day."

"Yes, but if someone's going to commit murder, he's not going to do it in broad daylight."

Some of the group had started eating again, having lost interest in the conversation. Mandolin music, evoking a distant land, came from some of the caravans.

"I mean, maybe a car drew up, opened its boot and . . ." Soneri insisted.

The man stretched out his arms again. "I didn't see a thing."

"Make one more effort. Ask them all. There's always somebody who sees something, but pays no heed to the one thing that turns out to be really important for us." As he finished, the commissario stretched out his hand and gave a smile of understanding.

The gypsy leader shook hands, relieved the visit was going to be over without too many complications. "I'm Omar Manservisi," he said, but his voice was drowned in the roar of a clapped-out car shooting off at speed down the road away from the camp. All the gypsies exchanged glances which Soneri could not interpret. Manservisi too became suddenly serious, but only for a moment.

"Did you catch sight of that car?" he asked Juvara as they set off.

"I only got the first half of the number plate, AB 32. There was another figure and two letters."

"Do you know the make?"

"An old Citroen XM, at least twenty years old."

"It seemed in a hurry."

"And in this mist . . ."

They passed the bins again and turned onto a side road. The commissario took a wide turn and one wheel bumped against the kerb, making the car shudder. The inspector jumped too. "Apart from the mist, they go and build these raised roads along the side of the canals," he said uneasily.

"It's because of the flooding; it lets you move about."

"Maybe so, but it's like a rodeo."

"There're bulls there too."

"Are you sure this is the right road?" the inspector said shortly afterwards.

"No," Soneri replied with a touch of anxiety in his voice, leaving the inspector in suspense. He realised as he spoke that he was not on the road he had taken on the way there. He had made a turning to follow the wheel tracks of the car which had sped out of the camp. It was all a matter of instinct.

"So where are we going?" Juvara asked.

"Let's go on a tour of the Lower Po Valley. Is that not a lovely idea? Try to imagine there's a girl here beside you instead of me."

The inspector made no reply and for a moment Soneri was afraid he had offended him. He would rather Angela had been there. It would have been more amusing with her and he would have enjoyed needling her.

"You see that?" said the inspector, pointing ahead.

"What?"

"Someone went onto the grass and nearly ended up in a ditch."

A wavy line in the mud marked the way forward for about a hundred metres.

"Do you think it happened only recently?"

"Looks like it."

"One of those bulls was most likely involved."

The commissario said nothing, but accelerated slightly, cutting confidently through the mist. He gripped the steering wheel tightly, ready to swerve. Shortly afterwards, the flashing blue lights of a police car made him draw up.

"A police cordon," Juvara said, relieved that Soneri was forced to brake.

When they came closer, they saw a car balanced precariously between a ditch and the side of the canal. It was the Citroen from the campsite.

"An evening full of surprises," Soneri said.

The patrolman was standing beside an elderly, somewhat dishevelled man. "He's drunk," the officer said.

The commissario nodded. "I did notice," he said, referring to the skid marks he had seen further back, but leaving the officer puzzled. "Who is he?" he asked, indicating the old man but not taking his eyes off the policeman.

"We're checking him out," the officer replied, pointing to his colleague on the car radio.

The man stayed silent, prepared for the worst.

"Is this your car?" the officer said.

There was no reply. The man continued to stare ahead into the mist in the background, as though he would rather lose himself in that nothingness.

"These are false documents," reported the other police officer who had been communicating the data to the control centre. "And the car is registered in the name of one Omar Manservisi, of no fixed abode."

"Oh great! Let's get this one along to the station," the patrol leader said.

The old man's attitude was surprising. For a few moments, he stood stock still in the same position, then turned towards the policeman who had taken him by the sleeve and stared at him with the expression of a bewildered child.

"Manservisi . . . Manservisi . . . I've heard that name, but I can't remember where," said the officer.

"He's one of the travelling people camped up by the dump at Cortile San Martino," Soneri informed him.

The officer looked at him in surprise. "The ones who lit the fire?"

"The very same. Manservisi is a kind of chieftain. I believe the old guy here took the car a short while back."

"Stole it? He stole something from gypsies!" The officer's tone was incredulous.

The commissario stretched out his arms, looking again at the old man who, judging by his expression, seemed sunk in a state of drunken depression. "What about the car? We can't just leave it here in case someone crashes into it."

The patrolman raised his visor and snorted: "Suppose not . . ."

"He's coming with us. You stay here until the pick-up lorry arrives," Soneri said.

This time it was Juvara who took the old man by the arm, and as he did so the man turned towards him with the same expression as before.

"You go into the back seat with him," Soneri ordered. "He looks like the sort who could do all kinds of crazy things. Keep your wits about you."

They set off and within a quarter of an hour they saw the milk-white glow of the first lights in the city. Ten minutes later they were turning into the courtyard at the police station.

"So, how come you took the chieftain's car and were going around with forged documents?" Soneri began wearily, reflecting on the bizarre conduct of this unknown figure.

The old man looked down at a point in the centre of the desk, avoiding Soneri's gaze.

Juvara cut in. "Would it not be better for us to leave him to Musumeci? He'll be here in about twenty minutes. We've got that other business to attend to."

The commissario shrugged. "The main thing is to get him to make up his mind to talk," he said impatiently. Just then, another officer came in to take the man's fingerprints.

"Look, it's in your own interests to put an end to this, eh!" Soneri said, raising his voice in growing exasperation at the man's indifference. "Could you tell us who the fuck you are?" he went on, tossing the false identity card on the table like an ace of spades. "That way we can clear this business up. You'll be charged with possession of forged documents, car theft and drunk driving, but you'll be treated lightly."

Nothing seemed to make any impression on the man, who was now sunk in a comatose stupor. The more the interrogation dragged on, the more absurd his behaviour seemed to Soneri. He was just concluding that he had a madman on his hands when the telephone rang.

"Not making much headway here," were Nanetti's opening words.

"Not surprising, with all that mist."

"It's not a laughing matter. This burned-out stump of a human being has nothing on him to identify him. He looks as though he's been on a spit."

"Have you searched around? On the grass verge?"

"You can forget the grass verge. It's been ploughed up by the emergency services. We'll come back tomorrow and comb the slope. The torches are no good in the dark."

"Alright. We can only hope you come up with something."

He was about to resume questioning the old man when Juvara and the officer who had taken the fingerprints came in.

"Commissario, there's a warrant out for this man. His fingerprints match those of Otello Medioli. He killed his wife twenty years ago. We've been on the computer and there's no doubt."

"This is some night for coincidences," Soneri said.

He turned to face the man: the suffering appearance, the watery eyes and the weary pallor made him an improbable murderer. He looked like an ordinary old-age pensioner, but no-one was more aware than the commissario of how

"You sound like a little boy who's just been told off."

"There are people here," he said by way of excuse, and in an attempt to conceal his state of mind.

"Is that what it is?" she said mischievously.

"No, I also wanted you to know . . ."

"Don't say it. There's no point. I understood everything from your voice and that's enough for me," she whispered.

"Yes, maybe it's as well if I don't talk. I've never been any good at finding the right words for moments like these. I feel ridiculous and I'll just end up ruining everything."

"Exactly. Anyway, both of us know what this telephone call is really all about."

He felt his hopes rising. He looked up to see Juvara staring at him incredulously. He smiled at him and Juvara pulled himself together. "We know a lot more about Dondescu," he told Soneri. "He worked for years as a peat digger, but he came down with something and the state gave him a sickness pension. When the regime fell, he was evicted and found lodgings for a while in some institute. He then lived without any fixed abode in various camps with travelling people, drinking too much and getting by as best he could. His pension was revoked some months ago, and it seems it was this decision which induced him to seek his fortune in Italy."

"So we have to feel nostalgic for the communist regime," Soneri said. "At least everybody had something to live on. Any relatives?"

"They told me he had a sister who was a lot younger. She was a dancer, but they've no idea what's become of her."

Soneri gave a gesture of impatience, and opened the newspaper to see a reproduction of the photographs the old man had had with him.

"Capuozzo wasted no time getting this news out."

On the opposite page there was an article about the

discovery of the body. "That was a real field day for the journalists and T.V. cameras, wasn't it?"

"If I may say so, commissario, I still don't see what connection there could be between a death by natural causes and a woman's burnt-up body," Juvara said, with some hesitation.

"I don't understand either, but I prefer to carry on believing in coincidences."

6

"THERE IS NO such a thing as coincidence. There is destiny," Sbarazza corrected Soneri. He was speaking about himself and about the particularly fortunate day he had enjoyed, and was saying it must have been written in some inscrutable horoscope of whose existence he was convinced beyond all question. On this occasion, he was seated in a place which had been occupied shortly before by a woman who emanated sensuality and good health: perhaps a bank manager. She had taken *anolini in brodo* and a little Parma ham. "It's rare for me to be able to have a first course," Sbarazza confessed. "Generally it's the main course that's left."

He was dressed elegantly and yet there was a nonchalance to his appearance, as though his clothes had been chosen carelessly from the recesses of a cupboard.

"What a woman," Sbarazza said dreamily. "The quintessence of femininity, voluptuous but with no loss of harmony, lovely hair, exquisite breasts, sensual in voice and manner. It was wonderful to make love in my imagination while her perfume floated around."

"A different one every day," Soneri smiled.

They were standing facing the church of the Steccata, under the monument to Parmigianino who was peering down on them with marmoreal irony.

"She was even kind enough to leave today's paper," Sbarazza said, showing it to Soneri, who glanced at the page with the two photographs. "Are these the two you're looking for?"

"By land and sea."

"That woman knew one of them. I heard her talking about her to the man lunching with her."

At that moment, the sun made a faint appearance through the mists and a ray of light glimmered in the sky. That too was a coincidence, or a sign of destiny, as Sbarazza would have put it.

"I must find this woman," the commissario said.

"I've no idea who she is, but if I saw her again, I'd recognise her. You can't get a woman like her out of your mind," he said, as though lost in a dream.

"Have you ever seen her before?"

"No, never. I trust she will come back here if it is written that we should meet again," he went on, still carried away by his private ecstasy.

"What happens if on that happy day she's starving and wolfs the lot?" Soneri wondered.

"Please!" Sbarazza spoke imploringly. "Spare yourself these banal thoughts. Have the courage to dream because therein alone lies our salvation. Take me. What would I be were I not able to play a part each and every day? A good policeman must know how to release the imagination and gain some insight into what might be."

"If that's what you mean, there's no shortage of people intent on making what doesn't exist appear."

"There you are mistaken," Sbarazza said reprovingly. "There's no lack of those who desire to be what does not exist, and so they prosaically imitate a model. On the other hand, the dream is life. It is a parallel universe, more noble than the world of things and of the multitudes that go about masquerading. Alceste's restaurant is always filled with such individuals. Trash . . ." he concluded with a dismissive, irreverent gesture.

"And what is your dream?"

"To be myself. I play the part of the man I was and can no longer be. I feel like a puppet abandoned at the bottom of a basket. I am poor and noble in a world of wealth and vulgarity. A splendid hoax, is it not?"

The commissario's silence implied agreement.

"Take my word for it, you will find that woman. I too long to see her again, but I'd be afraid of disappointment. It is we ourselves who make certain moments magic, not what we see. The same thing can bring either joy or sadness," he concluded with an elegant wave as he turned away.

Soneri watched him as he made his way slowly down the street which was illuminated by sickly shafts of sunlight. The commissario turned towards Alceste's restaurant, feeling like a hound in the wild on the trail of a strong scent.

"A bit late for lunch," Alceste said.

"It doesn't matter . . ."

"There's something left over . . ."

"You're taking me for Sbarazza?"

"He was up to his usual tricks again today, but with such a gentlemanly air that no-one bothered."

"It's because of him that I'm here."

Alceste became serious. "Has he done something stupid?"

Soneri shook his head. "He picked up something of great importance."

"In here?" Alceste, polishing off a plate of gnocchi, sounded amazed.

"I mean . . . the woman whose place he took."

"A real beauty."

"She knows the girl whose picture was in the paper today."

"The photograph found on the dead man in the coach?"

Soneri nodded. "I've got to find out who that client of yours was."

"I don't know her name. She comes here from time to time, but . . ."

"If she paid with a credit card, she can be traced."

"The man who was with her paid the bill."

"Makes no difference."

Alceste was drying his hands as the commissario was already on his way.

"What about the gnocchi?"

"I never say no to gnocchi. I'll have them in Sbarazza's usual place," he said, indicating the now empty restaurant.

"I've found someone who knows the girl in the photograph," Soneri announced later as he entered his office.

Juvara looked up in amazement. "How did you manage that?"

"I've already told you. I believe in coincidences. You can call it gut feeling if you like."

"I've got something to tell you."

"Fine, but first we've got to trace a certain Giuseppe Pianfarini. He was having lunch with the woman who knows the girl. He paid with his credit card, and his name is even written on the receipt."

The euphoria of his discovery had made him forget everything else – the woman whose body had been burned, his gloomy mood, and above all Angela. The moment she came back into his mind, something choked inside him and he became again prey to fear.

"Here you are, sir." Juvara surprised him with the news he

had to offer. "He lives at 15 Via Montebello and these are his various telephone numbers."

He passed a sheet of paper over to him with studied nonchalance, but in his attitude Soneri detected a trace of peevishness.

"We'll have a chat when you find the time," the inspector added.

"Yes, of course," the commissario said, as he dialled the number.

The man at the other end had the hoarse voice of a smoker.

"Commissario Soneri," he announced. "I urgently require to trace the woman you had lunch with today at the *Milord* . . . no, no, nothing very serious . . . just a bit of information . . . you know those girls whose photographs were in the paper . . . calm down, maximum discretion guaranteed."

When he rang off, he became aware that Juvara was ostentatiously displaying a lack of interest in that line of enquiry. "At least we're getting somewhere with one mystery," Soneri said, in self-justification. "I'm going to pay this Signora Robutti a visit. It seems she's a marketing director with some food company. I want to know how she got to know this girl."

"Talking about these girls," the inspector cut in, "the one who died was twenty-one or twenty-two years old and was three months pregnant."

An unpleasant sensation, like a symptom of the recurrence of a disease, assailed the commissario.

"Pregnant?" he stuttered.

"Nanetti was in touch a short time ago. He said your mobile's been turned off."

Soneri dived into his pocket for his telephone, which had indeed run out of battery, as happened often with him. He plugged it into the socket beside his desk and a few moments later a barrage of messages began to show up, accompanied by a symphony of identical notes. One was from Angela: *I see you have already forgotten everything we said . . .* He felt a second stab in the heart within a matter of seconds. The news that the girl was expecting reopened a wound that had never really healed. For him, that girl was Ada, that child his unborn son, and the burned corpse represented the irreversibility of things, like his lost youth and all that might have been but was not. He was for a moment overcome by an emotion which quickly turned to rage. He had to find who had killed her. It was the only way to exorcise his pain.

"You're right, Juvara. We must concentrate on this dead body. This must be our principal objective."

The inspector stared at Soneri in surprise as he flopped heavily into an armchair. He was so pale that he seemed on the point of fainting, but his telephone rang and brought him back to himself.

"I've been searching for you for hours," Nanetti said reproachfully.

"So Juvara has been telling me."

"I think this changes everything. Even if the fact that she was pregnant doesn't mean she couldn't have been a streetwalker, my nose tells me . . ."

"I would rule it out. Prostitutes take precautions."

"And what woman does not take precautions?"

"O.K., but it makes it less likely she was on the game. Anything else turn up?"

"Confirmation of what we suspected. She was killed by a very brutal blow, or else by a violent push. Four teeth knocked out and a broken jaw. She died instantly of a shattered skull. The body was burned and she was abandoned not more than one hour after the assault."

"So they set fire to her body not far from where she was found?"

"Somewhere in the surrounding countryside. In this temperature, her body froze quickly but not completely, because we found minuscule fragments of the bag attached to the skin."

"What about the baby?" Soneri asked, realising the absurdity of the question only when the words were out.

"Don't go there," Nanetti warned him, guessing what was going on in the commissario's mind. "You'll do yourself no good."

The commissario held back the rush of confused sensations which threatened to overcome him. "What has Marcotti decided to do?"

"The body will not be released for burial at the moment, but anyway no-one has come forward to claim it. The same with the other one, the old man. It's no accident they've been placed one beside the other."

"I might have found the girl in the photograph."

"Ah! Who is she?"

"I've still got to find that out from someone who knows her. You won't believe it, but this is all down to Sbarazza. I ran into him again, and it turned out he'd been sitting in the place of some woman who'd had the newspaper open at the right page and had been speaking about her."

"If you're so curious, why not give her a ring?" Nanetti said, but he sounded sceptical.

Instead the commissario telephoned Angela, but her mobile was switched off. Anxiety took hold of him again, but Juvara, unaware of what was going on and seeing him flare up, simply thought that colour was returning to his cheeks. Before they had time to discuss the new developments relating to the case, Musumeci appeared at the door.

"There's a woman here who wants to see you," he told Soneri.

For an instant he hoped it might be Angela, but when he went into the interview room he found himself facing a beautiful woman who answered fully to the description given by Sbarazza.

"Serena Robutti," she introduced herself, with a practised smile.

"I was going to call you," he said.

"Giuseppe told me you were looking for me, so I wanted to clear this matter up immediately."

"I was only looking for some information . . ."

"Yes, very good, but I'd like to make it clear . . ." Signora Robutti went on, with a steeliness in her voice.

Soneri gestured to her to continue.

"The girl was Romanian. Her name was Ines Iliescu, and when I first met her she was an illegal immigrant. You see what I'm getting at?"

Soneri thought this over for a moment. "You gave her work?"

The woman nodded. "As a housemaid. You know how it is. I'm always in the office, I travel a lot . . . For a while she slept at our place, but then she made other arrangements. But I assure you, I had every intention of giving her real employment. Since she was an illegal immigrant, I could not do things properly, but I was looking for some way to regularise her situation."

"You do know that's what they all say, don't you? Even on the buildings sites, as soon as someone gets killed in an accident they declare they were going to fix things up the very next day."

"I swear I would have done it, but I couldn't as long as she was not quite legal."

"So how did it all end up?"

"I'm not sure. One day, she quite simply didn't turn up. I

-72-

tried to call her on her mobile, but there was nothing . . . She just disappeared. Do you understand?"

"You are quite sure she is the one in the photograph?"

"Positive."

"What was she like?"

"She was very beautiful. The pictures don't do her justice. They're very poor quality."

"Yes, but I mean, what can you tell me about her?"

"I know she was a dancer. Folk dances, traditional Romanian dances."

"Anything else?"

"We didn't talk all that much. Apart from anything else, there was the language problem. She seemed to me a decent young woman, one who genuinely wanted to make a new life for herself, to lift herself out of poverty. Maybe a family . . ."

Soneri listened as though he had just gulped down a cup of boiling hot coffee. In every victim he found the frustrations of all human affairs, and for this reason he always felt close to them. The compassion he felt was an emotion which surpassed individual circumstances, but it was not so in this case, where there was something personal involved.

"If I knew where she was, I could offer her some assistance," the woman murmured.

"I'd like to know that too," Soneri said, leaping to his feet with one of those sudden movements of his. There were no more questions to ask, but he was left with a vague, insidious sense of foreboding.

Serena Robutti too rose quickly to her feet. "I hope what I've told you will not have implications . . . you know, for my work."

The commissario made a reassuring gesture. "All you've told me is that you don't know which clubs she frequented but she enjoyed dancing. It's something to go on."

"I don't think she went to discotheques. As I said, she did folk dancing. Gypsy dances, the gypsy tradition."

The interview ended on that note. Soneri shook her hand and watched her walk along the corridor without a backward glance. He went into his office and scribbled the name on a piece of paper which he handed to Juvara. "See if your friends in Bucharest can help."

Immediately afterwards, he dialled Angela's number but again without success. At that point, the unease he had felt shortly before changed into apprehension and then into fear – not the sort of fear which causes a surge of adrenalin, but one which burrows into the innards, like a worm under the skin. Angela was his security, the nail in the wall which keeps a person attached to life but which all of a sudden gives way. He wanted to talk to her, but had no idea where she was. The telephone in her home rang out, and after each futile attempt, the commissario felt himself gasping for breath in a hostile absence denser than water. He thought of her as though she was already far off, another possibility of life snatched away. This time, however, it was not the same as with Ada. Now he was no longer young, and starting out afresh would be much more difficult. His time was running out.

He decided to concentrate exclusively on the investigation, and left to go to the car park at the sports ground, which would already be packed with cars, vans and stalls and buzzing with unknown languages in a chorus reminiscent of a dirge or a lament. The sound seemed to him like life with its thousand faces or the many indispensable little illusions which coaxed it incessantly forward. At that point, desperate to shake off his disenchantment, he did not hesitate to plunge in head first.

7

THEY HAD TAKEN over the furthest part of the car park, making themselves almost invisible from the street. The Council turned a blind eye to the occupation because in the dead of night the foreigners did not bother anyone. Their trucks were lined up as if on a permanent campsite. One row marked the external border, closing off the area destined for the market, while inside it the various vehicles left free the passageways and a little clearing in the centre. Shrouded in mist, well away from the lamp posts in the car park, that little clandestine, extra-territorial community lived in semi-darkness. Some stalls stocked products newly arrived from Romania, while packages, perhaps even including unauthorised passengers, were loaded and unloaded from the trucks. It seemed impossible to recognise anyone in that faint light, but the whole operation was carried out as though in bright daylight. People greeted each other or shouted from a distance, and Soneri thought back to the times in the countryside where he was born when people endured the long, dark winter nights, or when in summer compassionate darkness intervened to put a stop to labour.

In the midst of the general bustle, he stopped to light his cigar. Pasquariello had been right. A sense of community was still alive there, and not only because some of the women were dressed in traditional costume and seemed to view the gathering as a sort of feast day for their patron saint. The commissario allowed himself to be carried away by the crowd swarming about him, but then quite suddenly the scene was lit up. A small stage had been erected in the centre of the market where a generator produced energy for half a dozen spotlights and for some amplifiers which were blaring out music of a vaguely eastern character. The lights in the centre and the trucks drawn up in a circle to close off the vital core of the community reminded him of the camps set up on the immense, snow-covered plains by earlier generations, arranging their wagons in a circle as defence and tending the fire to keep wolves at bay. That too represented an ancient link, never completely broken, redolent of long, silent journeys which saw fathers and sons shoulder to shoulder. On the stage, a few girls in costume were dancing, while about thirty spectators watched and applauded.

Soneri remembered that Ines had been a dancer so it seemed natural to ask about her. A man eyed him with evident distrust and without speaking a word pointed him in the direction of a corpulent figure standing on his own, keeping them under observation. The commissario went over to him. "I'm looking for Ines."

"Ines?"

"Iliescu."

"She's gone to Craiova."

"But she was here."

The man replied without looking Soneri in the face, never taking his eye off the stage. "Comes and goes. Many here like that."

"Anyone here know her well?"

"Everybody here know. All from Romania. Ask Roman. He make journeys, there and back."

The commissario moved away from that spot which was as bright as a hearth and plunged once more into the semi-darkness of the market. Roman's somewhat battered coach had seats for about forty people and he himself, in the midst of the ceaseless toing and froing all around, was engaged in negotiations with a family over a trip they wished to make. Goods from Romania were being unloaded and others – refrigerators, ovens, stoves, washing machines and packages containing various items – loaded in their place. The man overseeing the operation recorded everything in a notebook. Each item had a name and a destination, and only when it was loaded or unloaded did bargaining over the price take place. Nearby, women were queuing up at a stall selling Romanian foodstuffs.

The name Ines was known to Roman. "I took her to Craiova two weeks ago," he explained in reasonable Italian. "She stands out in my memory because she was so pretty."

"And she hasn't returned to Italy?"

"Who could say? There are so many ways to come and go. Apart from the established companies, there are lots of others. Here alone there are four. Anyway, I have not seen either her or her sister for at least two months."

"She has a sister?"

"She's pretty as well. Just one year between them."

"Ines used to dance . . ." Soneri went on, pointing over to the performance area stage behind him, nothing more than a spot of fading light.

"Yes, both did. But not in places like this," the man explained, hinting that their aims were higher.

"Where?"

The other became guarded, making the commissario realise he had gone too far with this line of questioning, and that Roman might well have previous experience of police methods. He gave a shrug, but made no reply.

"Do you get a lot of work?" Soneri asked, to change the subject.

"I don't charge a lot. The big companies take nearly twice as much. If I don't get people on board, I take goods."

The commissario looked around at indistinguishable figures moving about between the trucks, loading and unloading.

"Everything there costs less than here," the man said, before hurrying off to attend to some business and disappearing into the darkness.

Soneri lit his cigar, deeply conscious of being an outsider. It was odd to feel a stranger in your own city, and yet the names being shouted out, the pronunciation of unfamiliar diphthongs, the clothes, the faces emerging unexpectedly from the darkness communicated his non-belonging. One solitude merged with a deeper solitude, both interrupted by a signal from his mobile. It was a text from Angela which said simply: *I am interviewing*: three words conveying coolness, distance and a profound sense of alienation.

Quite suddenly, the atmosphere grew more excited. A name was passed from mouth to mouth, a name initially strange to the commissario's ears, but which gained in clarity, like an echo becoming more precise as it was repeated: "Gortan, Gortan . . ." At that moment, the headlights of a black B.M.W. shone on the vehicles and shortly afterwards a portly figure, accompanied by a woman who looked much younger than him, got out.

Soneri moved aside as lights were switched on near one of the vehicles. A decidedly suspicious looking individual, who had the look of a pimp with his favourite at his side, stepped forward. Six or so lackeys cleared a path for him, while several people hung about waiting to be received. He was plainly someone who had made his fortune, who now dispensed favours or work, and he was perhaps the most pitiless and ruthless of them all, Soneri thought, as he watched him pass in front of him, making his way towards the coach where he would receive the petitioners. The illusion of a happy community evaporated on the instant. In that area of mist he witnessed yet again all the familiar ways of mankind, but as he was falling prey to uncomfortable reflections, his telephone rang.

"Commissario, that Ines, she's not in the country now," Juvara said, with unaccustomed abruptness.

"I know. There's somebody here who says he took her back to Craiova about two months ago."

"Here where?"

"In the car park between the sports ground and the hypermarket, where the Romanians meet up once a week. They pick up some things here and send others off to their own country. They eat, dance, look for work and do deals. They reconstruct their own lives and then go their own way again. It's the destiny of all of us, isn't it?"

Not for the first time, Juvara was left baffled. "But if this Ines isn't here, who was the old man coming to look for?"

"I've been wondering that myself. Why do you think I'm taking an interest in this case?"

"Commissario, I cannot . . ." Juvara stuttered.

"For the reason that I believe in coincidences. On the one hand, a guy makes a hash of fleeing from the gypsy travellers' camp, on the other there's an old man who dies while searching . . . Behind every fact there is a certain scenario, and it's up to us to find out if the principal actors are not by some chance the same."

The inspector remained silent, so the commissario went

on: "Ines had a sister who was one year younger or older, I don't know which. The easiest thing is to believe that this sister passed herself off as Ines, and vice versa. You know how many immigrants take on multiple identities."

"I've found a colleague in Bucharest who speaks good English. I'll see if I can get him to explain this sister to me."

"Call someone in Craiova as well. The family comes from there." As Juvara was hanging up, Soneri added, "And try to trace that photographer, Dimitriescu. If he's not just a paparazzo who does snaps at weddings, maybe he can speak English as well."

The lights on the coach had been switched on, and the boss and his favourite were surrounded by people hanging around him like servants. The two were drinking calmly, while a group of people stood nearby, waiting.

The commissario turned away, his path taking him past fold-down tables placed alongside vans in which people were eating standing up and warding off the damp weather with wine. When he came to the clearing, the mist confused him and he was unable to find his bearings. He decided to follow the white lines of the car park. At intervals, a lamp post would light up a few metres around it, giving the mist a strange colour. A stronger light made him believe he was near the road, but instead of the roar of traffic he heard people talking and occasionally raising their voices. He walked across a flower bed and found himself at the back of the hypermarket, where a cluster of desperate people were rummaging in the dustbins in search of something to eat. Two had climbed inside the bins and were passing stuff out to others who added it to a pile on the ground, while others again divided it up and put it into old wheeled suitcases.

Soneri thought he made out a familiar figure standing on his own, and as he drew near he recognised Sbarazza, wearing an overcoat which was long out of fashion. "Destiny brings us face to face frequently," Sbarazza said.

"It is less elegant here than in the *Milord*."

"Undoubtedly, but here you are more sure of getting what you're looking for. Recently, the *Milord* has been very crowded and it's not easy to find the opportunity to . . . but here, there's always something to eat."

"But it's all refuse," Soneri said.

"No doubt, otherwise it would hardly be here, would it?" Sbarazza said with a little laugh. "But that is not the same as saying it's not edible. The things here are the same as products displayed on the shelves, but they have ceased to be products."

Soneri looked at him in bewilderment, drew in a deep breath but said nothing.

"Once there was no difference between food and products. Something could either be eaten or not. Not anymore. You see those tins of tuna fish with a dent in them? They are food but not products. No-one would buy them. Just as no-one would buy those packets of biscuits with a tear in the packaging, or those bags of over-ripe fruit, the blackening bananas, those lettuce leaves which would wither a little at the tips overnight, or even the confectionery past its sell-by date but still excellent. That is our good fortune," he said, pointing to the group of the destitute.

Some were already on their way, dragging their wheeled cases behind them. One came over to Sbarazza and presented him with a full holdall. He addressed him with the utmost respect: "Marchese, this is your share."

Sbarazza thanked him with a solemn gesture worthy of his ancient station. He spoke to Soneri in a whisper. "Tonight the Romanians are on the prowl, so we must move fast, otherwise they'll come and chase us off."

"You mean that they too . . ." Soneri said, indicating the dustbins.

"You can smell food a long way off when you're hungry. I had to learn quickly, but there's enough in there for everybody. You've no idea how much food is thrown away – enough to feed an army. That lot want to chase us because they'll sell off anything they can get hold of. There's no longer any solidarity among the poor. They'd cut your throat for a tin of mackerel."

Just then a shout was heard in the mist. "They're coming," he said in alarm, pushing his case aside. About twenty Romanians made for the dustbins and began emptying them.

"They'll have the night patrols down on us, and sooner or later we'll all be sent packing. The management of the hypermarket doesn't want us to take their refuse."

"Why?"

"This might surprise you, but I think we're upsetting their delicate consciences. It's a co-operative, you see. For them it's a worry to think there are people who have nothing to eat after they issued a guarantee of a full stomach for every person. They've turned into businessmen, but they still preach solidarity. In addition, they don't want to admit to themselves that they waste food, because they still remember what poverty means. Better to pretend it's all gone bad and then everybody's happy. We remind them of a mortal sin."

"You've got your share, so you've no need to go scrabbling about . . ." Soneri pointed out to him.

"I carry out other tasks. Let me put it this way: I look after the interests of these unfortunates and attend to bureaucratic procedures where knowledge, expertise and competence are indispensable. I am talking about subsidies, assistance, hospital appointments, medicines . . . They come to me and I make sure they're treated the same as everybody else. This also helps me to keep alive the memory of what I used to be. Fortunately, in the eyes of many functionaries I am still the Marchese, and my image is intact. None of them knows that I come here to rummage through rubbish and that in order to eat I employ elegant stratagems, like at the *Milord*. They see me as a philanthropist, someone who looks after his fellow man, a charitable person. That way I am taken for a wealthy man and a good Christian as well." Sbarazza gave a little laugh.

"Appearances are what counts," Soneri said. "Or rather, appearances are everything. At least you conduct yourself with class."

"These poor souls don't even have a piece of dirty floor to sleep on, ever since these foreigners turned up here. Young people with knives. For a bed in a dormitory, they wouldn't hesitate to stick it in your belly."

They were walking round the perimeter of the hyper-market, keeping close to the wall. When they reached the road they said goodnight, and Sbarazza, pulling his case behind him, disappeared in the mist.

The commissario continued towards the city centre, but even when he had reached Via d'Azeglio he had not managed to shake off the feeling of alienation which had come over him in the car park. He tried to free himself of it by telephoning Juvara. "The girl in the photograph is not Ines. It must be her sister," he said, with no preliminaries. He was following a hunch, but it was a hypothesis well-grounded in solid clues.

"I heard again from our colleague in Romania," Juvara said. "He has e-mailed the photograph to that Dimitriescu and has promised to get back to me."

"Want to bet he recognises the sister?" the commissario forecast, ending the call abruptly. At that point, a sudden recognition unleashed a rush of nostalgia which helped him shake off the feeling of alienation which had gripped him a short time previously. He was opposite *Latteria Numero 51*, one of the few of its type left in the city and once an afford-able meeting place for hard-up students: *caffelatte* and politics, *malvasia* and revolution. For the last couple of days, he had been resisting the temptation to seek out that lost Neverland which had been his hope as a young man, but now in front of the latteria he gave in. From the moment he pushed open the glass door with its over-embellished handle, he felt he was back home, all the more so when he saw Jole, now very old, behind the bar, and Libero Manicardi, nick-named "Picelli" after the historical hero of the barricades, seated at his table. An inflexible theorist who could tie even himself up in knots, Picelli represented that ideal mix of anarchism and communism which had set the city alight in the years leading up to the '70s. He had been a school friend of the commissario and they had maintained an intermittent friendship in the intervals between one journey and the next.

"Franco," he cried out on seeing him. He was one of the few who called Soneri by his Christian name.

They embraced under the delighted, tired eyes of Jole. "There's more chance of winning the pools than of bumping into you," the commissario said.

They took a seat and stared intently at each other like two lovers. Both wore a sad smile as each noticed how the other had aged. Libero was just back from a trip to Cuba, but he had abandoned all dreams of socialist paradises to come. He had moved from the revolutionary phase to oriental meditation and on to Latin American rebelliousness before ending up in a mood of cynical detachment from the world. He had no time for Castro – everything was going to the dogs.

"The only consolation is love," Picelli declared, raising his glass. "I'm with a woman who is twenty years younger than me, and it's like going back in time."

Soneri looked him up and down. The pockmarked face of a man who had lived life to the full, the long, nearly white hair still hanging down his neck, the clear eyes which shone against the leathery skin – all these things must have fascinated young women who in all likelihood saw in him a comic-strip hero.

"I am losing even that," Soneri said.

Picelli's face darkened. "That's serious, Franco. Very serious. Keep a glimmer of life open. And if something closes it down, open another one. We're not so old that we can't manage that."

"No, we're not, but at our age, after so many disappointments, maybe you don't believe in fairy tales anymore."

"When that happens, we really are old. It'd be as well to put an end to it all. What are you supposed to do in the world? Better a bullet in the head."

"I've even got a gun." Soneri laughed.

"When I think back to school days, to our scrapes with Fascists and teachers, you remember? If I had to draw up a balance sheet, I'd have to bring the books to the court. There's nothing left. Take a look at politics nowadays: two great bundles of what? Left and Right think the same way. One conformist line of thought with a ban on dissent and a mass of drivellers fucking about, looking forward to the weekend."

Soneri looked over at Jole getting on serenely with her own business: made of sterner stuff, the last generation with balls, a generation which had endured poverty and had lived during the war in close proximity to death. To people like that, even these vacuous years must seem bearable.

"And don't you dream of the weekend?"

"I have other problems. I'm in a relationship with a woman who wants to get married and have children. She's in her early thirties, she's religious and she's thinking of coming to live with me. I suppose she sees me as a conquest, not least because I've told her I'm an atheist and she wants to convert me."

"And has she?"

"I'm in love and that's more than enough. Everything else is bullshit. With her, I've at last escaped from loneliness, something I tried to do for years with my comrades, but with them I never managed to share anything that was genuinely me." Picelli got to his feet with a dramatic expression on his face. "Franco, the fact is no-one ever believed, really, deeply believed. The majority only wanted to do their own thing."

"Well, I always did mine, I always went my own way. You know how I cannot abide the herd."

"I always used to criticise you for that, and I cut you off for a while, but you were right to keep your distance."

"Anyway, here we are empty-handed, more than half our lives gone by and a sense of despair gripping us by the balls," the commissario summed up, looking out at the mist thickening in Via d'Azeglio.

Inside the latteria, he felt wrapped in a blanket as comforting as a mother's embrace. Outside, loneliness lay in wait. That was the root of his sense of alienation, and without the presence of Angela it would be total. Picelli had told him that there was nothing else: two souls seeking each other, feeling fully alive only when together in that ancient, arcane activity of striving to lose the self by clinging tightly to another person. He jumped to his feet as though galvanised by a new consciousness. He said goodbye to Picelli and did not turn back. He did not know if he would see him again. Only Jole understood it all, because she was in the habit of viewing the world and the destiny of the people in it without regret.

8

CONFIRMATION ARRIVED HALF an hour later. The girl in the photograph was not Ines but her sister Nina. "The Immigration Bureau checked the data supplied by the Ministry as well, and it turns out that more than one residence permit has been issued in the name of Ines in the last two years," Juvara called to inform him. He did not go any further, intimidated by Soneri's silence.

"Go on," the commissario said.

"In spite of having received these permits, Ines remained in Romania."

"So the old man on the bus was coming in search of Nina. But what's Ines up to?"

"From what I could gather, she works in clubs for foreigners in Bucharest. My police contact was a bit vague on this point, but you know what westerners are after in Eastern European night clubs. Ines is very pretty."

Angela came back into Soneri's mind and he felt a pang of anxiety over the time that had elapsed since he had last heard from her. He went into his pocket to find the Romanian girl's mobile number on the slip of paper Signora Robutti had given him.

"Nina doesn't use this number any more," the commissario said, in dictation mode. "I've tried several times, but the phone always rings out. See if you can find some lead from the record of calls."

He rang off and continued on his way to the courthouse. He had decided to wait for Angela to come out, but he had to be careful not to bump into some lawyer or magistrate who might recognise him, such as Dottoressa Marcotti who was in charge of the case of the girl whose body had been burned. What if Angela were to come out with the other man? Every time he thought of it, he felt unwell and keen to hear her voice, but he was irked by the telephone ringing out.

Having sent a couple of texts from which came no reply, he decided to wait a few hours under the arches or in a doorway. All the while, the mist sailed heedlessly past at walking pace. He felt ridiculous and guilty at the same time, ridiculous for harbouring the thought that at her time of life a woman like Angela could change her mind after some attempt to court her, guilty because he was shadowing her instead of dealing with the case of the dead girl. In addition, all this was taking place in the vicinity of the court to which he was answerable. Fortunately, it was nine o'clock, the city seemed asleep and everyone was free to spend their after-dinner time as they pleased.

He hung about for two hours, walking up and down the deserted lanes which were as silent as a graveyard. Towards eleven o'clock, the doors of the courthouse opened and a group of people, among whom he recognised Angela, the magistrate and a lawyer, emerged. The last two moved off in the direction of Piazzale Boito, while Angela and another man turned into Vicolo Politi, heading in the direction of Via Farini. That had to be him.

Soneri followed them until he saw them go into a wine bar. He knew he could not afford to do anything stupid since that would definitively compromise everything. He also knew he would not be able to do nothing, so his pursuit ended at that point, with him feeling so lost that he sought the protection of his own house, the only place that still had a familiar feel for him. He imagined her in bed with that man, or in the back seat of a car on a country road. He burst out laughing at himself, fearing that he was losing all his dignity, and this thought allowed impotent rage to take over from irony.

Angela appeared unexpectedly, as though ambushing him. Soneri had fallen asleep on a sofa and awoke to find her bending over him. He did not understand a word she was saying, but her voice was so gentle that the commissario forgot the scene he had witnessed. When he came round fully, he realised he was cold and ached all over.

"Come to bed," she whispered, taking him by the hand.

Soneri followed her, undressed and pulled the covers over him. She joined him almost immediately and took the initiative, almost assaulting him. The commissario's every sense was delightfully aroused, even if he still failed to understand, but when she crawled on top of him he suppressed all doubt and let himself go. Afterwards, as he relished the ardour they had shared, his eyes met those of Angela a few centimetres away on the pillow.

"Is this a wish that it would never end?" he asked, thinking more of himself than of his partner.

"Do you think it can produce these miracles?" she laughed.

"Sometimes partings can be very intense."

Angela shook her head but said nothing.

Soneri felt desperately in need of some confirmation. He wanted reassurance. He felt that something had burst inside him and was haemorrhaging, leaving him shaking with fear.

"Tell me what you want," he said finally. "Even if it will be terrible for me, I must know. I can't live with this uncertainty."

"If I were sure of what I want, I'd tell you, but I'm all mixed up. I need to understand."

"Whether to stay with me or with your other man?"

"I can't just live my life with someone as part of a settled routine. I'm trying to make out how strong the relationship between us really is, but I can only do that by questioning it. It's what you do when you're on a case and you get an idea in your head. You start to attack it, so as to understand. If it stands up, it means it's well grounded."

He knew well the methods of his woman. He had seen her too often at work in court and that made him fear the worst. "This is not a police investigation. Rationality has nothing to do with emotions. There is no way of measuring how unwell a person is, nor do I find it at all reassuring to hear that you're conducting a test."

She showed her awareness of what he meant by moving her head on the pillow. "I know. I'm asking you to live with uncertainty, to put up with my doubts, even if it's hard for you. It is for me too. After all, you ought to be used to the precarious nature of convictions, given the work you do."

"Exactly, and I've had enough of it. I'd like to have something solid in a world which is too liquid. I thought that you at least were a fixed point. Just today I met Picelli – remember him? I felt sorry for him. He's thrown everything up – him, the man who was intransigence made flesh. He's fallen in love with a thirty-something Catholic woman who wants to have children."

Angela shook her head in astonishment.

"He told me that emotions are one of the few things that matter. What's left? Every single thing that your head can think passes, but that obscure cluster of sensations that we call emotions endures. Maybe precisely because our heads can't really understand a thing about friendship, love, art . . ."

"He's not far wrong," Angela murmured.

"Maybe not, but we're running the risk of losing them," Soneri said, hoping that at that very second she would come back at him and say, no, that's not right, but she did not utter a word.

Both remained silent, thoughtful, heads on the same pillow.

The commissario broke the silence with a sudden outburst. "There's no point whining. Precariousness is the human condition. The difference is that very few people recognise it and the majority go blithely on." Anger had taken over from sadness, as it had outside the wine bar.

"But it's you I want. I am certain of this, if of nothing else," she said.

Soneri felt mildly relieved, and found the strength to go on asking questions. He was always enquiring, and for this reason it was often he who identified the villain, in police affairs as in life.

"Tell me if you've been to bed with him."

Angela did not reply. She stared at him seriously, with vacant eyes, and although not another word was spoken the commissario understood. It had never crossed his mind that she could hurt him so deeply. His phantoms took concrete shape and rubbed explosively against his subconscious and all it contained. His derailed thoughts careered off the tracks of rationality, and ran so completely out of his control as to leave him ashamed. He felt on the point of insanity. All the instruments he customarily employed to gauge things were out of kilter. Nothing could contain his pain or despair, nothing could save him from this headlong plunge into the void. All attempt at explanation, all dialogue would have been useless, and so the only partial antidote was a wordless caress from Angela. Her hand stroked his cheek, his neck, ran along his chest, washing away the pain for a few seconds.

"It has happened twice," she said after a few minutes' silence, "and perhaps will not happen again."

That "perhaps" only heightened Soneri's anguish. Angela did not dispel the ambiguity which was minute by minute eating away at him. They were engaged in an ongoing game of statement and denial and it was wreaking havoc on him.

He wandered mentally in a swamp of thoughts, then gave in. There was no point in seeking any reassurance from Angela as she herself was undecided. He looked at her without recognising her. For the first time, she appeared to him inscrutable, a stranger, and that was the most wounding sensation of all.

"You like that man, you find him attractive and perhaps he's going to be your future." Soneri sat up, yelling in fury.

She tried to keep him beside her on the pillow, but only managed to make him turn slightly to one side. "He's good-looking and clever, but you're more important. He knows nothing about the bonds between us, nor have I ever spoken about them. First and foremost there's you and me, and it will be you and I who will make any decisions," she said, with pitiless clarity.

The commissario sat with his back propped against the headboard. The investigation had reached its finale, the confession had been full and detailed, but the heaviest sentence would fall on him. He realised he had been at fault in having taken their relationship too much for granted, or perhaps, as Picelli had put it, for never having been able to get away from himself and open up to other people. He felt a lump in his throat which would not be removed by any words but only by the language of the body. He drew close to her, and they embraced, holding tightly to each other to maintain some equilibrium.

In spite of everything, he felt physically better when he left the house. He had not slept much and a multitude of thoughts were buzzing about in his head, but there was a spring in his step and in the mist which still enveloped the city he was breathing more easily. Juvara was a great believer in biorhythms, and perhaps he was right, or perhaps the body simply makes up its own mind when to respond to life and let everything else take care of itself, including the psyche.

In the police station, he found the record of the calls made by Nina. There was nothing that stood out: radio taxis, take-away pizzas, Signora Robutti, a car-hire firm and a beauty salon. The incoming calls were of greater interest. The list took up a whole page and there were some recurrent numbers.

"In great demand . . ." Soneri commented.

"They all say she was very pretty," Juvara said. "But not altogether in the clear," he added after a pause.

The commissario threw a questioning look at him.

"I've just been told she was wanted in Romania for a series of car thefts, but the impression is that she was small fry, used as cover for somebody or other."

"Have you made a fresh check on the missing persons list?" Soneri asked, changing the subject and referring to the case of the burned body.

"Nothing doing there. The forensic squad are engaged on a reconstruction of the face to produce a reliable identikit." He paused for a few moments, and then went on, "Do you know what criminologists say about bodies which have been set on fire?"

Soneri took the cigar from his mouth and shook his head.

"That normally they're people the murderer knew and with whom they had a relationship."

"A story, a love story . . ." Soneri said, accidentally plunging back into the pit of his discontent.

"Either that or a family connection."

For a moment Angela came back into his mind and he found himself overcome by feelings of rancour. He would have liked both to embrace her and get away from her. However, someone had wanted to eliminate the girl forever and destroy her with fire. Nothing had clear outlines in her case. It was a game of appearance and reality, an elusive dance of smoky figures or, better, of misty figures, since the cloak of mist was as heavy as ever and continued to weigh down on the city. Soneri paced up and down the room under the startled gaze of the inspector who seemed on the point of making some pronouncement, but after a little time the commissario wheeled round and their eyes met. It was Juvara who broke the silence. "Listen, commissario, I have a suspicion that this Nina . . ."

". . . is the woman whose body was burned." Soneri completed the sentence.

"I might be wrong. Maybe we've connected the two stories too closely and ended up with one jumbled up with the other."

The commissario shook his head, and resumed observing the coming and going of patrols in the yard. He heaved a sigh. "I don't think so. Do you understand now why I was so taken with the story of the old man who died on the coach?"

"You have a nose for . . ."

"No, it's just that I'm a bit older than you."

"If that was all . . ."

"Spending a long time with criminals makes you understand humanity. You get to a stage where you believe that evil is so familiar because it dwells inside us without us noticing."

He turned round again to find Juvara staring at him dumbfounded. "You and I too might one day become aware that it's part of our being as well, and this awareness almost always dawns when the evil manifests itself. And by then it's too late."

The commissario moved away from the window and changed the subject. "We'll find out if Nina is the girl whose body was burned when we have the identikit. It's only a matter of hours."

The telephone rang and Soneri rushed to grab it. He still hoped it might be Angela, but was surprised to hear Pasquariello's voice. "We've been interrogating that Mariotto, the gypsy."

"What did he have to say?"

"He's still saying he fell and bumped his head, but nobody believes him, even if technically it can't be ruled out."

"What do you make of it?"

"The Romanian and Italian Romas didn't get on very well. There's been a series of thefts. In my opinion, scores are being settled, but if Mariotto doesn't speak, we'll never make any headway."

The conversation with Pasquariello was interrupted by the ringing of another telephone. The head of the flying squad rang off immediately with the words, "I'll keep in touch."

Once again, it was not Angela. Nanetti, who grasped the commissario's disappointment, made a joke of it: "It could've been worse. It might have been Capuozzo."

Soneri said: "No, it's not that. It's just that . . ."

"Do you think I don't know? At least you might work something out with Angela. I've lost everything, but I'm plodding on. Meanwhile I'm getting more interested in lingerie."

"You're not becoming one of those men who make a collection of knickers?"

"Who do you think I am? Listen, colleague, do you remember the label between her buttocks that was saved from the flames? Well, there's a shop in Via Garibaldi that stocks only one brand – that very one! Do you understand me?"

"You are telling me she did her shopping there . . ."

"It's not the only outlet for that kind of underwear, but on the balance of probabilities it's likely."

"Right then. Since you've become an expert, would you like to pay them a visit?"

"Are you afraid they might take you for some kind of pansy? I don't do investigations. My job is to come up with proof."

"It was a joke."

"You're getting on my nerves, commissario. I've been there. It's the widower's syndrome, a sort of rancour that keeps you well away from anything that smacks of femininity."

"I'm already a widower," Soneri replied bitterly.

"Sorry, I've touched a raw nerve."

The commissario's mind was elsewhere, in a dreamland where the past and the present overlap, with the irreversible loss of Ada and the probable loss of Angela already a part of the landscape. That was what growing old meant – seeing parts of yourself and parts of a shared life fade away. As he forced himself to focus on the crime, memories of his dead wife and his unborn son merged with the image of the girl, producing a fresh surge of indignation inside him.

"I'm grateful for this lead. I'll go round myself," he said, cutting short the conversation.

Nina provoked a whirlwind of emotions because she brought back the trauma of the loss of Ada and the sudden disruption of his whole life. This case was running disturbingly parallel to the life he had known. He was unsettled by the realisation that people's experiences were not so very different and could be superimposed one on top of the other. Not even a solitary soul like him could claim originality.

"What idea have you formed of Nina?" he asked Juvara.

The inspector had nothing to say. The commissario envied his detachment. He was young and could dodge putting awkward questions to himself. There was time enough for that, and in the meantime it was better to let him live.

"The photographer, Dimitriescu, told me she was very shy, and she regarded her good looks as a problem," Juvara said.

"He confirmed that the photographs were his?"

"Yes. He even remembers when he took them. The first one at the end of high school and the second a couple of years later."

"They seem two different people."

"The photographer had the impression she had changed her lifestyle, but he doesn't know anything else."

Soneri contemplated the photographs in silence, but he became aware of a level of frenetic activity in the yard outside that was hard to reconcile with the rhythms of life in a sleepy town like Parma. Instinctively he thought of Nina as a naïve girl who attracted attention because of her beauty. Perhaps they had duped her and she had ended up in dubious circles. She reminded him of the fate of dogs abandoned on the motorways, acquired as fluffy toys when they were puppies and tossed aside the first time they peed on the sofa.

"What's causing all this commotion?"

"The maniac. Some serial rapist on the loose. He's been prowling after women in public gardens, in doorways, in parks. He's already raped three. They say he's a foreigner. Musumeci's in charge."

"He won't be operating during the day, will he?" Soneri said, looking at the grey skies.

"The city's completely neurotic. People are talking about nothing else. The switchboard's jammed. They're seeing maniacs everywhere," the inspector said.

Soneri was surprised he had known nothing about it, and put it down to the state he was in. "It'll be the same as with the bulls," he muttered, "but this guy knows how to keep out of sight a bit better."

9

"SEEMS LIKE THEY'VE got him," Alceste announced, as he put a plate of *anolini in brodo* in front of the commissario.

"Got who?"

"What do you mean – got who? The sex maniac, obviously. An illegal immigrant, or so they say."

"So now the witch hunt gets underway once again," he mumbled to himself as he blew away the steam from the dish. He could sense the opening of the tiresome ritual enacted so many times before: the Right railing in shrill tones against immigrants, the Left asking people not to make a mountain out of every molehill and the Fascists threatening to get their clubs down from the attic. Reality was always elsewhere, the facts denied, and he would have to deal with the consequences.

At least he could still enjoy the consolations of the table, the one pleasure left to him apart from walking in the mist and sitting at home with a book on autumn evenings. Such thoughts were running through his mind as he gazed at the rings in the soup, but they were interrupted when he found Sbarazza standing before him. His gait was so silent and discreet that it was easy to miss his approach, even for a trained eye like the commissario's.

"Thank goodness you're here, otherwise I'd have gone

hungry. There's not one free table and there's a queue of people waiting." Three women had just got up from a table next to Soneri's, and Sbarazza reached out to pick up a plate with an almost untouched chop. Another agile movement and a half-full bottle was placed in front of the commissario.

"A *dolcetto di Ovada*. Not bad," Sbarazza said

Soneri looked around in embarrassment, but no-one seemed to have noticed.

"Don't worry, commissario. The important thing is to possess the right measure of self-confidence and nonchalance. When you have these attributes, even the most crass gesture will not arouse the slightest objection, because you need a bit of pluck to make a fuss, don't you? And in this place," he added, looking around the restaurant, "who do you think has such pluck?"

The commissario thought again of the girl whose body they had found, and wondered if she had been particularly plucky. "A rare commodity," he said. "Did you fancy one of the women sitting there?" he asked.

"Each woman draws us into another world. When all's said and done, that's what seduction consists of. We're given a glimpse of the missing part of ourselves."

"Very much missing," the commissario replied in a dull voice, thinking of his own situation.

"We always lack something or other. In my case, time is running out. The man out there who is assaulting women lacks a partner, but these are all insignificant and transient passions, like a man complaining of hunger while facing a firing squad."

His reasoning was delicate and light. Listening to him, Soneri drew some consolation from his words.

Sbarazza went on. "I don't envy you, you know. For someone who considers the absurdity of our life, it must be frustrating to have to reconstruct the actions of those who steal and kill. If we were to reflect a little, we would all be forced to be good and to weigh every act, but we are such profoundly irrational creatures, governed by the passions. Our animal side always prevails. The wise man is the one who resists the pull of the passions and ensures that the brain triumphs."

"If only it were that easy . . ." Soneri muttered. "Look at you with women."

"Purely intellectual caprice, aesthetic diversion. Age is of assistance here," he said with a wink. "I can say that because it was not always thus. I was a fiery youth, and that was my ruination, yet I'd do it all again. The passions, even if they toss you about this way and that, impel you forward. It's because of them that we keep ourselves active. They move everything forward, transforming the world, perhaps into a repugnant mess, but somewhere in that shambles there'll be the spring of continual competition towards an ill-defined future." Putting his face close to Soneri's, he went on: "Wisdom is something for old men. And never believe it's a conquest of time. It's merely the decay of the body."

Inside himself, Soneri felt heartened. Any unhappiness over Angela was a sign he was still alive. Two police cars with sirens squealing passed by and he decided Sbarazza was right. The world was moved by the passions.

"Have they got him?" Sbarazza said.

"Looks like it," the commissario replied without much conviction, and before Sbarazza could ask him anything else about the maniac on the loose, the commissario got up so quickly that he seemed to be running away.

Refreshed and consoled by this conversation, Soneri set off for the lingerie shop in Via Garibaldi. En route he called Juvara. "So then, they got their sex maniac."

"If only! They arrested a Moroccan, but he was freed two hours later because he'd nothing to do with it. He was quarrelling with his girlfriend and somebody decided he was assaulting her."

"Give me some background. When did all this start?"

"Yesterday evening, a woman was attacked in Via San Leonardo, and the description of the rapist fitted one given by another woman who'd been assaulted in Via Solferino two days ago. It was probably the same man who also sexually assaulted a girl in Via Toschi."

It was true. Instincts and passions were what motivated people, and when these exploded outside the confines of law, he had to take over. He could hear sirens in the mist as the city attempted to cope with the tension created in its innermost being by an insidious virus capable of spreading and striking randomly.

The owner of the shop he went into shortly afterwards must have felt herself threatened, judging by the wary eye she cast on Soneri. She relaxed only when he introduced himself.

"Is there a Romanian girl who comes here?" he said, showing her the photograph.

"Ines. Certainly. A wonderful person."

Evidently she mistook her for her sister.

"Does she buy her underwear here?"

"She is a very faithful client. If only I had more like her."

"What kind of thing does she buy?"

"Oh, all kinds. Unlike other clients of mine, she doesn't have one definite style. One day she might purchase a very girly, matching set with lace and frills, and then two days later she would walk out with a much plainer outfit. Sometimes she would choose very sexy, see-through lingerie, but at other times she would take articles more fit for a young girl, with little angels embroidered into it. She would go from top of the range to economy items. In other words, there are no fixed rules with her."

"One of a kind, you mean," Soneri said, trying to make sense of what the woman was telling him.

"In general my clients have precise tastes and always choose the same type of article. Most times I get it right when I interpret their wants, but with Ines . . . in addition . . . such a beautiful young woman. I'm sure men go crazy over a girl like her."

"Did she ever come with a man?"

"Women never buy lingerie in the company of men, if for no other reason than not to spoil the surprise," she said flirtatiously. "However, now I think of it, I was once struck by seeing Ines get out of a dark car. There was a man at the wheel, but he stayed in the car and I didn't see his face."

"Do you remember what make of car it was?"

"I'm sorry, but I can't help you there. All I saw was a horse design on one side."

The commissario remembered Manservisi's account. It must have been the same sticker. "Do you have any idea where she lives?"

"Nearby, in Via Cavallotti, but I don't know the number. She didn't speak much about herself, and if the conversation turned to her, she would change the subject."

The commissario moved towards the door, and the woman followed him.

"Will you get him?" she asked apprehensively.

He looked at her generous figure, her enormous calves, her feet spilling out of her shoes and decided that she ran no risk of being assaulted. He shrugged and walked away.

A hundred metres further on he turned into Via Cavallotti, which in mid afternoon was deserted. He started peering at the nameplates like a postman on his first round, but there were so many names missing and those which were there belonged mainly to immigrants – Arabs, Moldovans, Russians, Albanians and Indians. Read in haste from top to bottom, the names sounded like the morning roll call in the Foreign Legion. At number 12, in a recently renovated block of flats, there were no names, only the numbers of the individual flats: 1/1, 1/2, etc. Instinctively he believed that Nina lived there, a belief suggested by the air of de luxe mystery hovering about the block and by its defensive, forbidding chestnut door with shining copper rings. He was tempted to go in, but elected first to obtain a search warrant from the magistrate Marcotti, who still knew nothing of his belief that Nina and the girl burned by the roadside were one and the same, with all that that involved.

The light was fading under the advancing front of mist enveloping one side of Via Garibaldi and wafting around the arches of the Pilotta as though a river had suddenly evaporated and was gushing down from the parapets. The sky darkened as if it had been coloured by the stroke of a brush and the whole city was plunged into shadow. He dialled Angela's number once more, but all he got was the voicemail. Seconds later, his mobile rang and he answered as quickly as a sprinter getting off the blocks.

"I've disappointed you yet again," Nanetti teased.

"Cut it out," Soneri said.

"You're waiting for a call, I know."

The commissario muttered something, but could not conceal his impatience. His colleague accompanied him along a street he had never liked. Like a tourist guide, he took note of every stage of the walk. He could not get Angela out of his mind, and still wanted her. "Anything new?" he said.

"We have the girl's identikit and she's very like the one in the photograph. I'd say there's no doubt," Nanetti said.

"I'll send Juvara to visit Signora Robutti and the haber-dasher who sold Nina her underwear to see if she recognises her."

"Haberdasher! The way you speak you'd think we were still in the Fifties. The place is called Intim Shop and it sells lingerie, not underwear. And it's not even correct to call it a shop. Where have you been all these years? It's a boutique!"

"Fuck off!" Soneri said. The air all around was filled with the sound of sirens. He snapped shut the mobile without saying goodbye as he watched a police car screech to a halt under an ancient plane tree in Piazzale della Pace. Esposito jumped out as though he were in an American gangster movie and raced over the grass in the direction of the foun-tain and the monument to Verdi. The commissario followed him, but after a few strides he realised how seriously unfit he was. The soles of his shoes slipped on the damp grass, and he lost ground with every step he took. The extra kilos made him almost bend double as he ran, but in spite of that after a few seconds he caught up with Esposito, who was himself out of breath and panting.

"Did you see him?" Esposito managed to gasp.

"Who was I supposed to see? I was coming after you."

"The bloody bastard," Esposito swore. Other policemen emerged from the mist. "There was a call to say that the maniac had been sighted harassing some poor girl."

"Ah well, if you don't slim down a bit, the only criminals you'll catch will be the lame ones. I gave you a hundred metres' start on a three-hundred-metre stretch."

"Hey, commissario, as if this life was not shitty enough, now you want me to stop eating."

In the meantime, a multitude of the curious had gathered round but they quickly showed their disappointment. "It's time you got this dirty Moroccan," yelled a heavily made-up woman with a crocodile skin handbag. Moroccans had become the whipping boys for all misdeeds committed by incomers.

"There's a psychosis abroad, and it's spreading," Esposito was heard groaning as he walked over to his car. "Thank God I'm not on night duty. Everybody sees monsters when the lights go down."

The two men stood in silence in the thick mist, getting their breath back.

"Alright, commissario. The fun's over," Esposito said as he got into the car and switched on the engine. At that moment Soneri's mobile rang, but he was once again disappointed when Juvara's voice came on. "Have you heard about the identikit?"

"Nanetti told me. Will you go over to Signora Robutti's for an official identification?"

"O.K., but I wanted to inform you that we have the details of the calls made to Nina."

"Recognise any?"

"There are lots of them, nearly all male."

"There's a surprise!"

"I mean, they're from people who don't seem to be the same age as her, mature men."

"Does it give their ages on the printout?"

"No, but if there's a lawyer or accountant who's got his own office, he can't be all that young."

"Are they all like that?"

"One phone number belongs to a company. I looked it up on the internet and I see it's a goldsmith's. It produces and deals in top-of-the-range items."

"Leave everything on my desk. I'll be there shortly and I'll have a look."

He felt that things were starting to come together, nothing that could be proved, just impressions, feelings and

window as he made his way through a group of excited officers. His calm stood out in the midst of all the euphoria.

He bumped into Sbarazza outside the *Milord*. "Nothing doing today." He shook his head and indicated the crowded restaurant. "There's an exhibition of Parmigianino's works on, but at this time of day the stomach takes priority over culture."

"That's very human," Soneri smiled. "Can I invite you for some salame and *torta fritta* at the wine bar down the street?"

As they walked towards it, the commissario was struck by the thought that this bar, a modern imitation of an old-style osteria, was becoming an obsession for him and he was continually on the lookout for excuses to go there. On this occasion there was no sign of the person he feared meeting, so he was able to relax. Sbarazza was a man who exuded good humour.

"You are one of the few who knows I am a tramp," he said, with the air of a man sharing a confidence. "I am known in this city as the 'Marchese'. Everyone respects me and they even raise their hats to me. If they knew how I really live, they wouldn't give me a second glance. They would despise me because here where everything is supposed to sparkle, they've no time for losers. But I haven't lost, on the contrary! They're the losers. I have won."

Soneri looked at him with a smile. Sbarazza seemed to him sincere as only those who have attained a high level of indifference to convention can be. "I imagine you feel extremely free – much more than previously, I mean."

"I am afraid of nothing. I am a true revolutionary. I try to live the life the priests preach, and since they avoid practising themselves, I do it for them. If you think about it, Christ was the greatest revolutionary who has ever appeared on this earth. A scandalous, unbearable creature, much more so than the communists, don't you think?"

"Do you suppose that's why they put him on a cross?"

"If we set theology aside, that's exactly why, no question about it. Just imagine what they'd do with him today. They'd call him an extremist, a fanatic, a troublemaker, and they'd use crueller means than nails to crucify him. They'd treat him like a madman, sneer at his preaching and ignore him. And that's what they'd do to me too if I didn't have this veneer of nobility to fool them. If I were a poor man I wouldn't be granted a permit to live in this town, but I am the 'Marchese'. It's like the label on certain products. They are valueless, deplorable, but they have the brand name and so they cost a lot. Or rather, they do have a value. That's the whole difference – in other words, nothing."

He spoke with no rancour and with an offhand casualness which revealed an enviable serenity.

"They all struggle for this nothing," Soneri said, looking around him at the tables of office-workers, lawyers and accountants, all in jacket and tie, all as indistinguishable from each other as pieces of macaroni churned out from the same processor.

"This is what we've become. You could be a stinking cesspit of a person, but the important thing is to keep up appearances." Sbarazza chuckled, making the commissario wonder whether appearances, the paradoxical appearances of life, amused him as much as any operetta. "And then this city, full of unreconstructed vermin strolling about bedecked in clothes worth a king's ransom, all to cover up their own vulgarity."

Soneri entertained the malicious thought that his rival

belonged to that caste. "You've got to make allowances. Their fathers shovelled shit in stables and they look on this past with shame. They do all they can to live it down."

"A big 4×4 with leather interior is the best remedy against the nightmares of the past, preferably with a bull bar, presumably to ensure defence against cows and their shit. I who had a father who was never short of money or women have been less fortunate," Sbarazza added, in another of his paradoxes. "I have discovered that what others envied in us was in reality the sentence we were serving. It is bad not to have wishes. The poor people I work with have many very human wishes: food, shelter, protection from the cold, surviving the slings and arrows. Everything ties them to the things which are of real importance, and sweeps away all that is superfluous. In this context, it does not take long to rediscover what is real in life. It has happened to me and each time I seem to be reborn. I look at all these people and laugh," he declared with a sweeping gesture, "because I behave like a mask and live on what they throw away. Then I turn up at the clubs with my aristocratic manners and enchant them as much as the pied piper. Believe me, that is real enjoyment − a fancy-dress ball, nothingness."

Soneri found this speech tragic. Unlike Sbarazza, he could not find anything exhilarating in the frivolity of life.

"There's no easy way out," Sbarazza went on. "You're either a believer, and in that case this world and all that's in it is short-term and of little importance, or else you're a non-believer and you'll arrive at the same conclusion, because nothing has any sense. Know what I've decided? To be a non-believing, good Christian. If there is someone up there, I'll take my chance on grace being doled out. It's better than being a hypocrite."

"You're not short of practical sense. You've been given a thorough grounding in prudence by poor people."

"That's not all. Finding a purpose in other people is the only way to have a role in life and to feel yourself loved. When all's said and done, is that not what we all want, to feel loved, ever since we were babies and screamed for our mother's breast and the soothing consolations of her embrace? It doesn't really matter if there are people out there who dispense love out of self-interest: all that's needed is one person who's sincere."

The commissario's instinct told him that Sbarazza was right. All he wanted was to have Angela near him. He looked at his watch and saw it was a quarter to two. He got up feeling reassured. Each time he spoke to Sbarazza was like a breath of fresh air. All in all, it was good to know there was someone who kept the lamp of hope burning, and he hoped the light was not the flicker of a funeral candle.

"Tomorrow I go to see the Chair of the Committee for Social Services," the old man said as Soneri was leaving. "I've convinced him to open another dormitory and a refectory. I'm a great actor!" And he executed a tango step and a half-pirouette.

Soneri too did a kind of pirouette when Angela seized him by the arm and pulled him to her as soon as he set foot in her office, and when they were face to face, he was thankful to see that her expression was not hostile.

"You were a complete shit," she said, but in a gentle voice.

"What was I supposed to do? Express approval?"

"It was only a coffee."

"And the rest."

She kissed him to cut off further discussion, but he was

waiting for a denial which did not come. There were no more words. They eased effortlessly towards that communication by gesture, touch and expression which characterises the boundless, soundless, shapeless world of the emotions. It was like a canal cutting through that chaos of fear and joy that bubbles inside each one of us, and is nearly always betrayed by words. In that way, it was possible for them to cling closely to each other even without having dispelled the rancour of betrayal, like two tigers making love while still biting at each other.

"Where are you with the case of the Romanian girl?" Angela asked him later when they had dressed

Soneri said only: "I had lunch with Sbarazza."

"Ah, the missionary," she commented.

"And an optimist, one who holds on to belief. I like his freedom of outlook in this world of rigid mindsets."

"And I like you when you get hot under the collar," she replied, taking him again in her arms.

The commissario remained passive. "Is that all you like me for?"

"I've been at work on your behalf these last few days," Angela said, pulling away from him. "I have a certain number of Romanian women among my clients, mainly young women assigned to me when I'm on duty in court. Some of them knew Nina and they all speak highly of her. They say she was a good person and that many men fell passionately in love with her because she was so beautiful, but she never took advantage of this to run off with their money. She wanted to marry an Italian and settle here, have children . . . in other words a normal life after all she'd suffered. She worked as a cleaner in several houses to put aside some money. A really nice girl."

The commissario heard her out and grew increasingly

frustrated over his inability to make headway in the case. He owed it to that Romanian girl, all the more so because she reminded him of his wife. "Maybe she was even sending some money home . . ."

"A nice girl undoubtedly, but don't go making a heroine out of her," Angela said quietly. "Your desire to rise above the vileness you deal with on a daily basis makes you idealise some things and some people too much."

"Criminals are sometimes better than a lot of the phoney people with their noses in the air that go about this city. The poor people Sbarazza meets show more solidarity. The Romanians who meet at the sports ground still have a sense of community, they help each other . . ."

"They help each other and they knife each other," Angela reminded him. "Because they're poor they need the protection of the clan. As soon as they become rich, they'll forget all that, even as many of us have. Affluence corrupts and there are not many who resist. Just a few, like Sbarazza, and they've had too much of everything so they can afford the luxury of living a grim life with perfect tranquility."

"Now it's your turn to overdo it with your dose of realism."

"Let me bring you back to earth. I told you I like you because you can still get indignant and angry. Affluence has done you no harm. You're still the wild thing you were when I first met you. There's something solid inside you, in spite of all your insecurities, something everybody always notices."

"O.K., you've brought me down to earth. In fact you've floored me."

She shook her head in good-humoured reproach. "There you go exaggerating again. It's not like that," she said, but she did not go on, leaving him once more without a full explanation. "See you tomorrow?" she said a moment later, another rapid change of mood.

The commissario gave a nod, but inside himself he felt disappointed. He was finding life trivial, elusive, anchored to the most fragile of intentions. A nothingness, as Sbarazza had put it.

12

AS HE TRAVELLED along the Cisa road, the bulls at Cortile San Martino came back into his mind. He wondered if they were still wandering loose in the Po Valley or if someone had managed to round them up. He hoped that instinct had driven them towards the woods on the Apennines and that they were living there in the company of the wild boars. He was still thinking of his own sun-baked mountains as he turned into the artisan district of Lemignano, with its workshops, warehouses and little villas. Suddenly, he caught sight of an oval bronze nameplate with the word GOLDEN in elegant italics. The atmosphere was typical of areas reserved for the prosperous. He rang and saw a light go on in the intercom. A woman's voice asked, "Who is it?" but she was drowned out by a chorus of dogs barking in a yard nearby. The C.C.T.V. cameras, the guard dogs and the reinforced doors all added to a sense of tension in the atmosphere, which would have been like that in the trenches in time of war, had it not been for the workers in overalls inside the workshops and the coming and going of vans.

The interior was welcoming: rugs, heavy wooden furniture and a pleasing scent of rosehip perfume. Soneri introduced himself to a secretary with a serious and sad demeanour.

Giulia Martini, who must have been in her mid-forties,

had the ascetic look of a mother superior. She was thin, short and sharp-featured.

"May I know why you are here?" she demanded.

"A Romanian girl has been murdered. You may have read in the newspapers . . ."

"What of it?"

Before replying, the commissario ran his eyes along the wall behind the woman, dominated by a portrait of the Pope. "Her mobile phone shows that there were some calls made from another mobile registered in the name of this company."

If the woman were at all disconcerted, she had no difficulty in dissembling. She paused only a few seconds for reflection.

"We did have a Romanian employee some while ago. She used to come in after six o'clock in the evening to clean the offices."

"Was her name Ines Iliescu?"

"Yes."

"Her real name was Nina. She was murdered and her body burned."

The woman did not betray the least sign of discomposure. She kept her thoughts to herself and said nothing.

"Don't you think you have some explaining to do? When did she come here?"

"She came until a few weeks ago."

"And then?"

"We neither saw nor heard anything further from her. She simply disappeared."

"The telephone calls continued until a week ago," Soneri said.

"We carried on trying to reach her. She was very good and it's not easy to find reliable people nowadays."

Soneri gave a smile which was more of a smirk as he looked at the samples of sacred vessels arrayed inside display cabinets.

"Whoever was trying to reach her did find her," he snapped. "Twenty-one minutes of doing their best to convince her."

The woman was growing impatient. She adjusted a plait behind her ear and glowered at the commissario.

"When I dialled that number, a Roberto Soncini replied," Soneri said calmly. "Is your husband responsible for personnel matters?"

"My husband takes no part in running the business. He's good at selling, and that's his field," Giulia Martini said.

"You mean he does the round of the curias, the bishop's palaces . . ."

"We don't sell only sacred objects. We deal in jewellery as well. Look, commissario," she cut him short, "I can tell you for a fact that we have nothing to do with the death of this girl. You ask me for explanations, and I accept that that is your job, but I assure you that any explanations relate exclusively to the personal sphere. Do you understand me?"

"Perfectly. This girl was, or used to be at one time, your husband's lover," the commissario said.

Signora Martini looked at him coldly, leaving Soneri unable to decide if that look was meant to convey hatred or merely expressed the need to work out a strategy.

"You are well versed in the ways of the world," she began again, by way of resuming control of the conversation. "My husband often conducts himself with great superficiality," she said, never taking her eyes off him.

The commissario got the impression that she had already written him off. He looked hard at the woman and thought that Soncini was not entirely to be blamed for turning his attention elsewhere. Apart from anything else, she must have limited interest in the emotional sphere of life, but at that moment declaring herself a woman betrayed got her out of a tight corner. She seemed to be challenging him: yes, my husband has a lover, and so what? Should that bother me?

"Did you know about this affair?"

"She wasn't the first and she won't be the last," she replied, with conspicuous irony and detachment.

"With the cleaning lady . . . a bit vulgar, don't you think?"

"Men are pigs," she stated in a fatalistic tone, gazing at the commissario as if to make it clear that she included him in that judgment.

"Did you sack her? In such cases, that's generally the outcome . . ."

"Not at all!" she said, shaking her head. "I've told you. She disappeared. Anyway, as far as work went, she always performed well. Her defect was to be very pretty and I believe that if she stopped turning up, it was to avoid distressing consequences."

"Your husband has no hand in running this business, do I understand correctly?

"No. He's one of our employees," she stated firmly. Just then, with remarkable timing, a door opened behind her and there appeared a slender girl with long chestnut hair and a dark dress reaching below the knees. She too had a severe appearance. She approached Soneri, holding out her hand coldly. "Micaela Soncini."

Perhaps because the walls were lined with sacred objects, Soneri thought that there was something nun-like about the girl.

"Micaela, the commissario is here about the death of the Romanian girl who worked here for a time," Signora Martini said, throwing her daughter a look of complicity and then proceeding swiftly to change the subject.

"I was explaining that my daughter and I are the sole owners of the company."

The girl had gone over to the armchair where her mother was seated and had placed her arm on the back of the chair, taking up a fashion magazine photo shoot pose. "I am responsible for the day-to-day running of the business and for customer relations," Signora Martini explained. "My daughter deals with the economic and financial side of things. She studied at Bocconi University."

"And your husband does the sales . . ." the commissario butted in, attempting to bring the conversation back to where he wanted it to be.

"Exactly," the woman confirmed, raising her voice.

"He gets a fixed salary and commission, I suppose."

"He spends money like water." This time it was the daughter who spoke. "My mother . . ." she said, glancing at her before going on, "will no doubt have explained to you that if it'd been left to him, the company would have gone bankrupt long ago."

"The mobile from which the calls were made to Ines Iliescu is for your husband's use alone?" the commissario asked, turning back to her mother.

"Yes, but for that phone we have a pay-as-you-go contract," she said.

"Now if there's nothing more we can do for you . . ." Micaela interrupted.

Soneri got up, aware of the full force of their hostility. He had the feeling of being somewhere between the crypt and the sacristy, and this made him uneasy. Even the rows of workshops and villas facing him as he came out seemed more welcoming. He climbed into his car and turned back towards the city. On the way, he tried to contact Angela, but without success. He got her voicemail both at her office and on her mobile.

"Do a bit of research on these two," he told Juvara when he got to his office. He handed him a sheet of paper with the names of the mother and daughter, the joint owners of Golden. He then asked: "Has all the fuss over the arrest of the monster died down?"

"They're interrogating him. If you ask me, Musumeci will be completely insane by midnight."

"And he might end up raping Capuozzo," Soneri said, riled by Angela's silence.

"Listen, commissario, I'd do anything I could to help you, but I can't make head nor tail of this entire business."

Soneri almost felt a surge of tenderness. Every so often, with the impetuous spontaneity of a young hunting dog, Juvara surprised him with one of these generous outbursts.

"Neither can I," he replied with a smile. "We need a stroke of luck. In this case, coincidences have been important, and maybe there'll be one more. When all's said and done, Parma is a small city, isn't it? Sooner or later, you bump into everybody."

"Well," Juvara muttered, "I've been around for a while, but I still haven't found what I'm looking for."

"That too is a matter of coincidence, you know. However hard we try to construct our lives for ourselves, there's not much we can do against chance. This poor Romanian girl was pursued by men because she was exceedingly pretty. She could have had a good life if she'd given herself to the highest bidder, but she wanted to build her own future, even if that meant breaking her back cleaning toilets and offices. She wanted an ordinary life, a husband, children . . . and along comes some madman who murders her."

"Are you certain that's how it went?"

"What else?" Soneri raised his voice. "Do you think a woman takes on work as a servant light-heartedly? Washing underpants, making beds and changing pillowcases?"

"I meant to say that sometimes . . . in other words, in certain cases, I've had occasion to see things change so quickly that I was left dumbfounded."

"I know, but for the moment I see it in those terms, and that's what makes me so furious with myself for not yet getting my hands on whoever killed her."

The inspector stared at him, partly intimidated and partly sympathetic. After a while, he said: "You're forgetting about the text."

"What text?"

"The one here in the printout. Didn't you see it?"

There were several texts, all except one with the numbers of Nina's ex-partners. He had not read the list thoroughly enough, and had taken too much for granted. He immediately attempted to make a call, but the reply was the usual recorded reply. "Do you know whose phone this is?" he asked.

"I've written it out for you underneath," Juvara said. "It seems to have been stolen about a fortnight ago from a certain Giorgio Pagni during a burglary at his house. He'd left the mobile in a drawer when he went to the seaside for a couple of days and he only noticed the theft when he got back, so there was a delay in blocking the account. It's all set out in the statement I got the people in the crime report office to forward to me."

"And in those two days, only one text was sent."

"Just the one you see."

"Yes . . ."

"Come, everything's prepared," Soneri read aloud. Then he added: "What mast is the phone connected to?"

"You were talking about coincidences, so here's the funny thing. The text was sent from a telephone transmitted by the mast at Cortile San Martino."

"This really and truly is a step forward," Soneri exclaimed.

"I wouldn't be too sure," Juvara cautioned. "All the conversations from a good stretch of the autostrada and from a huge swathe of the Po Valley, not to mention the local hypermarket, go via that relay station. And remember the fairground was operating at that period and the text was sent at half past six on a Saturday evening."

Soneri groaned and his enthusiasm drained away. As though by magic, what had seemed a promising lead turned out to be a dead end. The same dead end as before. Once again, anguish overwhelmed him. It had been dark for some two hours, the days were slipping past and the investigation was making no progress. He took out his mobile and dialled Soncini's number. He should have done so earlier, he realised, when the other answered, in no way put out by the call he was receiving.

"I know you've already seen my wife and daughter."

Soneri noted with alarm he was losing his touch. He had not paid heed to that different number in the printout, he had failed to read Juvara's notes and now he realised that Soncini had already been alerted by the two women to the possibility of an interrogation. In all probability they had agreed on their stories so as to ward off suspicion. His mind was not focused, as the magistrate Marcotti had gently suggested.

"I need to talk to you," the commissario said. "Could we meet at the wine bar in Via Farini in an hour?"

"Alright," Soncini agreed. He showed a surprising degree of compliance. Only when he had rung off did Soneri realise that he had fixed the meeting for dinner time. Out of scruple, he tried to call Angela. He very much wanted to go round to her place but would have preferred to receive an invitation from her. The mobile was switched off, but the office phone rang. Just as he was beginning to fear hearing the recorded message, she picked up the receiver. "You got me by pure chance. I was on the way to the prison."

"Can we meet later?"

Angela hesitated a few moments before answering. Soneri detected an embarrassment which was now becoming all too familiar.

"I think I'm going to be tied up for a bit, and I'm already feeling very tired."

He did not know whether to believe her or to view her reply as a diplomatic lie. It would have been easy to check up since each had the keys of the other's house, but he had no wish to go snooping and he was in any case afraid of what he might discover.

He was about to ask her what she was doing in the prison when she said: "Anything new on the Nina story?"

Now it was his turn to remain silent for a few moments. He wanted to talk only about the two of them, but he felt so low that he launched into an account of his visit to Golden.

"It can't have been nice talking to those two harpies," Angela said.

"Do you know them?"

"Signora Martini found making money her only raison d'être after her husband's many betrayals. She takes revenge on him by making him aware he's nothing more than a hired hand."

"Why doesn't she dump him?"

"You must be joking! They're a deeply Catholic family and she works with priests. If she was separated or divorced, she could kiss goodbye to her dealings with the bishop. She cares more about her business than anything else. She's turned her daughter's wedding into a commercial deal."

"Why? Who's she marrying?"

"The eldest boy in the Dall'Argine family. You know, the ones who manufacture engines and hydraulic pumps."

"Ah!" Soneri said distractedly. He did not understand why they were talking about weddings.

"I see my information fails to interest you," Angela said. "I don't know when I'll get back but send me a text before you go to bed."

"I wanted to talk about us," the commissario mumbled. "We should be making decisions, shouldn't we? How long do you intend to keep me dangling?"

"I am not keeping you dangling."

"You're still seeing that other man. You can't make up your mind."

He heard a snort from the other end of the line. "Listen, we'll talk about this later. I'm not up to it at the moment."

As the conversation ended, the commissario felt short of breath and experienced the now customary agitation which made him feel he needed air. He left the office to seek relief from that state of quasi-asphyxiation but found his lungs filling with the dead miasma of the mist.

He dragged himself to the wine bar where he had arranged to meet Soncini, but he noticed his rival's Mercedes parked with two wheels on the pavement, and when he approached the door of the bar he made out, in the half light of the portico, a tall, trim figure. The other man slowed down, but when he saw Soneri turn the door handle to go in he changed direction slightly, with the gentle movement of a boat in a regatta, and walked on towards the far end of the road.

The commissario was sure that he had been making for the wine bar, and that his being there had made him change his mind. Perhaps that was where he was to meet Angela and he preferred to avoid unpleasant encounters. Soneri watched him move off, speaking into his mobile phone. Suspicion prompted the idea that he was calling Angela to change their rendezvous.

He had no more time to think about it before Soncini arrived. He recognised him instantly even though he had never seen him before. The idea he had formed of him corresponded perfectly to the man he now found standing before him – long hair, greying, smoothed down with gel, dark moustache, tall, lean, slightly stooped, skin suggesting exposure to a multiplicity of tanning lamps, all combining to give the impression of fragility, like a crumbling tower. He told him he had once been employed as a model and had worked on the catwalks in Milan. Perhaps it was there he had met his wife, a woman with money and anxious to show if off.

"Were you recently Nina's lover?" Soneri adopted the inquisitorial tone from the outset.

"Our relationship had been ongoing for some time, with ups and downs," Soncini replied, with irritating detachment. "We separated several times but always got back together again."

"Did you get to know her when she was working at Golden or earlier?"

"No," he said with an ironic smile. "Earlier. It was she who wanted me to find her a job. Ines was very keen on her independence and wanted a normal life. She spoke a lot about marriage and children."

"You were in no position to guarantee her these things."

"No," he said, shaking his head. "But she was young and she had time on her side. And we were very close. She went off with other men, but in reality we never separated from each other."

"Indeed," the commissario murmured, thinking of his own situation. "In the last few weeks, had you got back together?"

"Yes. She said she'd never have hesitated about getting married to me if I'd been free. She didn't care about the difference in age. Believe me, we were very much in love."

"Why was Ines not with you on the night of the crime?"

"I was busy. I was with a lawyer friend. There was a problem over an order for some goldsmith's work. Then we went to a bar on Lake Como. I don't know what Ines was doing that evening. She told me she'd be going out with some Romanian friends I didn't know."

"What's the name of your lawyer friend?"

"What's going on? Do you want verification?" Soncini sounded astonished. "Look, I'm not telling you lies. But you can call him, he's Arnaldo Razzini. Check with him."

"It's my job to double-check."

"Then go ahead," Soncini declared brazenly. "I'm an entrepreneur. I don't go around assaulting women the way these foreigners do. Ines told me all about what goes on in Romania."

"You say you are an entrepreneur, but your wife might take a different view," Soneri said maliciously. "She tells me an employee paid by commission . . ."

Soncini glowered at Soneri with deep resentment, but he could not hold that look for long. He was obviously a spineless human being, a man of straw.

"Well then, say that I'm a manager, will that do? I'm a good salesman, and nobody can take that away from me. Not even my wife." He spoke of her as though she had the right of life and death over him.

The commissario stared at him and thought of Giulia Martini. A couple who hated each other but were held together by business interest, exactly like members of a board of management. She kept him in exchange for being able to sell to bishops and cardinals the outward display of married life, while he moved from one bed to the next, deceiving young foreign girls. The commissario delighted in the opportunity to disrupt their minuet and cause trouble. "Your wife and your daughter tell me you spend money like water . . ."

Soncini gave the slightest of shrugs, as though bored. "My daughter used to love me a lot, but she's come under her mother's control."

The distance between them seemed to bother him a great deal, but everything in Soncini appeared improbable. He was a man who must have dabbled in everything, but who had so completely wasted everything life had offered him that he was incapable of even one authentic emotion. The commissario looked hard at a face that could in another age have been Casanova's, and had the displeasing impression of seeing in front of him a man embittered, exhausted and dissatisfied, let down by his body and by age. Quite suddenly, Soncini was transformed into a ghost.

"I've nothing more to ask you," Soneri said, anxious to be free of the man.

Soncini rose slowly to his feet. He had maintained a kind of fading, early autumnal attractiveness, and his walk as he left the bar had the slow deliberateness of an elderly gentleman.

Soon after, Soneri too went out. The discussion with Soncini added nothing to what he had already known, but did leave him with some impressions he could not yet manage to decode. And no-one knew better than him how important impressions were when everything appeared inexplicable.

13

THE NIGHT WAS a time of peace for the commissario, when the inexplicable ceased to torment him. The darkness of the *borghi* in the old town set itself up as a natural obstacle to anxiety, leaving it no option but to slink off. Momentarily washing his hands of his problems offered great relief and gave Soneri, as he strolled about in the mist, a break from his nightmares.

It did not last long. Once more the sirens blared out in the labyrinth of streets around the Duomo. Excitement exploded and transformed itself into a mob. An ambulance raced by, pursued by the curious on foot. They made for the Vicolo del Vescovado, but the entrance was blocked by a pair of police cars. In the midst of things, he made out the figure of Musumeci and immediately afterwards saw a flushed woman being taken by the arm by Esposito.

"We've made a cock-up of the whole thing," Esposito shouted.

"You mean it wasn't him," the commissario said, meaning the Moroccan now being crucified as the Brute of Parma.

"No, no way. Oh, don't get carried away. He was no saint, eh! He did try to hassle that girl."

"Him and how many others, Esposito? There are

thousands of potential rapists, especially among respectable, apparently innocent fathers of families."

"Maybe so, commissario, but this is one weird human being," he concluded with an eloquent gesture of his finger.

Musumeci was conducting interrogations and a number of people were lined up along the wall of the Bishop's Palace. There was something blasphemous or even perhaps deliberately provocative in raping a woman in that place. A symbolic coincidence, and Soneri had a continuing interest in both coincidences and symbols. A new piece of information crackled out on a radio held by one of Esposito's colleagues. A man whose description fitted the rapist had been seen under the Portici del Grano at the City Hall. After a challenge to the spiritual power, it was the turn of the temporal power. Two cars sped off with tyres screeching. The commissario followed them on foot. A few metres on, some boys went racing past him, and he too broke into a run, abandoning himself to a puerile excitement that reawoke memories of leaping from stone to stone in furrows created by water or by tractors, and of boyhood competitions on sun-soaked paths lined by poplar trees, and at the same time contemplating how pitiless is time in burning us up.

Soneri stopped in Via Repubblica, in front of the police station, unable to decide if his breathlessness was due to emotion or exertion. He had the impression that, quite suddenly, that night he had begun to make some headway. Something must have been happening under the mist which seemed to be continually rolling over the city, even if to all appearances everything was returning to its customary stillness and to the subdued sounds of the night-time hours. He walked along Via Mazzini, and observed the faint lights on the far side of the river pierce the darkness, while the bells of the Duomo rang a quarter to midnight. He leaned on the parapet of the Mezzo bridge and looked over at the river only a few metres below but almost silent. He was finally floating with a lightness he had been experiencing for some time, nothing more than a bubble released from the graceful hand of a child, rising without wind, tossed slowly about before bursting, forgotten.

The ringing of his mobile brought him back to earth. "Commissario," the voice of Pasquariello's deputy came booming out, "we've got the car you described to us, the black B.M.W. Remember?"

"The one with the horse on the side? Of course I remember."

"Well, you won't see much of the horse, because there's a scrape on the side of the car, but we think this is the one you're after."

"Where is it now?"

"Here with us."

"Who was driving?"

"Two Romanians. We've checked with the vehicle registration office, and it turns out the car's stolen."

Soneri muttered something incomprehensible. "When?"

"Couple of months ago. But that's not all. The pair who were in the car are underage. The guy who was driving is seventeen and the other one's sixteen."

"How did you apprehend them?"

"They crashed into another car at the Crocetta and ran off. A squad car gave chase until they turned into a cul-de-sac. There may have been a third person who got away."

"Don't let anybody touch the car, and first thing tomorrow morning call in the forensic squad. I want that car examined," Soneri ordered.

Shortly afterwards, he was at the police station. On the way he tried to get through to Angela, but without success.

He sent her an ambiguous text: *I don't know if I'll go to bed tonight. What about you?* He saw the B.M.W. parked in the courtyard, not the most recent model, but one still in vogue. It had a long scratch on one side, but the galloping horse could clearly be made out.

"Where are the two you've arrested?"

A custody officer escorted him to the interrogation room, but before they went in he warned him: "I think you're wasting your time. They won't open their mouths."

They were young, but they had the look of having been through a lot.

"You stole the wrong car," the commissario began. "Anyone in possession of it is in deep trouble, facing much more than a straightforward charge of car theft."

The two remained impassive. They seemed not to have understood what was being said to them. Soneri turned back to the officer.

"Do these two understand Italian?"

"They understand perfectly well. They're bluffing."

"It'd be better for you to come clean, much better," the commissario threatened. Not a muscle on the face of either man moved.

"Even if you are underage, a murder charge is no trivial matter," the commissario said.

Only at that point did the two exchange a brief glance, but still did not say a word. They gave the impression of being in a waiting room rather than a police station, and the idea of ending up in jail seemed not to have crossed their minds. They stared straight ahead impassively, with an inexpressive, almost obtuse look on their faces. The commissario wondered how they could maintain that pose except by anaesthetising the brain, leaving it dulled during the hours and hours of waiting, with no other aim than to let time pass. He would have liked to punch the pair of them and shake them out of a silence he found deeply irritating.

"Where are you from?"

No reply. Soneri looked questioningly at the officer.

"They had no papers on them, commissario. We're making enquiries with the immigration office."

He peered at the two young men impotently. Although in a fury, he did no more than take a seat opposite them, attempting to intercept any glance they exchanged. Their clear eyes darted about like lizards', but when they were still they had the fixed vacuity of a pane of glass.

"I don't understand why you're so keen to make trouble for yourselves! Ruining your lives before they've really begun." Addressing the officer, he added, "The car was the one used in the Iliescu murder."

He hoped to make some impact on the boys, to shake them out of their apathy, but they were plainly hard cases. Or simply two lads who had been trained in a code of blind obedience to the clan, imposed by beating after beating. Or else they were terrified. Only once did the younger of the two display a sign of concern, throwing his mate a glance which the commissario read as a willingness to yield, but immediately afterwards everything settled back as before: the same apathy, the same immobility, the same lizard-like looks.

The commissario cut short the interrogation. "O.K. You'll be spending the night in the cells."

He got up and walked slowly to the door. As he squeezed past the custody officer, he stopped and turned round for a last look at the two Romanians staring into the void, as impassive as ever.

In the corridor he bumped into Pasquariello, who had the grim expression on his face of a man dragged out of bed in the middle of the night.

"So? Where are these two little shits?"

Soneri nodded in the direction of the room he had just left. "It's a waste of time going in. They're like two statues."

They both went into the office of the head of the flying squad. There were three officers at work on the case, but at that moment the commissario felt the absence of Juvara and his computer skills.

"The car was stolen from some firm," one of the policemen announced.

"Which firm?" asked Pasquariello.

"It's called Golden. It's a goldsmith's firm based in Lemignano."

Something clicked in Soneri's mind, even if he would not have been able to identify the connection which was suggested. Unquestionably he was facing another coincidence: he had just been talking to the irreproachable family which held the reins in that firm.

"Do you know it?" Pasquariello said.

The commissario nodded. "Nina Iliescu worked there for a while and then she became the lover of the owner's husband."

The chief of the flying squad gave a malicious grunt. "So the skin trade was part of it after all. Who would have guessed it? What about these two Romanians? Can we put a name to them?" Pasquariello asked the officers.

"No. Either they're illegals or else we're going to have to do lengthy research. Meantime, we've taken their fingerprints."

"Have a look in the camps of the Roma travellers. It's likely they come from there," Soneri suggested, remembering Medioli's ill-fated flight.

Pasquariello agreed. "Maybe you're right. Running off with a car with no licence is typical of them. It wouldn't be the first time."

"There were some Romanian Romas at Cortile San Martino in the clearing near the rubbish dump. They left a couple of days ago and who knows where they've ended up? I requested help to trace them, but we'd need the collaboration of our cousins," the commissario said, referring to the carabinieri.

"Is there no way to get them to talk?" Pasquariello asked.

"No, and even if they did, they'd give a false name. Who knows how many aliases they have," Soneri said.

"And how many expulsion orders . . ." added one of the officers, his eyes still glued to the computer screen.

"Anything found in the car?" the chief of the flying squad said.

"A quick search didn't reveal anything, but maybe tomorrow Nanetti will come up with something," Soneri said, as he left with Pasquariello.

"Do you think these two clowns have anything to do with the murder?" Pasquariello asked.

Soneri shook his head. "I don't believe so, but who knows? They could set us on the right track."

He turned away without saying goodbye. As he walked under the archway which led to the Borgo della Posta, he heard the bell on the Duomo strike one. Immediately after, the mobile in his pocket vibrated. *Perhaps I won't either*, he read on the screen. He knew she meant she would not go to bed that night any more than he would. A state of agitation once again overcame him. These few words could indicate either that she had complex work in hand or that she would not be going home.

He felt the need for some slices of Parmesan and a good, dark Lambrusco, always the best remedy at moments like these. He was about to head home but had to jump aside to avoid a squad car arriving at top speed. The car stopped in the archway, lights flashing and sirens blaring, until the officer raised the barrier. Two other cars also arriving at high speed came in behind the first.

Soneri rushed back into the courtyard. In the absence of Parmesan and Lambrusco, throwing himself into the thick of the action could well be the best way to keep worried thoughts at bay.

"We got him! This time we caught him with the mouse in his mouth," shouted Esposito, hauling out a man of distinguished appearance but plainly distraught.

Soneri watched him go past, ashen-faced, head bowed, dressed like an executive: jacket and tie, finely fashioned knee-length overcoat, English shoes, elegant trousers with flares. The commissario followed the short procession into the offices and it occurred to him that this was the night of the reckoning. He left to his colleagues the satisfaction of the first interrogation and went off to pour himself a coffee from the machine. At that instant, he felt once again refreshed. All the clamour around him seemed to him a vacuous, grotesque pantomime and for that reason, with that coolness which follows disappointment and disengagement from spent passion, he succeeded in seeing the world in a wholly new light.

Pasquariello appeared at his side. "Why don't you come in as well? We're going to interrogate him."

The man was called Vincenzo Candiani, a professor fairly well known in the city. Soneri tried to imagine the reaction of Parma's *bien pensant* society when they discovered that the Brute was not a foreigner, nor even some poor addict, but a respected professor of Law. Observing him now, seated on a plywood seat in the police station, leaning forward on his elbows like an ancient elm tree blown over by the wind, made him an almost pitiful figure. The commissario saw reflected in the man all the instability of humanity. Only the most shadowy of boundaries separated the professor revered in the lecture halls from the depraved, rapist ogre. "A nothingness," as Sbarazza had said in support of his view that everything cohabited in every man in a turmoil continually churned up by circumstances.

Esposito whispered into Soneri's ear. "He was in a doorway in Borgo Scacchini, with his prick in his hand, ready for use. We were phoned by an old woman of ninety-odd years, the most alert in the building. At first we couldn't believe it. A professor like him. Just imagine, we've seen him so often in court."

"We're not sure of anything yet, Esposito. Human beings can take as many forms as the mist," the commissario said.

Esposito looked at him without seeming to understand a word. He said nothing then turned away to give orders to his men.

"Professor, what are we to make of this?" Pasquariello began in a menacing tone.

"I lost my head . . ." Candiani kept on repeating. He had opened his coat and loosened his collar because of the heat, making him look like a man who had fallen asleep fully dressed on the settee after lunch. He looked around at the policemen with a kind of candour, as though he wanted to apologise for what he had done, but did not really think he had done anything particularly serious.

"You could have had any woman you wanted," Pasquariello continued. "What's going on?" he said incredulously, shaking his clasped hands back and forth.

"I lost my head," Candiani repeated again, but this time he added, "It was all because of one woman. It all began there . . ."

It all seemed unbelievable, and yet that man seemed genuinely possessed by an obsession, a toad lurking deep in his guts. His eyes were sparkling brightly and his face seemed to be twitching like a bird's. He was in the grip of a febrile agitation which would calm momentarily before flaring up again as he faced the questions put by Pasquariello and Musumeci. He gave every impression of having surrendered completely and even of being happy to be free of a weight, as had been the case with Medioli in that same room days earlier.

"Have you any questions for him?" Pasquariello asked Soneri, leaving Candiani in the custody of Musumeci until the magistrate arrived.

"Not now. I don't know if he has anything to do with my investigations, even if Parma's a small town and everything links up."

He had thought of contacting Angela to ask her about the professor, but he would not have been able to cope with a switched-off phone and the conlusions which that would have provoked. All his fears and conjectures merged into the one image of his beloved making love to that other man, with all that might be obscene or noble in lovemaking.

He went out to light a cigar, and in the still, heavy air of the courtyard he rediscovered some peace. The whirlwind of arrest after arrest had disturbed him, causing him to feel the need to let his impressions settle and pass through the sieve of his memory. This he could do only by drawing apart a little from the throb of the action, and looking on from a distance.

As he was going over all that had happened that night, he heard footsteps behind him. He turned and saw Juvara approach with his stumbling walk. He had a scarf round his neck and the dreamy air of someone who has overindulged.

"You look as though you're just out of a discotheque," Soneri greeted him.

"I was at a party," the inspector said in self-justification. "There was such a racket I couldn't hear the phone."

"You can go to bed. Nothing's going to happen as regards our investigation before tomorrow morning."

"What's been going on? There's such a frenzy . . ."

"They've picked up the rapist and it turns out he's a well-known university professor. But what matters for us is that they've arrested two teenagers driving the car from which Mariotto was seen dumping the body of Nina alongside the autostrada. We're not going to find out much more until tomorrow. We'll have to wait until Nanetti looks it over."

"Was it them?"

"I doubt it. They're just boys, and the car was stolen two months ago at Golden. That's the most intriguing aspect."

Juvara nodded. "And this rapist?"

"He says he lost his head over a woman and from then on he went haywire. Want to bet it was Nina?"

"She was well capable of it. He obviously wouldn't have been the first."

"It wasn't her fault if men went running after her, nor if they lost their heads over her. All they wanted was to screw her, but then they got in deeper than they expected, and that's all there was to it. Was that her fault? She was looking for a man to marry, but the ones she found wanted her as a toy. They ended up whimpering when she moved on."

"No, I just meant . . ." Juvara, stung by the commissario's exasperated response, stuttered incoherently. Each time Nina's name came up, a conditioned reflex provoked him into an outburst.

"Get to bed. That's what I'm going to do," Soneri said, calming down. "I've got nothing more to do, not this evening anyway."

He watched the inspector turn away before he moved off himself. He wanted to be on his own, perhaps at a table in an *osteria* with a half litre of wine in front of him, but there was nothing open at that time. Night life was reduced to a series of squalid clubs and no-one was out after dark anymore, perhaps because it was too hard to put up with the silence.

The silence was broken in Via Saffi by his mobile ringing, producing the same effect on the commissario as an alarm clock on someone fast asleep.

"Are you still awake?" Angela said.

"I'm not even home yet."

"Who did you go out with?"

"Are you kidding? It was you who went out, not me."

"If that's what you think, you're off the mark. Let me warn you it doesn't seem to me the ideal way to make a fresh start."

"But I never finished! I still don't understand why you wanted to put me through all this. It's hard to bear when your most ferocious torturer is the person you love. I don't know what to make of you, you're tormenting me . . ."

He realised that for the first time he had let himself go, speaking out without caution or discretion, and it seemed that Angela was deeply moved by this fact. Soneri had overcome the reserve ingrained into men from the mountains where he was born. It had dissolved in the slow heat of the passions bubbling in his soul. "But perhaps you've finished with me," he said, his voice breaking slightly.

"No, that's not the way it is," Angela contradicted him with sudden gentleness. "I was at the prison for an interrogation until half an hour ago. I didn't go out with anyone."

"But you might have done."

"I could have," she said drily.

"And it was only work that stopped you?"

"That had a lot to do with it." Her reply was delphic, keeping him on tenterhooks.

Soneri could no longer put up with her frankness. He was thinking he would have preferred a merciful lie when it occurred to him that this desire for security was absurd.

"I'm going to bed. It's nearly three o'clock," he said, after waiting a few seconds in vain for her to speak.

"If it weren't so late . . . Come tomorrow to my office," Angela proposed.

"So we're not meeting any more in the evening?"

She deflected the question. "I like our encounters over the lunch break. They're less predictable."

"What have you got on in the evening?"

He heard an impatient snort from the other end of the line. "Is that you off again, the interrogating policeman act?" Angela raised her voice. "You know it's the wrong approach."

"What do you want me to do? Keep my mouth shut while you're being unfaithful?"

"Oh God, unfaithful! That's the way people spoke half a century ago."

"You can use any term you like, but I prefer to speak plainly."

"Come round tomorrow," Angela invited him once more, this time in a more wheedling tone of voice.

"I'll tell you all about Professor Candiani."

"What has our great academic done?"

"He's been raping women."

"Him! There were some rumours about a female student. When did you pick him up?"

"An hour ago. In flagrante. In Borgo Scacchini."

"He's an advisor to the court and a friend of a lot of lawyers."

"Including Paglia?"

"I think so. They meet in an equestrian club in the hills, near Traversetolo. I believe it's called Cerreto."

The mention of horses touched a chord in Soneri's memory.

"A police patrol unit stopped the car used to dump Nina's body in the ditch," he said.

"So you're home and dry," Angela exclaimed.

"Not quite dry, but we're on the home run," Soneri said, as Angela repeated her invitation to lunch the following day.

14

HE AWOKE ABRUPTLY and sat bolt upright in bed. His bedroom seemed to hold on to the darkness of the night, and he searched vaguely around until his eyes located the phosphorescence of the alarm clock. Nearly nine o'clock. He groped on his bedside table for his mobile phone, but then saw something shining on the floor. He could not remember putting his mobile on vibrate, but the pulsating movement must have caused it to fall off.

"I've been looking for you since seven," Nanetti grumbled.

"I was up till three," the commissario said.

"Good sign. It means you're coming back to life."

"Go to hell. I was working. They'll have told you what happened while you were asleep or reading crime fiction."

"I've never read any such thing in all my life. I know real detectives like you . . . ."

"Do you want me to tell you again to go to hell?"

"It'd be better than being where I am now. There's a stench in this car that would make a python throw up. They must have been using it for the delivery of take-away fry-ups."

"Oh God, the smells are getting to you now! Have you found anything worthwhile?"

"Not so far. The fingerprints belong to the two boys, as

well as to an army of other people. No trace of Nina's, if that's what you want to know."

"And that's all?"

"There's a till receipt," Nanetti said off-handedly. "I don't think it's got anything to do with the Romanians. They'd rather take things without going near any till."

"What kind of receipt is it?"

"A computer shop, called Elettronica Sauro, in Borgo Regale."

"Did they spend much?"

"No, two hundred euros. Maybe an accessory, who knows?"

"Is there a date?"

"Six months ago. It must have fallen and ended up under the seat. Anyway, I'll stick it in an envelope and attach it to my report. There's nothing else of any interest."

Soneri dressed hurriedly and grabbed hold of his mobile. There were seven unanswered calls. Juvara, Nanetti, Musumeci and Angela had all called, but the only one he was interested in calling back was Angela. When he was greeted by the familiar voicemail, he went into a rage which almost drove him to smash the mobile against the wall. He left the house and set off for the police station with the unpleasant feeling of not being abreast of developments.

The first person he met was Musumeci, who looked weary but euphoric. "I've had compliments from Capuozzo," he said.

"Let me add mine," Soneri said with a tired voice. The opinions of the chief of police were of no interest to him.

"The newspapers have only managed to get it into 'late news', but you've no idea the uproar it's caused!"

"That way the good people of Parma will learn to consider themselves as living in the best of all possible worlds," Soneri said. "What extenuating circumstances has our professor of Law given?" he asked, realising only as he asked the question just how extraordinary it was that the holder of a Chair of Law should break the law so outrageously.

"Commissario," the inspector began, drawing closer to Soneri with an air of complicity, "he's up to his eyeballs in cocaine. We found some in his house, and since it was a fair amount he's facing a charge of drug pushing as well."

"Who would have believed it, eh?" Soneri exclaimed sarcastically. "He said he lost his head over a woman. Did he say who she was?"

"A Romanian woman," Musumeci said. "He said her name is Doina, and that she dumped him without any warning, and I think I can understand why."

The commissario lit a cigar and as he inhaled, he saw the inspector standing silent and embarrassed before him.

"And?"

"These are unconfirmed stories," Musumeci said, in an attempt to play things down. "We've heard from a couple of the professor's ex-girlfriends and, you see . . . it seems his tastes were a bit on the perverted side, if you get my meaning."

"Seeing what he was up to, he could hardly be called normal, could he?"

"Certainly not," Musumeci said quickly. "It all fits. I just couldn't find the right words," he went on, his embarrassment increasing while Soneri struggled not to laugh out loud. He had frequently heard the inspector use scurrilous language when speaking to the men in his division, and here he was almost blushing in front of him. A question of rank, no doubt, but Soneri also knew that yet again age was a factor.

"You don't need to go into details. I can imagine them for myself."

He thought it was perfectly reasonable of Nina/Doina to leave him. She seemed to meet only men who wanted to keep her as a toy, or a doll, in Goretti's words, but one so beautiful as to make grown men, seemingly sure of themselves, lose their heads.

These thoughts were in his mind as he made his way along the corridor leading to the office of the road patrol.

The moment he saw him, Juvara gave a start as though he had been caught in the act of committing some crime. "There you are at last! Dottoressa Marcotti has called several times. She needs to talk to you."

"About what?"

"The carabinieri have caught up with the Romanian Romas who were camped at Cortile San Martino."

"Where are they now?"

"At Suzzara. That's why Marcotti was looking for you, but in the end she had to decide for herself. I explained to her that you were running late and that . . ."

The commissario cut him short with a wave of the hand. "Get over there as soon as you can. With Musumeci. He's half gypsy and he'll take no nonsense from these people."

"Yes, but Marcotti also ordered the carabinieri to identify the two car thieves."

"We'll see if the Romas will talk. There's no way of knowing if this pair belong to the same group. And who cares anyway? This is our investigation and the bold boys in the carabinieri have no idea what's behind it all."

Juvara got up, a picture of confusion. Soneri was already on the way out and took no notice.

The inspector called him back. "One thing, sir. I've found out who owns the flat in Via Cavallotti."

The commissario gave him a quizzical look.

"It's an accountant, name of Gino Aimi."

"The name doesn't mean anything to me."

"Nor to me, at first, but then I checked up Traversetolo on the company list at the Chamber of Commerce and discovered he's chairman."

"You see where coincidences lead?"

"There are getting to be a lot of them," the inspector said.

"That's a good sign."

A moment later he was in his Alfa and heading for Golden. He needed to speak to Soncini, and more so to his wife.

The countryside around the city looked strangely like a black and white photograph. Even the wheat, which was past time for harvesting, was so soaked by the rain that it had a grey cast. The plane trees lining Via Spezia seemed turned upside down, with the bare branches dissolving into the mist and looking more like roots exposed by running water. The last trace of colour vanished totally when he turned into the street leading to the industrial zone of the city. Every time he ended up in one of those places, he wondered how it had been possible so totally to eliminate every hint of beauty.

The sight of the pyxes, chalices and crucifixes in the offices of Golden did nothing to raise his spirits after such ugliness, particularly since he also found himself confronted by Signora Martini's decidedly unwelcoming expression. However, the woman herself was too conformist to allow herself to voice her displeasure. She restricted herself to coldness and to that blank expression she must have put on in response to setbacks in a dull life.

"I trust you are not the bearer of bad news," she said with a scowl. "Policemen . . ."

"Good news. We've found your car. A bit scraped but intact."

She showed no emotion other than a forced smile. "Where was it?" was all she wanted to know.

"It was being driven by two teenagers: two of the Roma community."

As had happened on the previous occasion, the daughter came in and took up position alongside her mother in a prearranged pose under the portrait of the Pope.

"Who had the use of that car?" Soneri said.

"My husband. He's the one who does the travelling. My daughter and I have smaller cars."

"Is your husband available?"

"Micaela, go and call your father." Signora Martini gave orders in the tone of one accustomed to being obeyed.

"We'll get rid of that car," she said. "The lease was nearly up and we'd have changed it in any case."

At that moment Soncini came in, followed by his daughter, meaning the whole family was now lined up in front of the commissario. Each one wore a different expression, as though they were passengers thrown together by chance on a tram. Soncini looked nervous and bereft of the *bon viveur* self-certainty he had previously displayed, his wife gave the impression of keeping the situation under control while waiting patiently, and the daughter glowered at the commissario with unconcealed malevolence.

"I've read the witness statements about the B.M.W. It was stolen from Via Cavallotti some time after ten o'clock at night. At that hour I presume that it was not there for reasons connected with work . . ." Soneri began.

"You presume? My clients do not necessarily see people during office hours."

"Priests go to bed after Vespers, or else are at their prayers," Soneri said.

Soncini was about to reply when his wife interrupted him.

"He was with his lover." She cut him short so peremptorily that there followed a few moments of silence which no-one dared to break. "That's what you were getting at, weren't you, commissario?" she went on. "They already know the Romanian girl had a flat in that street," she said, throwing a reproachful look at her husband.

Soncini said nothing. He seemed relieved to let his wife take the initiative.

"You didn't report the theft until ten o'clock the following morning," Soneri continued, in an inquisitorial tone.

Giulia Martini turned to her husband with what seemed like a challenge. She appeared to be inviting him to get himself out of trouble.

"I only noticed the following morning when I went to pick it up," Soncini said.

"Commissario," his wife intervened with her customary brusqueness, "it seems to me that we have cleared this matter up, don't you think? The car was stolen two months ago, and what happened thereafter is no concern of ours."

She was in charge, as was evident from the subservient expressions of husband and daughter. It was her task to defend the family, the business, the veneer of respectability.

"Do you know Gino Aimi well?"

"Of course," Soncini replied. "He's a good friend. I don't see what . . ."

"Was it through him that you found the house for Iliescu?"

The man was at once embarrassed and his wife looked on, savouring the spectacle.

"It's logical to turn to friends . . ."

The woman gave a devious smile, but her attitude upset Soneri more than it did her husband. It announced that she feared nothing and that his questions in no way unsettled her.

He, on the other hand, was aware of having no other weapons in his armoury.

"The good old-fashioned male complicity," she remarked sardonically.

The commissario ignored her. "However, it's very curious that your lover was tossed into a ditch after being hauled out of a car similar to yours."

Signora Martini's face darkened slightly.

"You did say 'similar'," Micaela intervened determinedly. "We're hardly the only ones in this city who have a B.M.W."

Soncini stopped her going any further. "Commissario, there's something important I haven't told you. Nina was burning her bridges with her relatives. She wanted a life of her own, where she wouldn't have to be accountable to any family members. Do you understand me? One side of the family was mixed up with the Roma people, and I don't have to tell you what that means. They never leave you alone. They're always trying to screw cash out of you. Over and above that, they were trying to decide her future for her, arrange a marriage. She rebelled, and they made her pay. They tried so many times. To them, I was a thief, someone who took the community's women away. For that clan, Nina was a licence to print money. Like her sister."

What left Soneri most dumbfounded was observing Soncini's wife listen impassively to her husband's account as though it involved a complete stranger. Micaela likewise betrayed no emotion. They were the real clan, untouchable, calculating, hardened to a state of indifference. Thinking of his own anguish over Angela's betrayal, Soneri envied that tough-minded woman.

"Commissario," Soncini's voice interrupted his reflections, "I have no way of proving it, but I am pretty sure that those Romanians tried to frame me too. What could be better than to steal my car and then use it to murder the woman with whom I'd been having an affair? Maybe they wanted to do it immediately after the theft but had to put it off because . . ."

"How could they know you wouldn't report the theft?"

"They've managed to put me under suspicion. Proof of that is your presence here."

"You have a poor opinion of us, but our sins are not a matter for criminal law," Giulia Martini said, once again throwing an accusatory glance at her husband.

"As for your sins, you can attend to them yourselves." Soneri was curt because he was tired of the conversation. The whole range of Golden's sacred objects lying nearby made the room look like a sacristy. He felt nauseous as he rose to his feet and observed the triumphant expression on Micaela's face. As before, when he went out he felt the mist to be a comforting and friendly presence. It was good not to see too far ahead and to lose himself in it as though in sleep.

He drove back to the city with a vague, troublesome ill humour weighing down on him. En route, he received a phone call from the prosecutor Marcotti to inform him that the two Romanians arrested for car theft were still taking advantage of their right to remain silent. As for the camp they came from, she was still waiting for the report from the carabinieri. In due course, he would receive fresh news from Juvara and Musumeci, who had gone to Suzzara to find them in their new campsite.

When he got to the office, he found the membership list of the equestrian club at Traversetolo left for him by Juvara. It included the majority of the people most involved in the case, and Nina seemed to be the focal point around which the whole lovers' comedy rotated. The slightest change of perspective could give a new slant to the whole story, which was itself as changeable as its participants, who in their turn differed every time in their continual denial of their role.

There was no knowing what angle would be revealed by that receipt for Elettronica Sauro found in the B.M.W. by Nanetti. He had decided to stop at the shop when he noticed that it was gone one o'clock. Getting up late meant drifting through the day, as his father had always warned him. Right on cue, the mobile rang.

"So, are you coming or have you had second thoughts?" Angela took him by surprise.

"You're like a cat. You decide when to purr."

"Do hurry."

It was yet another very intense encounter, and Soneri abandoned himself to it with the bitter conviction that the ardour was not really aroused by him. But soon all thought faded away and everything was transformed into pure instinct and desire, with all rationality irrelevant. Sex could have the same narcotic effect as sleep, with the difference that it did not last as long.

Then the reawakening, followed by the return of the familiar spectres. It was no doubt the same for someone coming round after taking drugs: the same withdrawal symptoms after the injection-induced high.

"Angela, have you made up your mind about us?"

He heard a brief snort at his side. "Why must you always ruin every beautiful moment?"

"I have a need for certainty, an absolute need."

"You know there can't be certainties, don't you?"

"I would be happy with the illusion."

"Even if I spoke reassuring words, even if I were to tell you that I'll stay with you always, you would still leave here as doubtful as ever," Angela whispered to him. "One moment later, you'd have forgotten what I said. And you know that's true, you're sure of it, so I don't understand why you go on like this. I don't want to deceive you and show contempt for what you are and have always been. Your own rationality rebels against yourself. Haven't you always claimed that you detest people who allow themselves to be dominated by instinct? Haven't you always said you'd never let yourself go that way?"

"Goddammit, Angela, I only want to know if you want to stay with me or would rather go off with the other guy. I'm not asking for an everlasting pledge!"

"You know perfectly well that things have to be constructed day by day."

"Constructed day by day? What drivel is that! Everything has fallen apart, Angela. Everything I believed in since I was a boy – my profession, my marriage, the son I never saw, my dreams . . . and now you and I are going to pieces as well. I'm broken up inside, and I can't take it any more."

Angela gave him a hug, but in that gesture he thought there was more tenderness than real feeling.

"If we feel all this, it means we have still a lot to give each other," she murmured in his ear, all the while holding him tightly and communicating a pleasing sense of warmth.

"At least I'm happy about one thing," Soneri said. "There's no sign of that pity for the other that sometimes comes out with two people who have been together a long time."

Angela pulled back to look at him more closely and more intensely, then said simply, "No, no pity." Somehow a phrase which could have been wounding sounded, on the contrary, gentle.

Shortly afterwards, as he was on the doorstep, the commissario felt a moment's confusion. "You were supposed to talk to me about Candiani," he said.

"I can ask about him if you like, but maybe you'd rather not."

"Why not?"

"The other man," she said with evident embarrassment, "he's a great friend of his. If you want, I'll call him and try to ask him . . . He wouldn't refuse."

"Forget it. I'll see to it myself," Soneri said, before dashing down the stairs to escape the anguish which threatened to overwhelm him yet again.

15

ELETTRONICA SAURO OCCUPIED some thirty square metres, divided between display space and workshop. Giorgio Sauro, the young man in his thirties who was manager, seemed to have wagered everything on it. He was plainly a courageous individual since, apart from anything else, he had not given his shop an English name. This was enough to make Soneri take to him immediately.

"I do know Signor Soncini. He's been here a couple of times and I've added his name to our client list. I keep him up to date by e-mail."

The commissario produced the till receipt which Nanetti had given him. "Could you identify what this referred to?"

Sauro examined the date and the amount. He opened a drawer and pulled out a sort of ledger. He was exceedingly punctilious, and it crossed Soneri's mind that he and Juvara would get on well.

"It's to do with the repair of a laptop, a Sony. He had problems accessing the internet from it."

"Would that be Signor Soncini's own laptop?"

"That I couldn't say. If it was his, he must have another one seeing as he's never come back to collect it."

"Have you still got it?"

"Yes. He paid me and then said that a friend of his, a girl, would come and pick it up, but she never turned up. I called him a couple of times and he always said she'd be along soon. As you can see, I'm a bit short of space and I can't keep too many things."

"Has Soncini been here on other occasions?"

"A couple of times in the last few months," Sauro replied after consulting his ledger. "The last time was a few days ago."

"What was he here for?"

"Problems with the hard disk on his office computer."

Soneri registered this information without having any idea what it might mean, and when Sauro tried to explain, he said: "Save yourself the time. I won't understand the first thing."

"I thought the police . . ."

"Not all of them, not the older ones, not me."

"It's all a question of familiarity. I've got a customer in the police force who could teach me a thing or two."

"Is his name Juvara?" Soneri said, with no doubt in his mind.

"You see? You guessed right away. You might not understand much about computers, but you've got a feel for things."

"It's very famous, that feel," Soneri said as he was leaving.

In the short time he had been in the shop, the afternoon light had faded. Darkness was advancing between the houses of the *borghi*, but there was still the bustle of daytime. Soneri turned into Via Farini and came out on Piazza Garibaldi. The clock on the Palazzo del Governatore showed ten past four, but the lights in the windows on Via Repubblica had already been switched on. The gathering dusk strengthened his sense both of the importance of his investigation and his remorse towards Nina, due to more than the desire to find the truth. At certain moments, the thought of this young woman

– pregnant, murdered and consumed by fire – moved him deeply, and each time the thought came back to him it set his nerves jangling. Something similar had been happening in the city since the papers had screamed out the news of Candiani's arrest. Parma, a hive of gossip and rumour at the best of times, was already beginning to take the development on board, partly relieved that the Monster had been identified and partly already exorcising the memory by picturing Candiani as a deranged outsider in an upright, hard-working community.

The city was digesting everything with a smile and a satisfied belch, he thought to himself as he walked through the door of the police station. Juvara, however, had the expression of a man whose lunch was lying heavily on his stomach. "Were there bulls running free at Suzzara as well?" Soneri enquired.

"Commissario, those Romas are not the most friendly of people. There were two of us against seventy of them."

"I didn't expect you to challenge them to a pitched battle."

"They don't like us! They'd rather see a herd of bulls than have a visit from us."

"Who does like us? We get sour looks even from people who come whimpering to us when their pockets have been picked. The Left accuses us of being too right-wing, and the Right accuses us of being too soft."

The inspector made a resigned gesture. "Well, the upshot is that we didn't find out very much."

"Still, it was worth trying."

"The carabinieri went one stage further. They searched the camp. Maybe that's why the Romas were so pissed off."

"What did they come up with?"

"Gold. They're specialists in thefts of gold."

"That's hardly news."

"Not true. Thieves today go in for copper. The price has gone through the roof, and it's not hard to find – building sites, warehouses and even electrical wires. I saw some statistics on the internet . . ."

The commissario silenced him with a wave of his hand. "Find anything else?"

"That they hated Iliescu."

"Hated her?"

"The moment we mentioned her name, they went berserk and started spitting on the ground. 'Whore' was the mildest epithet they used."

It all fitted in with Soncini's story. Nina must indeed have been lonely and desperate in her effort to defend herself, fought over by her various lovers and by a ruthless community, but for precisely that reason the girl seemed to him all the more admirable. For him the investigation was breaking down more and more barriers and becoming more than a simple act of duty.

"Listen, Juvara," Soneri said, changing the subject. "What's this Sauro like, the guy with the computer shop? I know you're one of his clients."

"I've only been there a couple of times," the inspector said.

"Juvara! You're a policeman! You've no need to be so defensive. If anything, it's your job to put the questions other people have to answer."

"I thought for a moment he'd been up to some funny business."

"Not at all. One of his other customers is Soncini, who's been to him a few times with some problem with his laptop and with something else I couldn't understand. Anyway, he never went back for the laptop. He told the guy that a female friend would be along for it, but she never turned up. It might be Nina, but you can't be sure with a man like Soncini."

"You see now that computers can be excellent leads?"

"Don't kid yourself. If there'd been anything compromising on that laptop, do you really think they'd have left it with your friend?"

"He's not a friend, but he's good at his job. And I believe he's honest into the bargain."

"O.K., could you work on him a bit? You know, one expert to another? By the way, I liked him too."

Just then the telephone on his desk rang.

"Commissario, at long last." It was Dottoressa Marcotti.

He was about to defend himself but the investigating magistrate came straight to the point. She was a woman with no time for small talk and invariably in a hurry, another reason why she and Soneri got on so well.

"I have requested authorisation to tap the phones of all of Iliescu's lovers. I hope the judge will agree in all cases. Meanwhile, your colleagues have sent me an account of the C.C.T.V. footage shot near where our car thieves were operating. Not much help, I have to admit. The only worthwhile thing is that the older one turns to the younger and says they'd been set up. It's a sentence that could mean everything or nothing."

The commissario gave a groan and nodded, but before he could say anything, she put him on the spot: "Tell me, have you by now come up with a theory about what's been going on here?"

He did not know what to say. Each time he began to develop a hypothesis it was overturned a moment later, and he had failed to translate that complex of impressions continually whirling about in his head into anything coherent. "Not yet," was all he said.

He heard a laugh at the other end of the line. "We're doing a great job! Neither one of us has a clue!"

"It won't be like this for long," he said.

"I do hope not," Marcotti said. "With every case, you have to go through a period of darkness when you don't know which way to turn, but we've cast so many nets that sooner or later some fish will get tangled up in them, you'll see." The prosecutor was an incurable optimist.

At that very moment, Soneri would have happily asked her to marry him. Having a woman like that at your side was the equivalent of a transfusion of ginseng. Angela was made of the same stuff, and that was one of the things he liked about her – always assuming she chose not to leave him.

He lit a cigar and decided to go out. It was rush hour, the time when employees left their offices, the admin staff and managers all dressed in the standard, starched-and-scented uniforms. He felt a pang of nostalgia for the sight of house-wives carrying shopping and shouting in dialect to each other from opposite sides of the road, or workmen with cloth coats thrown over their overalls as they cycled home from factories still located inside the city and not ten kilometres into the hinterland, like Golden.

His mind was still on the squalor of those lots out at Lemignano, where the asphalt and the factory buildings had devastated fields and vineyards, when he came across a noisy procession of cars decked out in white ribbons. He watched the parade as it turned into Via Cavour, opened specially. He was going in the same direction, as far as the junction with Strada al Duomo. Just ahead, he saw the square overflowing with vintage cars and the cathedral precinct crowded with people done up in all their finery. Security guards manning the barriers prevented onlookers from drawing too close to the festivities. Official cars and company limousines swarmed busily about, as though the Duomo were the Grand Hotel.

The mystery was solved when a woman's voice squealed

out: "It's the wedding of the eldest of the Dall'Argine family."

That name clarified everything. The eldest of the Dall'-Argine line was marrying Soncini's daughter. The wily, emerging dynasty was forming a union with a scion of the patriciate, thereby ennobling their line. Soneri moved off, in search of fresher air he could breathe in solitude. Never till that moment had he felt himself so proudly anarchist, with a will for freedom and the purity of a young wolf.

He wandered about aimlessly until hunger and curiosity brought him back to the wine bar. He went into the dining room and looked from table to table, simultaneously fearful and hopeful of spying his rival, but Sbarazza was already seated at the table where he had last seen him. He got up and with an elegant gesture invited Soneri to sit beside him.

"So now you're laying on receptions," the commissario said.

"It's getting harder and harder at the *Milord*. Too busy. I have to adapt. This evening I had no appetite for tinned tuna," he whispered confidentially.

"No problems here?" Soneri said, pointing to the bar.

"Bruno knows me. A good man, like Alceste."

"But they're nearly all men here."

"Not so. There were several couples."

"Was there a couple sitting here?"

"Yes, having a light meal."

"Do you mind if I ask what they looked like?"

Sbarazza stared at him, clearly taken aback. "You want a description? He was tall, distinguished-looking, well turned out. She seemed very lively, not exactly beautiful but with character, if you get my meaning."

Soneri hesitated for a moment, and as he was about to answer he became aware of Sbarazza's baffled expression fixed on him.

"What is it? Does that correspond to the identikit of two suspects?"

"No, not at all. I was just thinking how vulnerable we all are."

"Ah," Sbarazza smiled. "We are eggs with fragile shells, or better, we are fragile, full stop. We don't even have a shell."

"Rather than having no shell, right now I feel as if I have no gravity," Soneri said.

"That might be an advantage."

"Like being in water without fins or in the air without wings."

"Don't be such a pessimist. The mistake we make is to be always engaged in a search for certainties. We need certainties, we demand them, we never resign ourselves to being what we are. If we were to face up to our condition we'd be more serene and might even see opportunities rather than frustrations."

"Facing up to what we are is itself a certainty, is it not?"

"Alright, I grant you that, but it's the only one: the certainty of not having certainties. That has to be our starting point."

"That's very much the reasoning of a police officer, you know. They teach exactly that to beginners: given a case, never start out with a preconceived idea. But in fact a commissario has the facts in front of him."

"You know better than me that facts are never objective! Take history. What we are convinced of today will have no value tomorrow, and the day after that something different will come along. We die each evening and wake up afresh the following morning, and so the world renews itself minute by minute. The essence of our being is changeability, not stability, and every man who aims at coherence is nothing but a self-deluding fool. The point is to accept what we are and open ourselves to the great flourishing of possibilities which time continually offers us. The acceptance of the world, that's the secret. Do you remember Nietzsche?"

Fortunately Bruno came over to the table at that moment. "What can I get you, Commissario?"

"I'll have some *culaccia* and Parmesan shavings."

"Marchese, would you like something else?" the waiter asked with absolute seriousness.

"I'll borrow something from the commissario. He's the only man with whom I would share a plate."

"And bring us some red Lambrusco," Soneri said. He needed a drop of strong wine to wash away his thoughts. As he was being served, he raised a slice of *culaccia* to his mouth as though officiating at some rite. "These are my certainties," he announced, his tone doleful.

"I see you've understood. Life is like a game of cards: you must always wait for something good to emerge from the pack. Look at me. I once had a mansion and a family endowed with coats of arms and emblems evoking battles won and honours received. The most absurd thing is to imagine you can actually leave something behind you. They drummed this into me ever since I was a boy by showing me portraits of my forefathers in the corridors of our ancestral home. The genealogical tree is a load of bollocks."

Sbarazza seemed to be on the edge of delirium, but Soneri could not dispute the force of his logic. His thoughts went back to Angela and those passionate lunchtime rendezvous, but for the moment he had drawn from the pack the card he had, and to ask for anything else for the future was futile.

He poured himself a glass of Lambrusco the colour of black pudding. "That couple, the one that was here . . ." he began hesitantly, with the unpleasant feeling of possibly occupying the seat recently occupied by his rival.

"You haven't got it, have you?" Sbarazza interrupted him with good-natured authority. "You're still after the confirmation I do not wish to give you. What does it matter to you if you know or don't know? All it would do is poison your evening. Have you any idea how many things are happening at this moment in your favour or to your disadvantage? Dozens, but you don't know. We live in a constant state of unawareness, and this is both our salvation and our damnation. It leaves open the doors of our emotions but makes us as volatile as an alcoholic scent."

The mention of alcohol made Soneri throw back a glass of Lambrusco in one gulp, looking for that mild euphoria which would keep him afloat. "It may be destiny that I have some very unforthcoming witnesses," he said.

"I think I understand your situation. It's one I've been in many times myself." Sbarazza had assumed a more serious tone. "If the person you're fond of has already decided to leave you, there's nothing you can do to convince her otherwise. If on the other hand she is unsure, the only thing you can do is be gracious. The only salvation lies in graciousness towards your neighbour because what all humans, even the most atrocious criminals, seek is to be loved. We are all orphans, after all, are we not?"

Soneri nodded thoughtfully, going over in his mind the criminals it had been his lot to encounter in his work as commissario. Yet again, Sbarazza was not wide of the mark.

"It may seem not worth much to you that all we can do is exchange feelings of unhappiness. I'm aware it's a bad deal, but that's all there is. Unless . . ." Sbarazza broke off abruptly.

"Unless what?"

"Unless you turn to God."

"That's a different matter altogether," Soneri said. "In any case, He does not seem to take much interest in human affairs."

"Please! Don't come out with bar-room arguments. I expect better of you."

"It's just that not even by having recourse to God do I find any sense in things."

"You are an incurable rationalist. You search for meaning in things so as to draw some reassurance, but God is beyond the boundaries of our reason. We dance on the edge of a waterfall, waiting to be finally washed away, ignorant of where we'll end up. We can't choose: life overwhelms us. Others have written the script and if it's a question of God, then it all comes back to what I was saying a moment ago. Listen, pick a card from the pack and resign yourself to your choice. At the end of the day, we'll all get the same pay-off."

"I'm playing more than one game," Soneri said.

"I understand. One is that girl whose body was burned, is it not?"

"I've been drawing cards from the pack for some time now, but I never get the right one."

"Sooner or later you will. You'll see. My advice is still the same. Let events follow their own course and take every opportunity as it presents itself. All you have to do is recognise the opportunity when it comes."

The commissario heaved a deep sigh and again sought refuge in wine. It would have been good to end the evening on that note, with the right flavours in his mouth, but he knew that any time now the bar would fill with noise and laughter loud enough to exasperate him. In addition, Sbarazza had not entirely endeared himself to him for the reticence he had shown earlier. He still had a lingering doubt over whether Angela and the other man had really been there, but the descriptions fitted. Here too his policeman's frame of mind was becoming a burden. Events were getting on top of him in spite of his obstinate determination to put them in order.

"I must go and see my old ladies and gentlemen. It's dinner time at the hostel, and that will be followed by a bit of socialising," Sbarazza said, with that light irony which marked his detachment from the world.

"You're not going to the wedding feast then?" Soneri asked, referring to the Dall'Argine–Soncini ceremony.

"Money provides no remedy against vulgarity," commented the old man with a smile of kindly commiseration.

16

THERE WAS SOMETHING profoundly vulgar about the profanation of the night which had transformed Piazza Duomo into an *haute couture* bonanza. In clothes alone, the wedding must have cost thousands of euros, before taking jewellery and limousines and vintage cars into account. The chatter among Benedetto Antelami's marble sculptures clashed with the notes of the organ as they swelled out through the wide-open doors of the Cathedral. Perhaps the chalice used to give communion to the newly-weds had been manufactured by Golden.

Soneri detested solemn ceremonies. He found them phoney and was always afraid of laughing out loud when faced with such pantomimes, but what he saw unfolding before his eyes outdid anything he had ever previously seen. It verged on being a display of ostentatious marketing, degenerating into a senseless replay of society functions of the sort recorded in glossy magazines in a hairdresser's salon. In spite of that, he stood there, leaning against the wall of the old Fiaccadori bookshop, staring, glued to the spot, incapable of dragging himself away. He was, as Sbarazza had advised, letting events take their course.

And events did indeed take their course. As the couple emerged to a flurry of rice and flashbulbs, the noise rose in volume, the cheers bounced off the noble stones of the Duomo rising in a crescendo until they deafened the golden angel on the cusp of the belfry somewhere beyond the curtain of the mist, and even awoke Correggio's little *putti* in the neighbouring church of St John. But then in a sudden diminuendo the piazza fell silent and the commissario was aware of the shudder which precedes movement, as when a train is about to depart. He realised that something must have happened to change the evening's programme, and he felt no displeasure at seeing that exhibition disrupted.

Pasquariello's voice on the mobile brought him up to date with what had happened. "A bomb has gone off at Golden."

"Was anyone hurt?"

"No, it wasn't a big bomb, but if it had gone off when the workers were around . . ."

"Yet another problem!"

"Two idiots. The carabinieri picked them up in the vicinity. They're Romanian."

Soneri could not help thinking that this was another point in favour of Soncini's hypothesis. The Romanians really were out to take revenge on him.

"How did they find them?"

"The idiots didn't notice the security guards doing their first round. The guards heard the explosion and raised the alarm, and our two lads ran straight into a carabiniere patrol."

The piazza was emptying. With the occasional explosion of back-firing engines, the vintage cars made a juddering start one after the other. A different sort of explosion ten kilometres away had brought the festivities to a premature end.

Juvara called shortly afterwards. "Do you want me to come and get you, Commissario?"

The thought of returning to Lemignano was dispiriting, but he hoped the mist would have blanked out the ugliest parts of the district. "Alright. I'll meet you in Via Cavour, but watch out you don't crash into the Nuvolari car."

"Commissario, the days of the Mille Miglia are long past."

A few minutes later, the police Alfa Romeo flashed its lights from Via Pisacane. "These people are mad!" the inspector shouted. "They nearly ran right into me. What's going on? Is this some costume drama?"

"Nearly," the commissario laughed. "The party's been ruined and that's why they're going off their heads. Tomorrow they'll be on to the Chief about law and order and dangers to public safety. And you can be sure that blame will be laid at our door. Again."

"What party was ruined?"

"You obviously don't keep abreast of the goings-on in high society in this city! It was the wedding of the century."

"Don't tell me those cars were there for the Dall'Argine . . ."

"You see, you knew after all. You obviously read the glossies in the hairdresser's."

"You're kidding. It was in the papers today. Two whole pages."

"Instead of printing something serious . . ."

"Now I get it," Juvara said. "The Dall'Argine boy was marrying the Soncini girl and that's why they put a bomb in the Golden workshop. At about the very moment the daughter was saying 'I do'."

"Right," the commissario said.

"A terrible business," Juvara said as they got out of the car in the darkness at Lemignano, but it was not clear if he was referring to the dynamic of events or to the large black mark on the factory wall where a fire had briefly blazed, shattering the windows.

The investigating magistrate, with her blonde, flowing locks standing out in the headlights as clearly as the phosphorescent jackets of the carabinieri, arrived within minutes. Maresciallo Santurro of the carabinieri had taken charge because of the success of his detachment in making the arrest, and he directed operations like a little Napoleon. Soneri had little to do except observe what had happened and absorb any suggestions of the kind invariably prompted by a crime scene. While Marcotti went to speak to the maresciallo, the commissario turned in the direction of the Golden offices, and there he found Soncini gazing at the burn marks on the wall with the concentration with which another man might have looked at a painting.

"I was right," he muttered without turning round.

"The facts are on your side," Soneri said drily. "Thus far, at least," he added, reminding himself of the changeability he had discussed with Sbarazza. "Anyway, they've got them in custody, so you can relax . . ."

"With those people, you can never relax. They never give up and there are so many of them. This is a warning shot. Next time . . ."

"There won't be a next time."

"You should've done something when I told you they were threatening me," Soncini said angrily. "I have the right to protection. And then . . . the business . . ." Soneri could have sworn he all but said "my business".

"They'll not try again for a while. They're not that stupid," the commissario reassured him. "To change the subject, I know you came to the station to identify your car. It seems there are no doubts, is that right?"

Soncini nodded. "It's mine alright. They wanted the blame to fall on me."

"Where are your wife and daughter now?"

"Where do you think!" exclaimed Soncini arrogantly. "At the reception. They could hardly walk out on the guests!

What would the Dall'Argine family have thought? These things make a lasting impression. Even if we were the victims, mud sticks."

The commissario began to feel so exasperated with Soncini that he was tempted to give a brutal reply. What did he have to be afraid of? The wedding had taken place and it was too late for the Dall'Argine family to have second thoughts. However, he remembered his position as a public servant and merely said: "People forget very quickly."

Marcotti came over and took him aside. "Did you know the judge has refused permission to tap the phones of Iliescu's lovers? He said there were not sufficient grounds."

Soneri stretched his arms wide, all the while thinking that had he been in the judge's shoes, he too might have been cautious. There was nothing concrete to point to them as likely murderers. They had gone to bed with Nina and had left part of their hearts with her, but nothing more.

"What do you make of this bombing?" she asked Soneri.

"It's another piece in the jigsaw, but we don't know where it fits."

She laughed. "We're still pulling in the nets and something will come to the surface. However, I have to warn you that tomorrow the newspapers are going to go wild. This time somebody has trodden on the toes of the high and mighty. It's no longer just about some poor Romanian girl."

As he went back to the car with Juvara, Soneri reflected on that obscure threat. "We're going to have the questore breathing down our necks," Juvara said.

"The city demands an explanation of the disturbing events occurring all around us," Soneri said in a sing-song voice, mimicking Capuozzo and the next morning's headlines. "As long as everything's covered up they'll all sit tight, fooling themselves they're in the best little city in the world, but the moment the dirty washing appears in public, they start screaming about it all being a terrible scandal," the commissario bellowed.

Juvara said nothing until Soneri had calmed down.

"Tomorrow," Soneri said, changing tack, "pop along to that friend of yours who sells computers and make him give you Soncini's P.C. Take it home and have a good look inside it – although you'd better talk to Marcotti first. If you can't get hold of her, try to persuade that Sauro."

"Do you think there'll be anything interesting in the laptop?"

"No, but you never know."

"A couple of days ago you told me Soncini needed something for his office computer. What was wrong with it?"

"You know perfectly well I never remember these things. It must have broken down or something . . ."

"Forgive my saying so," Juvara began timidly, "but I think you should get to grips with this field. It's fundamental for our work to—"

"I know, I know," Soneri interrupted in annoyance more than anger. "But I'm too old now to learn new tricks and I'm going to carry on with the tried and tested."

"What do you mean? You're still young. You're suffering from nothing more than mental laziness. Did you know that even Capuozzo is taking a course?"

"Well I never! He should really be taking a course to raise his I.Q., but unfortunately there's no such course available."

"And it would be a good idea for you to learn some English."

"Juvara, that's enough. You're getting on my nerves. You know what you're going to do next? You're going to come with me on a visit to the Campo San Martino Romas to see if the bulls have all been rounded up."

"In this mist? And it's nearly ten o'clock," said the inspector hesitantly.

"They can have a long lie-in tomorrow."

They took the narrow roads along the Lower Valley, as they had done the time before, when it was all starting up.

"If this is a punishment, it seems to me over the top," Juvara grumbled.

"Don't talk nonsense. I want to hear what Manservisi has to say. I think we might be given the right cards by our good friends, the Italian gypsies."

"I don't follow."

"Doesn't matter. It's a coded language I learned from Sbarazza, a highly eccentric aristocrat."

Juvara made no reply. He was relieved the commissario was not angry with him.

Soneri missed the signs to the dump and the U-turn he executed brought the inspector out in a cold sweat. Nothing much had changed in the clearing apart from the fact that there was more rubbish than ever and now it was piled alongside the huge bins. The encampment was deserted and the fires almost out. All that remained were a few tongues of flame on a bed of ashes. Some televisions flickered inside caravans. The commissario parked and walked over, with Juvara at his heels. The heads of several children appeared at windows and some doors were hurriedly opened and just as hurriedly closed. A moment later Manservisi, cap on head, came to meet them with the relaxed gait of a man without a care in the world.

"Good evening," he said, drawing up in front of Soneri. In the background, the mist took on a yellowish tinge in the lights of the service area and hypermarket. There was no music playing. Perhaps the fairground had moved on.

"I take it something serious has occurred to bring you out in the mist at this time of night. Another death?" Manservisi enquired.

"We just wanted to know how Mariotto is getting on," Soneri said.

Manservisi gave a raucous laugh. "You must be joking."

"By no means."

The gypsy put on a serious face and grew tense.

"Now it's you who must be joking," Soneri said.

"Me? Mariotto has already told you all he knew. We've told you everything too. What more can you want?"

"That you don't piss me off with that story about a bull goring him. You know very well it's not true. Mariotto was beaten up."

"Commissario, in the mist people see all sorts of things that never happened. Go and ask him for yourself."

"Don't talk shit. There's no doubt he was threatened, and it was probably you who ordered him to keep his mouth shut. In addition, no judge would credit a witness who is mentally defective."

"I have not ordered anybody to do anything. I defend my community, that's all I do."

"And you think you'll defend it by not talking? Why did the Romanians rush off so suddenly? There must have been a huge row between all of you."

"This is a big world. There's room for everybody," Manservisi said, implicitly confirming what Soneri had suggested.

"Not big enough, to judge by all that's been going on. They dump a burned body in front of the encampment, one of your lot runs off after a ridiculous theft, and another one is beaten up and it's passed off as his being gored by a bull. That's a lot of coincidences."

"So what are you getting at?" Manservisi said impatiently.

"That you know much more than you've told me."

Manservisi grunted, while somewhere behind him there was a rustling sound and a snort. They must have caught one of the missing pigs and put it in a pen.

"Anyway, the carabinieri did a search of your ex-neighbours and they came up with piles of gold. A magistrate could order the same thing here," Soneri said, knowing his threat was a bluff.

"Go ahead," Manservisi said with total confidence. "We don't touch that stuff. The people here go to work and our children go to school."

"What became of the Romanians' gold?"

"How should I know? If you had valuables in your possession, what would you do with them? Not any old stuff, but stuff that had a name and address."

"Like a painting," Soneri reflected.

"But you can give gold a new identity. You can't do that with a painting."

"That's true. Gold comes in many shapes and forms."

He remained where he was for a moment while Manservisi moved off with the same self-assurance with which he had arrived. Juvara was by the fire trying to get warm.

"Let's go," Soneri called to him, as he got into the car. Juvara ran awkwardly to the car, and there was no concealing his relief that they were leaving.

"What do you think he meant by that last remark?" the commissario said as they drove through the mist.

"I think he meant that objects in gold are easily recognisable by the person they were stolen from, but they can be melted down and transformed into perfectly anonymous items."

"Well done. I see you're beginning to develop an investigator's mind. Tomorrow I want you to go to Suzzara and see if there's been a rise in the number of thefts of gold. And persuade our colleagues to tell you if there have been robberies around Cortile San Martino."

As they reached the city boundary, one of their mobiles rang. Juvara fumbled about for a while before he located the correct one. "It's yours. They both have the same ringtone," he said.

It was Marcotti. "Soneri," she began, "I've had the two bombers moved to prison. I wanted to let you know that if you plan to interrogate them, I'll be there tomorrow morning at nine."

"Are they talking?"

"No different from the other two: not a word. And they too say they've been fitted up."

"We'll have to find some way of making them talk. Maybe they could be convinced . . ."

"Forget it, commissario. I've got experience in dealing with gangs from Eastern Europe and it's not only the Italians who practice *omerta*."

"Then we have only one card to play."

"Which card is that?"

"Medioli. I invited him to cooperate, and perhaps he will. He's not one of the Roma community and doesn't subscribe to their rites. We could look on him as an infiltrator."

"And you really believe he'll help? He doesn't seem to me quite of this world."

"Let's have a go."

He dropped Juvara off at his house.

"I'll be in the office first thing tomorrow morning and I'll get to work on the internet to do the research we were discussing."

"Internet, internet! Wouldn't you be quicker going round in person to the officers responsible for investigating thefts? Their office is only two floors up. It's always better to talk face to face."

"Whatever you want, commissario, but you really are too dismissive of computer technology."

"Enough, Juvara! And don't forget your friend Sauro. You can drive each other crazy with all this talk."

The inspector made a sign that meant 'I will obey', and shut the car door. The commissario accelerated away in the direction of Angela's house. He wanted to see her and spend the night with her. He parked underneath her residence and called her, but the telephone in the house rang out. Her mobile was switched off. He sank from desire to frustration and on to unhappy thoughts, and then began to think like a policeman and assess all possible hypotheses concerning his partner's silence, coming inevitably to the worst possible conclusion. He was tired of forever banging his head against forces that refused to yield up their mystery, first in his work and now in his emotional life. Sbarazza had been right: for him it was all too much.

He decided to go home, but then could not bring himself to drive off, so he chose instead to smoke a cigar and walk off his anxiety. He went along Via D'Azeglio with the mist ahead of him and swirling at his back. From time to time groups of Arabs and Africans emerged from the nearby neighbourhoods, their raised voices cutting through the silence of the deserted street. He came to Piazza Garibaldi and crossed into Via Farini before turning into Vicolo Politi in the direction of the court. There were still cars parked in front, perhaps belonging to magistrates. Angela might be busy inside, perhaps questioning a witness. He hung about for a while, and then saw Marcotti, the chief prosecutor, Capuozzo and Maresciallo Santurro go out. There had been a meeting no-one had told him about, and that promised nothing good for him, unless the agenda had been limited to the explosion at Golden.

He went away certain that there would be trouble the following day, but he did not want to think about it. He was tired, disappointed and frustrated. He could not take any more. The moment he got home, the telephone rang.

"Were you looking for me?" Angela said.

"You talk to me as though I were president of the society of lawyers."

"Sorry. I'm out of breath. I've been working late and I'm extremely tired."

"So am I. And not only because of work."

"What does that mean?"

"That I can't stand any more of this. I can never find you, I can't reach you to talk to you, and when I do you're very cold."

"I've really got a lot of work on."

"And I'm telling you that this is no way to live. You'll have to make up your mind, Angela. One way or the other. I know you're still seeing him. You were in the wine bar with him tonight."

There was a pause. Soneri would have given anything to hear her deny it, but instead she came back at him, totally composed. "So you're playing the policeman with me again, are you?"

"You're wrong. It was pure chance. But I believe in coincidences."

"You've already said that. You'd be better to keep your imagination in check, considering the job you do."

"Angela, I'm serious. I can't go on this way. This situation is causing me too much pain."

She sighed. "I'm sorry, I don't want to hurt you, but I'm not ready to decide. I'm too confused."

He would have liked to tell her to let events take their course, as Sbarazza counselled, but he stayed quiet and it was she who murmured: "I still want to see you."

Soneri could understand nothing, but at the same time he was aware that there was nothing to understand, that there was nothing for it but to live for the moment, savour it and take everything he could from it without wondering what would happen next.

17

JUVARA HAD BEEN at work a full two hours before the commissario arrived at the office.

"You were right," Juvara told him. "There's been quite an increase in reports of thefts of gold and jewellery in recent weeks, but the really interesting facts are contained in the data provided by colleagues who investigate theft and robbery. In the area around Cortile San Martino a lot of houses have been burgled and they've lost count of the number of cars broken into in the parking area at the autostrada petrol station."

"A whole industry!"

"And another thing. They've not spared the churches either."

"The churches?"

"Four parishes have reported thefts in the last two months, and in every case sacred vessels in gold have been carried off."

"Did this happen in Suzzara as well?"

"Apparently not, but that could be because they've only been there a short time."

A few minutes passed and then the telephone on his desk rang.

"Commissario Soneri, I've got Dottor Capuozzo for you,"

announced the questore's secretary. It seemed to Soneri there could be no worse way to start the new day.

"I'm phoning about the Iliescu crime," Capuozzo began. "I'm worried about this investigation because, unless I am very much mistaken, we're not even within sight of a conclusion."

"It's a particularly complex case, Dottore. Initially the identity of the victim was unknown, and then we established we were dealing with an illegal immigrant who was using her sister's passport, and then there was the case of the old man whose body was found on the bus."

"All that is understood, but we're going from bad to worse. Now we've got bombs going off. What are we going to tell the city?"

Soneri struggled to stop himself letting out a roar. He assumed that following the uproar created by the disruption of the wedding, some local grandees had been in touch to complain. These were the people to whom his superior was accountable, certainly not the city as a whole.

"We're working on it." Soneri said. "Neither Dottoressa Marcotti nor I will rest until . . ."

"I've called a meeting with the Prefect, the Mayor and the President of the Province for this afternoon. We must send out a bulletin."

The usual comedy with a cast of bureaucrats, Soneri thought to himself. He saw cameras and notebooks clustered around two dozen authority figures, reporting the "tireless work of the security committees". Perfect for a world which thrived on appearances.

"I hope to have good news for you soon." Soneri made an effort to be diplomatic. "Sooner or later we'll draw the right card," he said, realising as he spoke how deeply that expression had lodged in his mind. As he replaced the telephone, he felt his anger and unease return. Calls from Capuozzo were utterly vacuous, but, like an alarm clock about to go off, they always induced a state of anxiety.

"Did he tell you about the meeting?" Juvara said, as he got up to go out.

"You knew about it?"

"His secretary called this morning as soon as I got to the office, but she told me there was no need to pass on a message because she'd call back. I thought it better to spare you a half hour's bad mood," the inspector explained, before hurriedly adding, "I'm on my way to see Sauro now."

Soneri signalled his approval with a wave, but without looking up. He was thinking about the meeting. He had no wish to waste time on prattle, the only purpose of which was to command some column inches in the newspapers and give the impression of what the politicians would call "putting all arms of government on an emergency footing". He decided he would absent himself once again, even if that would do nothing for his relations with Capuozzo. If he was not going to the meeting, what would he do with his afternoon? He attempted to find a motive to justify his absence, but all of a sudden he found his head empty, as though he were about to faint. The only thought that troubled him related to Angela.

He considered telephoning her, but pride and self-respect held him back. It was up to her to make the next move, although he was aware that there might well be no move at all. Everything might be frozen in the final checkmate.

And then, without knocking, Musumeci burst in, providentially bringing Soneri's mind back to the investigation. "I've got a report here from the Romanian police which arrived a couple of hours ago. Our translator has just finished working on it."

"Report on what?"

"They've found Iliescu's sister. She works in a lap-dancing club in Bucharest, and finally we know the identity of the old man who died on the coach."

"And who was he?"

"The grandfather, but there are gaps in the report. He had something to do with the Romas. In fact it seems he was one himself."

"What made him risk his life coming to Italy?"

"The sister was very worried about what might happen to Nina, because she had heard from various sources that the Roma community here were out to get her."

"Soncini explained the reasons why they were after her, but I've no way of knowing if he told me everything."

"The fact is her sister claims she spent a long time begging their grandfather to come to Italy and try to make peace and stop anything worse happening. According to what she says, she gave him a lot of cash and paid for his journey."

"He must have drunk the cash or else someone cheated him out of it. The old man was down to his last penny when he died."

"It's likely it went down his gullet. The guy was a notorious drunk. Anyway, he didn't succeed in his mission."

"Leave this report with me. I'll read it later."

"I've given you the substance of it," Musumeci said.

There was a knock at the door and a good-looking policewoman, who drew Musumeci's appreciative attention, came in.

"Today's papers, commissario," she said, placing the bundle on his desk.

"We've made great strides in the quality of our staff," Musumeci observed, but the commissario ignored him. He was already flicking through the pages to find the local news.

The reporters had gone overboard. There were four pages

devoted to the wedding and how it had been disrupted by the bomb planted at the Golden factory, followed by an array of dramatic photographs and a rosary of indignant interviews with the well-heeled of Parma society, each one "dismayed by the escalation of violence", and some requesting "whoever is in charge" to take all steps necessary to prevent "the decline of civic standards". The heads of the Dall'Argine and Martini families had declined to make any comment. They restricted themselves to showing expressions of outrage to the photographers who captured some images of them as they emerged from the Duomo. Soneri imagined they would have used their influence behind the scenes, putting pressure on senior officials and perhaps stirring up a storm in the press by telephoning the newspaper proprietors directly. Soncini alone had given an interview overflowing with righteous indignation, thereby exposing his inferior status and putting himself on the same level as councillors, chairs of committees and the city's resident intellectuals. There was also a piece devoted to the investigation in which details were given of the various leads being followed by the investigators, but making it plain between the lines that the police had no idea where next to turn.

The commissario threw the papers on the desk in a rage. He found the hypocrisy of Parma more and more nauseating. All those people preaching respect for the law and then going about their business as though they were above all reproach. He regretted the loss of the city's democratic soul, which had always shown itself ready to scoff in public at local bigwigs and bien pensants, perhaps with a biting, satirical scrawl on walls near the houses where such people lived or with a salacious slogan on the porch of the Regio theatre. In those days, Parma could kill with a jibe.

The telephone rang on a couple of occasions and each

time the commissario dashed to pick it up. He was burning inside during that impotent wait. He had already put in a request to interrogate Medioli, but it would take some time before the final authorisation came through. He had no idea how to fill his time.

Mercifully Juvara came back and took his mind off the various pieces of bad news.

"It was the hard disk," the inspector told him.

"Whatever that may be," Soneri said.

"It's the core of the computer, where all the data end up. It's a bit like our mind and memory."

"Soncini had broken its brain?"

"Not quite. It wasn't broken. In fact it was working, and perfectly."

"So?"

"Sauro told me Soncini had asked him how to go about deleting all trace of the operations executed by that machine."

"And Sauro replied that he had to change the . . . what's it called?"

"It's the only way. Everything is stored on the hard disk, and any technician worth his salt would have no problem reconstructing the life of the computer and all the operations carried out on it."

"At last, something interesting."

"You see what you can do with technology?" Juvara said enthusiastically. "You can set up whole lines of enquiry with the help of computer technology."

"Did he change the . . . whatever it's called . . . for him?" Soneri interrupted Juvara, but he was beginning to feel guilty for having underestimated his colleague's skill.

"Yes, but he told me he only changed the hard disk after a couple of days. Soncini came back to say it didn't have enough memory and he needed a more powerful computer.

In other words, he now had different requirements, and that was another reason why Sauro didn't bother too much about it."

"Did he hang onto the old dish?"

"Disk. He's afraid he threw it out. He doesn't have a lot of space, but he'll have a look and let us know."

"If he has thrown it out, we've wasted a lot of time."

"We'll know this afternoon."

"Listen, if that thing turns up and is of any use to us, I swear I'll buy myself a laptop."

The inspector smiled. "I'm sure you'll fall in love with it."

"Meantime, let me buy you lunch. I haven't eaten properly in days."

"I'm sorry, I'm on a diet," Juvara said, pulling out a plastic box containing an assortment of lettuce leaves, diced carrot, sweetcorn and slices of tomato. On the top there was a sachet of oil which had to be squeezed to produce a dressing for the whole concoction.

"That stuff would disgust even a bunny rabbit," Soneri said, staring at the transparent packet with an expression of sheer nausea.

Juvara apologised, patting his stomach to indicate *force majeure*.

When he was on Via Repubblica, the commissario felt the need of someone to talk to. It was a new sensation for him and gave him the measure of his depressed state of mind. Loneliness had never held any fear for him: in this regard, he was like a cat. Perhaps this was one of the effects of his crisis with Angela. He asked Alceste to prepare him a bit of space in the kitchen, so he could chat to him while he was doing the cooking. He enjoyed watching pots boil, waiters running about and steam forming the same shapes under the ceiling as the mist outside. It was the kind of day that called for a plate of *anolini* accompanied by a good Bonarda. He counted on the calories to set him up for an afternoon which threatened to be grim.

The warmth of the wine and the pasta, the aromas of the prosciutto and salame had the desired effect, and when he was on his way back to the police station he already felt better. The good humour lasted until he reached the piazza and saw from the clock that the time was two-thirty. He felt a lump in his throat. Angela had not called, and between her hostile silence and his proud indifference their post-lunch appointment had passed. By the time he got to the office, his foul mood had returned. Juvara avoided speaking first.

"Any news?" the commissario said.

"Nothing yet."

"Have you requested printouts for the mobile phones of Soncini and his friend Razzini?"

"I have, but you know what these companies are like. They go at their own pace. I called back this morning to ask them to get a move on. Dottoressa Marcotti called as well but . . ."

The telephone rang. Soneri feared the worst, and in fact it was Capuozzo's secretary. "The questore would like to know if you intend to be present at the meeting," she said. She had the perfect voice for cajolery.

"Tell him I'm very sorry, but no. I'm waiting for the results of a crucial line of enquiry. I can't leave the office. I have to be here just in case."

The secretary said she would pass on the message. Fortunately she made no effort to put Capuozzo on the line.

"And what will you do if Sauro doesn't come up with anything?"

"It means Capuozzo will remove me from my post, and

when all's said and done, it wouldn't really upset me. But let's hope we pull out the right card. So far, we've only been dealt the occasional face card, but you can't really believe, can you, that we could go through the whole game without getting one ace?"

"I don't know much about cards. What game are you talking about?"

"You don't even know how to play *briscola*? Every time I talk to you, you make me feel Neanderthal."

The conversation fizzled out under Juvara's embarrassment and Soneri's black mood, but the silence which fell in the office was even more oppressive. The two were like castaways on a drifting raft. The telephones remained obstinately silent. Finally impatience got the better of Soneri and he could wait no more. "Give me Sauro's number."

The inspector wrote it on a scrap of paper and handed it over.

"Hello? It's Commissario Soneri here. I was anxious to know if you'd managed to locate that hard disk," he began, pronouncing the English word impeccably. "Ah, you have? You were just going to bring it over. No need. Inspector Juvara will come and pick it up from you in Borgo Regale."

He replaced the telephone with a satisfied expression. "We'll need to play this hand right."

"I'm on my way," Juvara said

"I'm coming with you," Soneri replied, grabbing hold of his duffel coat.

While Sauro and Juvara starting combing through the memory of the hard disk, the commissario felt left out. The two communicated in computer-speak, a dialect unknown to him. The words he heard seemed to belong to a language with no verbs and with no connection to anything he understood.

"We've struck it lucky," Soneri cut in. "If you'd thrown it out . . ."

"I nearly did, you know. In fact I should have. Soncini told me to."

"What made you hold on to it?"

"A customer came in looking for a computer for his son. The new models were too expensive so he asked me if I had a second-hand one lying about. It was then I thought about recycling the hard disk. It wouldn't cost me a thing. I know it wasn't strictly correct, but I've only just started up and the debts are mounting."

Soneri burst out laughing. He thought of Sbarazza and his theory that chance offers us thousands of opportunities every day: the problem was to know how to recognise them.

"If we ever get to the bottom of this story, it'll be all due to coincidences and chance," he said with a smile, addressing Juvara.

Sauro looked at both men without understanding. He decided it did not matter and turned back to the computer.

Soneri watched the two of them intently. On the screen, sequences of numbers, questions and windows with lists began to appear. Every so often Sauro and Juvara would exchange phrases which were incomprehensible to him. After half an hour, boredom forced him to start walking up and down the room, but then it began to seem too narrow and he felt himself suffocating. He needed to get out.

"Call me when you come up with something," he said.

Once outside he lit a cigar and began walking around the *borgo* between Via Farini and Via Repubblica, already cloaked in the gathering dusk. He realised that for the first time in his career he was reliant on the work of a younger colleague. Until now, Nanetti and his forensic colleagues had always seen to the scientific part of any investigation, but he was a contemporary and he could take that from him. Juvara was of a generation light years younger, and belonged to a world alien to him. He wondered if he should indeed learn a little English, especially now that even Capuozzo was going on a computer course. Never had he felt so completely washed up as at that moment. A hardened peasant, by-passed by time, an old coin forgotten in a piggy bank.

Such was his gloomy frame of mind that when Juvara called from the shop, he did not even react to his good news. "Commissario, we've made some very interesting discoveries. I told you computers—"

"I'm being converted," Soneri said.

"Soncini has done a bit of surfing, using different search engines."

"What do you mean, engines? Juvara, talk clearly. For me engines are things that drive cars."

"Search engines are used to find information on particular subjects, and in general you consult them via a key word."

"Like the one you used to access the terminal?"

"Nearly. With search engines, a key word is used to find texts which contain that word."

"What words did Soncini use?"

"Oh, he used a lot, but for half a dozen searches the key words were 'woman', 'burned', 'autostrada'. Speaks for itself, doesn't it?"

Soneri shook off his gloom.

"It certainly does. When was he doing these searches?"

"In the days immediately following the murder," the inspector said, choosing his words with care.

"Juvara, you've won your bet. Tell Sauro that one of these days I'll be over to invest in one of these devices. I trust you'll give me advice about which one to choose."

"I'll be your consultant and I'll teach you how to use it. Then you'll be able to reply to Capuozzo when he sends you an e-mail."

The commissario mumbled something intended as light-hearted. "Pick up the disk and let's go to the questura."

As he turned away, he thought again about what had been found in the computer, and his initial enthusiasm waned.

"There's no way Soncini can wriggle out of this, Commissario," Juvara repeated several times once they were back in the office.

"It's only a clue," Soneri cautioned. "Don't forget that Nina was Soncini's lover and she was an illegal immigrant. It wouldn't have been possible to do a search through official channels, so he had to use his internet to find out if a local paper had carried some report."

"Then there's the car . . ."

"Stolen by the Romanians." The commissario shook his head. "On the basis of the information we have, both the Roma revenge theory and what we've just uncovered remain possibilities," he concluded. Juvara weighed up this verdict with evident disappointment.

"Maybe the printouts will tell us which lead to follow," Soneri said.

"I'll be sure to get them tomorrow morning, even if I have to present myself in person at the office of the telephone company," Juvara said grimly.

"You need to be patient. Reality is extremely complex. Computers are so fast because they deal with numbers, not human beings."

"This seems to me a really barbaric story. Is anyone going to be saved out of all this?"

"Have we ever had an edifying story to deal with?"

"This one seems more savage than any other."

"I'd save only Nina. She was one of life's unfortunates, doing her uttermost to escape from poverty and from the miseries of those around her."

18

HE STAYED ON in his office pretending to work until Juvara too started making preparations to leave, not before asking hesitantly: "If there's anything you need, Commissario . . ."

"On you go," Soneri said, with a grateful smile, but the moment he was on his own he grew dispirited at the prospect of the empty evening ahead of him. He decided not to go out until later when there would be fewer people about, apart from some lonely souls like him.

He went into the wine bar without seeing the people he feared. He ordered from Bruno a portion of Parmesan shavings and some slices of *coppa*, then he made for home, taking the long way round. On winter evenings, in spite of all the vandalism which had been wreaked on its inner spirit, Parma seemed to him simply beautiful. Its straw-coloured patina survived intact, indifferent to the torrent of vulgarity which threatened to drown it. Soneri still carried inside himself the city he had once known and attempted to locate it in the doorways, in the façades and in the irregularly shaped attics in the roofs on the far side of the river. He descended slowly into that malaise called memory, while simultaneously keeping a tight grip on his mobile in the hope of receiving a call in the present. But perhaps, as Angela's persistent silence on the future of their relationship implied, she too would soon belong to the realm of memory.

He walked in the direction of Piazzale della Pace where, in days that now seemed far off, he had taken the call from Juvara that had initiated the investigation. He thought back to that moment before his life had fallen apart, as it had now. He was reliving that situation when his mobile, in a curious reprise of the other occasion, rang again. It was Musumeci, wanting to update him on the developments concerning the rapist. The woman who had driven Candiani out of his wits *was* Nina.

"Commissario, this woman was a real demon with men!" the inspector exclaimed. Soneri thought about the more colourful expressions he would have employed with his fellow officers. "To keep up with her, they had to be forever snorting some substance or other."

He had never thought of it in those terms. Many of her lovers were cocaine addicts, but that was not altogether unusual in the circles of wealthy men in search of new emotions. Everything was becoming complicated again. There were too many men who wanted that girl and too many who ended up frustrated. He quickened his pace. Once again, there was nothing for it but to let events take their course.

And the following morning they did, in fact, take their course. The printouts of the calls made by Soncini and Razzini on the night of the murder were at long last delivered. Soncini had switched off his mobile around 22.00 and had turned it back on about two hours later. The mast to which his phone received the signal was the one at Cortile San Martino, while the last call had been routed through the transmitter station near Lodi. Razzini, on the other hand, had received half a dozen calls and texts via a mast some-where south of Lake Como. Soncini's alibi would not stand up. It was clear he had been with his friend until a certain time, and then they had gone their separate ways.

"That ties it all up," Juvara said. "And this too is down to electronics," he let fall after a moment's silence.

Soneri did not immediately reply. "There's still something that doesn't add up. In this whole business, every time you seem to be getting to the heart of things, new doubts jump out at you and you're back to where you started."

"I was sure we'd found the ace this time. At least I hoped we had," Juvara said.

"The car. That's what doesn't add up. The stolen B.M.W."

"Commissario, that's all based on the evidence of a drunk."

"Yes, but he's also a fanatic who knows all there is to know about cars."

"It could've been another car of the same make."

"You're forgetting the horse on the side."

"The symbol of the Cerreto equestrian club."

"Did you get a membership list? Have a look and see if one of the members has a B.M.W. like Soncini's."

The commissario got up and went over to Juvara's desk and picked up the folder with the documents. He began flicking through them.

"Can I help you?" Juvara said.

"I'm looking for the Cerreto number. Call that bar on Lake Como where Soncini claimed he spent the evening with his friend and ask the owner how Razzini got home."

"In what sense?"

"If he left in his own car or if he got a lift from someone else."

Without waiting for an answer, Soneri took hold of the telephone and dialled a number. Juvara watched him act with the determination he showed at his best and assumed he must have formulated a precise theory, but then he noticed that, on the contrary, he was calling Nanetti.

"Listen, what model was the B.M.W. stolen from Soncini? What was that? A turbo diesel 520, year of make 2005?"

Next, without even replacing the receiver on the cradle, he dialled another number. "Hello? Is that the Vehicles Registration Office? This is Commissario Soneri. Could I speak to Ronchini, please? . . . Ciao, how are things, Eugenio? Listen, I need you to do me a favour. Could you run a check on all the cars owned by Arnaldo Razzini? That's the one, the lawyer."

As he waited, he turned to look at Juvara but saw that he too was on the telephone. A few minutes later, he called Ronchini back. "What's that? A Fiat Punto and a B.M.W. turbo diesel 520 convertible? Thank you. That's a great help."

Soneri and Juvara hung up at the same time, but before the inspector had time to open his mouth the commissario picked up the phone again. "Musumeci, go and find Razzini, in his office or at his home. Have a good look at his B.M.W. It's a black turbo diesel 520 convertible. What I want you to do is check if it has a sticker with a galloping horse attached to one side. Let me know right away."

"Commissario, do you suspect . . ." Juvara stuttered.

Soneri nodded. "I suspect that Nina's burned body was not dumped from Soncini's car but from his friend's. They're identical, and that would mean that Mariotto was not mistaken."

"At the joint on Como they told me Razzini went home with an acquaintance. He was a bit tipsy and was seen getting into a car with this other man, an habitué of the place."

Soneri confirmed this version. "In fact Razzini must have had a lift, because that evening Soncini took his B.M.W."

"This time you can't say there are any doubts."

"We've reached the first solid point in the whole story," the commissario conceded, "but there are still doubts. Bear in mind that there's never any closure except in a judicial sense, but that'll do us."

Their satisfaction lasted no longer than the delivery of the newspapers which fired off a fresh round of accusations, aimed equally at the police and the civic authorities. The prefect was quoted as saying he was "on the side of the people" for the "restoration of law disrupted by recent events".

"A bunch of arseholes," Soneri yelled. He was heartily sick of such drivel in a city given to preaching, as if the much-vaunted "civil society" was made up of saints. "They go around shitting in the streets like their pet dogs and then complain about there being dirt everywhere," he shouted, banging the papers down on the desk. To make matters worse, he had heard that Capuozzo was furious with Soneri for deserting his post the day before.

"Don't get too worried," Marcotti tried to calm him down over the phone. "Until somebody decides otherwise, I'm coordinating this investigation and I'll decide who to put in charge of the case. Capuozzo can jump up and down all he likes."

Here at last was a woman who dispensed reassurance, the commissario thought to himself, reflecting again that she was the one he would have chosen to marry.

"I would like a warrant to search Signor Razzini's car. I have reason to believe it was the one used for the murder."

"Could you give me the background?"

"Soncini carried out some internet searches with compromising key words at a time when very few people could have known about the murder. In addition, Razzini owns a car identical to Soncini's, with, as I believe, the same emblem on the side. We've learned from the owner of the bar where Soncini and Razzini say they spent the evening when Iliescu was murdered that Razzini was given a lift home by an acquaintance. Am I making sense?"

"Perfect sense. In this regard, I meant to tell you that the head of the Romas arrested at Suzzara in connection with the theft of gold has admitted that the boys driving the car have nothing to do with this case, and said he'll provide the proof soon."

"So let's wait a bit. Dottoressa, will you take it on yourself to inform Capuozzo? Right at this moment, our relations are not of the best."

"Certainly. I'll see to it," she said. The commissario would have liked to kiss her.

At last he felt at peace. He looked up at Juvara and saw him looking in his direction. "This is the moment to put the noose round Soncini's neck," Juvara said.

Soneri's mood darkened once more. "But what made him do it?"

The motive, one of the fundamental elements in a murder case, escaped him. Did Nina want to leave him? She had had so many other relationships. Or did he plan to leave her only to find he could not get rid of her? But she was not the type of woman to entertain regret, even if accompanied by threats of blackmail. No matter from which angle he examined the question, he could not make out what had led Soncini to kill her.

Musumeci's call disturbed his reflections. "Commissario, I can confirm that the B.M.W. has the emblem of the equestrian club on its side."

"Stay where you are. I'll send Nanetti over to join you."

"But we need a warrant."

"You'll get one."

He called Marcotti immediately. "Dottoressa, there is a horse on Razzini's car as well."

"Carry on. I'll sign the warrant at once."

He then telephoned Nanetti, who said to him: "You sound in good form. That means that everything is coming to a head."

"I might have found the person who murdered Nina."

"Is that all? I thought it was something else entirely. That's just routine for you."

He would have liked to tell him to go to hell, but the moment was not right.

Two hours later, the first results came in. Traces of petrol were found in the boot of the car, perhaps spilled from the container of petrol used to set fire to the body. In addition, luminol had shown up traces of blood on the rugs, even though it was evident that the car had been valeted with immense care. Tests would establish whether the blood was Nina's.

While having a sandwich in a bar in the city centre with Soneri and Nanetti, who had spent the morning working on Razzini's car, Dottoressa Marcotti set out her own conclusions. "It's clear to me that the proof is overwhelming, but I have to warn you that in the present situation that proof is only circumstantial. That's sufficient for me to lock him up, but it will be a different kettle of fish when the case comes to court."

The commissario was the first to share her doubts and feel dissatisfied. He thought he had had Soncini in his grasp, but instead he only had him by the hem of his coat. The affair still looked murky. It stank, but like something which spreads foul air all around without anyone being able to determine its source.

"If you want my advice," she said, shaking her magnificent blonde hair, "don't stop working on this case. We haven't got to the bottom of it yet. Anyway, you know what the next step is."

"Soncini," Soneri said.

"Come to my office and I'll sign a warrant for his arrest here and now."

It seemed as though he had been waiting. Possibly Razzini had managed to make a call before the police arrived, but Soncini had the complexion of a man who had been ill. His face no longer showed that world-weary look which the commissario had found so unsettling. Two days' growth on his chin, greasy hair straggling around a head which suddenly appeared small and pointed, wrinkles in the leather-coloured skin of his cheeks, all combined to give the impression of a man who had grown old overnight. The combative manner which the commissario had been confronted by in the first interviews was gone, and he now looked like a man resigned to letting himself go without even the slightest attempt to fight back.

"This is not a happy situation," Soneri said, after a silence in which he pretended to be reading through some documents. In fact, he knew every word by heart, yet took his time so as to keep his adversary on tenterhooks. He expected Soncini to deny the charge or seek some way out but against all expectation he murmured: "Yes, I know."

The lawyer who had accompanied him, a young man about Soncini's daughter's age, was also surprisingly reticent.

The commissario took that meekness as a sign of assent,

and went straight to the heart of the matter. "Why did you kill her?"

"I didn't mean to. It was an accident," Soncini said, in a whisper.

"Bollocks!" Soneri threw back at him in an explosion of anger which surprised even himself. The figure of Nina pregnant appeared in front of him, with once again the memory of his wife superimposed.

"It was obviously premeditated," he said, trying to control the words which were tumbling out of him in real fury. "You borrowed the car from your friend Razzini so that you could incriminate whoever had stolen yours. Maybe that was because you knew exactly who *had* stolen it."

"It all happened by sheer chance," Soncini protested. "Razzini was drunk. Nina had called to ask if we could meet as soon as possible. That was why I borrowed my friend's car, and anyway he was in no state to drive. Do you really think I'd have planned to use a car the same as my own?"

"It was the best way to ward off suspicion."

"It was an accident, I tell you. I left the place on Lake Como before ten o'clock. I don't deny that. Nina was pestering me with calls, so I arranged to meet her in Parma in a bar not far from the toll booth on the autostrada, and after a short while I switched off my mobile. She sounded extremely agitated and kept on saying she had something very important to tell me."

"Agitated in what sense? Terrified?"

"No, no. Highly emotional. Excited. She seemed happy and afraid at the same time. When we met, she threw herself into my arms, like a teenager, and told me . . . well, she told me she was expecting a baby. She'd just got the results from one of those kits you can buy in the pharmacy."

"And you were none too pleased."

Soncini looked at him with the ghostliest of smiles. "No, I didn't take it well at all. You can understand that. I'm a married man."

"That doesn't seem to have stopped you playing about," Soneri said bluntly.

"No, but there were no babies involved."

"You mean there was always a clear agreement?"

"Nina had always told me there would be no problems. And then with the life she led . . . I couldn't even be sure it was mine," he said indignantly.

"So, you could take any liberty you wished, provided your affairs remained out of sight. It's a sad old story, a little bit of philandering on the side. Even your wife went along with it, I imagine. From what I've picked up, there was nothing much between you."

Soncini nodded slowly. "The fact is that Nina wanted to keep it," he burst out as though this was the greatest monstrosity imaginable.

Once more Soneri had to make an effort to contain himself. The interview was touching more than one open sore, and he was tempted to punch Soncini's face. "Do you think it's easier for a woman to have an abortion than to keep the baby? For a woman like Iliescu, I mean, with the life she was leading?"

"She wanted us to get married. She wanted me to throw everything up," Soncini sobbed. That too seemed an outrage in his eyes, that she would ask him to give up exclusive clubs, luxury holidays, moneyed friends.

"So you made up your mind to be done with it all, mother and child in one fell swoop," Soneri cried, cutting the air with his hand like a guillotine falling.

"No, I keep telling you it was all an accident," Soncini protested. Even the lawyer began to show signs of impatience.

Soneri made a sign to both of them to remain calm. "Explain to me how it happened."

"We'd been talking a long time and it got quite heated. Nina would not budge. She said she was tired of living that way, that she was young and wanted a normal life. I told her she had cheated me and that it took two to produce a child. Then she started insulting me, saying that I'd taken advantage of her, that I had a good life while she was struggling to get by. We both lost our tempers and people in the bar started giving us funny looks. Next thing we got into the car and drove around a bit until we found an out-of-the-way place, not far from Lemignano. I gave her an ultimatum: either she had an abortion or else it was all over between us. She could say the child's father was one of the other men she'd been seeing, or else she could say, for instance, she'd been raped by Candiani. What did it matter to her? She could take him to court and make herself a bit of money. Everybody knew she'd been seeing him. But she wouldn't have it. She wanted me. She wanted to ruin me. Well, I started hitting her, not too hard, just enough to keep her under control and make her see sense. But she jumped out of the car and started running away, shouting in the mist that the whole city would find out because she was going to tell everybody. She seemed to have gone off her rocker. I ran after her. I thought I'd never catch her, but next thing I found myself on top of her. We had both run into a fence which you couldn't see in the mist. She kneed me in the balls, and I lost it. I won't deny that I went too far that evening. It was pure instinct and maybe I lost it. The fact is I landed a punch on her, the sort of punch you would give a man, and she seemed to fly backwards, as though she'd been carried away by the wind. I'd got her full on, under the chin. She fell with her neck against an iron railing. It had all happened so quickly that when I stopped to draw breath it seemed unbelievable, in the stagnant mist, the utter silence ... I knew right away she was dead. I was scared out my wits. I had a couple of grains of powder with me and I took them. What did it matter any more? I was done for. There was no hope. However, the cocaine cleared my head and I started to think. I dragged the body into a field. Then I went to the workshop and got a container used for solvents and a sheet of canvas used for packing. I filled the container with petrol at a self-service garage, and went back to get Nina. After about a quarter of an hour I bundled her into the boot of the car. I returned to the workshop and went round to the yard at the back. It gives onto a ditch there where they often light fires to burn the crates used by a transport company. I had an hour before the arrival of the night guards on their midnight round. The petrol makes quick work of everything. It flares up quickly, burns a few minutes and then dies down. With all that mist around, there wasn't much chance of anyone seeing me. I waited for the corpse to cool down before I could wrap it up in the canvas again. That didn't take long with the temperature what it was. I laid the body on the back seat and drove onto the autostrada. I knew there was an encampment of Romanian gypsies at Cortile San Martino, and since Nina was an illegal, I thought of leaving the body there. An autostrada is the most anonymous place in the world. The whole world uses the autostrada! However, I couldn't have foreseen that there would be a pile-up at exactly that point. But for that, the body wouldn't have been discovered for ages."

Soncini collapsed on a chair as though he were on the point of fainting. He appeared more distraught and unnerved than before. Soneri allowed the silence to emphasise the gravity of the confession, but his mind went back to the farce played out in front of him a few days previously by Soncini, his wife and daughter, and his fury increased. In comparison,

Nina, no matter how casual with men, seemed to him like a lost soul trying to stay afloat in a sea of filth. The thought of her helped him nurture a little hope that he would not sink into that slime.

"It would have been better for you to keep the baby and pretend to be a caring partner. Perhaps even, for the first time in your life, you would have assumed responsibility for something. And you wouldn't be where you are now."

"Please," the lawyer intervened, "avoid making judgments. It's not your role."

The commissario threw a contemptuous look in his direction. "You're quite right. It's up to the judge to do that." He turned once more to Soncini. "You forgot to add one thing."

Soncini looked up, giving him a quizzical look.

"You'd have had to resign your position as a kept man."

Soncini bowed his head again and said nothing.

19

AFTER HE HAD signed his confession, they took him away.
Soneri watched him being led off by two officers followed
by the lawyer, done up like a mannequin, and wondered why
at that stage murderers appeared to him always so banal, so
bereft of all pride, even of the pride of malice. He invariably
found himself confronting unremarkable faces or insignificant people who were nothing out of the ordinary. It was
impossible to see them in the role of killers. He recalled
substantial mafiosi who looked like pensioners, serial killers
with the appearance of admin staff, rapists who could have
passed for seminarians and pitiless female poisoners with the
features of a doll. Never had there been one with the surly
expression of a cut-throat, the menacing eyes of a basking
shark or the insolence of arrogance.

As he reflected on this, he felt his disquiet grow. There was
something artificial in Soncini's submissiveness. He might
have been playing a part. If it all went well for him, he might
indeed be able to show it had been an accident and perhaps
even get off with a sentence of a couple of years' imprison-
ment. He might claim he had acted under the influence of
cócaine, and that burning the body had been a reaction of fear
produced by the drugs.

All these doubts were swept aside for the time being by a

flood of congratulations, starting with those of Capuozzo, who knew that this way he was guarding his back against public opinion and laying the groundwork for the parade of the following morning's press conference. The newspapers were guaranteed to write that the investigators had done their job, and the political bigwigs would express their renewed faith in justice. Even Esposito phoned him from his car: "Well done, Commissario. We've pulled it off. You're the pick of the bunch."

Soneri was pleased, but he found it hard to show his satisfaction in public. He was uncomfortable with compliments because he never knew what to say. Fortunately the investigating magistrate, Marcotti, who was very like him in this way, restricted herself to a vigorous handshake and an eloquent look which said it all. The thought occurred yet again to him that if they had been contemporaries, he could easily have fallen in love with her. Juvara, who had been gazing into the middle distance for a while, apparently wrapped in thought, attempted to bring him back to earth. "Don't forget your promise, commissario."

"What promise?"

"The computer, remember? If we've solved the case, it was all down to the hard disk."

"It was down to chance. And self-interest. Young Sauro thought he could make a bit of money from a machine he should have put out. He did it because some guy had asked for a computer at a giveaway price, so he was acting in his own interests."

"That's a very reductive analysis. Sauro could have kept quiet, told us he'd thrown everything out and fitted the hard disk to another computer," Juvara objected.

"He had just opened up and needed customers. He might have decided it's always a good idea to stay on good terms with the police. Anyway, what did he care about Soncini? You're a much better customer."

The inspector surrendered. "You're always too pessimistic. Anyway, the case is solved and that's what matters."

"Solved? Mmm . . . You know what bothers me? That note, the one at Nina's house, covered with insults. Whoever wrote that must have known Nina's intentions regarding Soncini, and presumably before finding out about the baby."

Not knowing how to reply, Juvara threw up his hands helplessly, but at that moment the telephone on Soneri's desk rang.

"Commissario, Dottor Capuozzo has called a press conference for tomorrow morning at ten and would like to invite you to come along," the usual secretary announced.

"Unfortunately I can't be there. Please give the questore my apologies," Soneri said perfunctorily.

The secretary was by now accustomed to Soneri's refusals, and acting almost mechanically she assured him she would tell her superior.

"I'm going out for a breath of fresh air," he told Juvara.

He wandered about in the city centre and dropped in to a couple of tobacconists to buy cigars and the wooden matches he continued to use in preference to a lighter. He detested those bright little implements which produced fire with no smoke, these being two elements which should always go together. He made his way back to the questura, but when he was in the courtyard under the fir trees, he realised he had no wish to shut himself up in an office, so he got into his car. He had a vague idea of where he would like to go. He would like to drive across the plain towards the first of the Apennine slopes and from there climb above the mist. On the road towards the hills, the skies would gradually clear, the sun would begin to peep out, but then he would briefly plunge once more into the last of the white mist before everything would finally brighten and the world would change. At times it was only a matter of a couple of metres. He would be happy to warm his bones over lunch in a trattoria on a hillside, looking down at the plain under its sheet of chilly mist.

Such thoughts were in his mind as he got to Via Spezia but instead of proceeding in the direction of Cisa, he turned at Lemignano towards the industrial zone. He did not know what had made him abandon the idea of an outing to the hills, but he soon understood as he parked in front of Golden. He was missing Angela. Once in the hills, he would be reminded of their days away from the city, and that was what had made him turn back. He had no wish to invite pain. Better to face the hostility of Giulia Martini, who was even now staring resentfully at him. The commissario preferred to tussle with another person rather than with himself.

"Did you manage to visit your husband in jail?" he said.

"No, and I don't care to. As far as I am concerned, you can keep him. That man has been my ruination."

"You could have left him, if you hadn't been slaves to a *bella figura*."

"All my life I've had to put up with his affairs. The man is an inveterate womaniser," she said, without restraint. "After a while, I told myself I didn't care about him anymore and he could do what he liked. Once my daughter had grown up, she understood. However, I could not tolerate the idea of him breeding a litter of bastards. There is a limit."

"Don't go any further. That unborn baby had very little to do with it. What mattered was your self-interest. You're not defending respectability, just business."

The woman seemed about to assault him. The commissario savoured his own mordant lucidity and was indifferent to any offence he gave. He stood in front of her, throwing down the gauntlet with words she had never wanted to hear, words which stripped her naked.

"For years the two of you were happy to play the part of the united couple, just so long as it kept the business turning over. It was of no concern to you if your husband went after other women in nightclubs, because the thing that mattered was to put on a brave front for the people who placed the orders, the ecclesiastical curias. A fine marriage, a flourishing company, a daughter who marries into the Dall'Argine family, a veneer of dutiful Catholicism . . . a model family," he said sarcastically. "And all to display an irreproachable image, a guarantee for the bishops and traditionalist clients who buy the gold and jewellery from you. And then a Romanian girl turns up and it all gets serious. She wants a family. You know perfectly well she'll not back off and so you threaten her, you send her threatening letters, but the girl holds fast. At that point, you take to blackmailing your husband: either you stop seeing her or I'll cut off your allowance. No more *dolce vita* as kept man, no more women, no more clubs and expensive cars. And when you find out she's expecting a child, you deliver your ultimatum. He's got his back to the wall, forced to choose between the playboy life and giving up Nina, and he opts for the second, but he didn't reckon with her sheer grit. She really did want an ordinary life with the man she loved most of all of them. So she had to be got rid of. After all, what was she but an illegal immigrant from Romania? Who's going to go looking for her? And in fact nobody did go looking for her, except one old grandparent who set out for Italy to act as peacemaker between the girl and the gypsy community, but the bus journey finished him off. End of story." By the end of his story, Soneri found himself trembling with rage.

"You're a visionary!" Martini screamed, hissing like a

cobra. "You can believe anything you like, but she was no more than a common whore. She gave herself to one and all, and I'll tell you something else. She had a great talent for getting men all worked up. She knew how to appeal to their weaker side, playing each one in a different way. She sniffed them out like a snake, and then drew them into her trap. I can't help laughing at your portrait of her as a victim. A vulgar prostitute! A slut!" She was yelling at the top of her voice, all pretence at being *una vera signora* cast aside.

Soneri stared at her in consternation. At that moment for the first time he grasped just how venomous to each other women can be, and to a degree unimaginable in a man. Her eyes expressed infinite ferocity, and her snarling mouth twisted by hatred could have torn off chunks of meat with a single bite. The commissario took a step back when she screamed at him to get out of the office. He felt sick, and as he left he was glad once again to breathe in great, reviving gulps of fresh air. He felt himself growing lighter and lighter, less bound to life and for this reason more pitiless in his judgments of it.

He sat behind the wheel of his car and when he got to the turn-off for Via Spezia he contemplated for a moment which direction to take, Cisa or the city. He remembered it was time for lunch and thought it would be a waste of time to go looking for the sun when the sky would already be taking on the colours of dusk. In the mountains in winter, only morning counts.

When it was almost two o'clock, anxiety began to take hold of him again. He was still hoping for some communication from Angela, but he sensed that she would not call that day. He decided to go to Alceste's, once again looking for refuge in food and drink. With a wry smile, he recognised that there was not much else available to him.

There were not many people there, but Sbarazza had had the luck to find one table which apparently three women had just left.

"You've chosen a place where there's not much for you to eat," Soneri said, coming up behind the Marchese.

"Man does not live by bread alone," Sbarazza replied. "I was very taken by the lady who was seated here."

The outline of her lips had been imprinted on the serviette in crimson, and Sbarazza gazed longingly at that trace of femininity. "I can smell her perfume and the seat still has the warmth and the very form of her body," he said, as if in a dream.

The commissario smiled. The old man was one of the few people with whom at that moment he was happy to spend the afternoon. There was something profound and consoling in his conversation.

"I hear you've solved the case of that unfortunate Romanian girl," Sbarazza said. "So did you finally draw the right card from the pack?"

"It did finally emerge, although I was on the point of despair."

"You see? Never give up. Never lose faith."

"For the last few days I had been thinking I would never get a good hand."

"It's when it seems that nothing can happen that chance does its work for us. Even at this moment while we're here eating, absorbed with nothing more than flavours and scents, perhaps something which concerns us is occurring. A billiard ball rolling into a pocket can be the result of a thousand cannons," the Marchese chuckled.

"Maybe you're right," Soneri said as a plate of *tortelli di zucca* arrived at the table. "Maybe something will cannon off something else in my path this afternoon and change the prospects for me. This morning . . ." He tasted the first *tortello*.

"What happened to you this morning?"

"I was making for the hills when, on an impulse, I changed direction. I made a choice, there and then. If I'd gone the way I first intended, I'd have spent the morning quite differently. For a start I wouldn't be here talking to you, and instead of having a plate of *tortelli di zucca* I'd be having a plate of *gnocchi ai funghi*."

Sbarazza made a sign to him to stop. "Don't go down that path. It'd be an infinite process and finish up in complete nonsense or with the conclusion that everything you do is wrong because there's always a more promising possibility."

"So? Is that not true to life?"

"I prefer to believe that if a choice has been made, there's a reason for it. You could call it providence, or determinism, but in both cases our will is only in part responsible. The rest is something obscure that we are not permitted to know, whether it's transcendent or immanent," the Marchese declared, in philosophical mood.

"I deal with much more banal but all too human causes: money, sex and the passions which spring from them."

"Those are only effects. Don't muddle them. If you think about it, that obscure, pre-eminent cause which directs our lives conducts itself in such a way that killing or loving are, when all is said and done, on the same level of potentiality, but then, in time, the balls cannon off each other in a certain way and produce now one outcome, now the other, or both."

The commissario savoured another *tortello*, and then muttered his dissent: "Do you know why I enjoy your company? You make me feel an optimist. I can't resign myself to the thought that we're all machines controlled from long range. Neither one of us can rule out the possibility that we might become murderers, but the fact is that we are not. The majority of people are not."

"From fear, only from fear. For a minority there's also an element of awareness."

"What is this awareness? Morality?"

"A conquest, a point of arrival. When someone in thought or deed falls to the very lowest point of humanity, he begins to be aware. Then and only then, after dabbling in evil, can he choose. Other people draw back from fear of the reaction which wickedness arouses, but life with its limitless sequence of possibilities could entice them to say yes to even the most nefarious acts."

"Are you one of the fellowship of the aware?"

"Don't you know I've done all sorts of things? And you too are a member of the fraternity, after all you've seen."

The commissario smiled and got up. "I do see so much that is appalling," he said, thinking of his most recent meeting. "And I see no end of it."

"Seize every opportunity. You know what to do."

"Well . . ." Soneri said. "I'll go and face whatever the afternoon brings."

The first thing was the authorisation to interview Medioli. Soneri arranged to see him in the evening, and hoped he had decided to talk. He was seeking some enlightenment on the world of the Romas. All those years spent in the caravans could not have been in vain.

The second thing to arrive was news brought by the beguiling policewoman who had made such an impression on Musumeci.

"There's someone here who wants to talk to you. Looks like a gypsy," she told him.

In the commissario's mind, the Roma camp and the man asking to see him fused into one.

"Send him in."

The man was dressed like the old peasants in the Apennines, in the modest but dignified elegance seen in ageing prints. He said his name was Floriu and he must have been in Italy for some time, for his Italian was fluent.

"You've come from Suzzara?"

The man nodded. "From the camp."

"If it's about the gold, you'll have to go and talk to the carabinieri."

"I know, but that's not why I'm here. I've come about those two boys."

"The ones in the B.M.W. stolen from Soncini?"

He nodded once again. "I wanted to tell you they had nothing to do with it. They were just showing off."

"Are you the father of one of them?"

"No, but I'll take responsibility for what has happened. I stole the car. I came to give myself up, provided you let the boys go free."

"I doubt if it really was you who carried out the theft, and anyway the legal system does not allow exchanges of that sort."

"They had nothing to do with it," the man repeated forcefully. "The car was in the camp to be dismantled and sent off to Romania. There are lots of our people going there and back. They would have reassembled it over there. It's the safest way, but those two pinched the keys and went out for a run. That's all there is to it."

"Are you telling me this to get revenge on some family enemy? Why otherwise would you give me a tip-off like this? To save two boys who'd be let out soon in any case?"

Floriu straightened up, betraying his embarrassment. "No

vengeance, and no tip-off. It's the first car we've handled. I know others do it, traffic in cars, but in our camp it's the first time it's happened."

"Why should that be? You've decided to branch out?"

"No," the old man stammered. "There'll be no trafficking in cars."

"Well then, explain yourself more clearly." Soneri was growing impatient. "None of what you've said so far makes any sense to me."

"It was those four. They did it."

"Which four?"

"The ones who were involved in stealing the gold. They took the car, even if they've never done it before. I don't know why. One night they came back with it. There are honest and dishonest people among us. Like among you Italians."

"Now you're making more sense," the commissario said. "The four found by the carabinieri with the gold are the same ones who stole the B.M.W. Is that what you're saying?"

The Romanian nodded, but without much conviction.

"But you insist you've never stolen a car?"

"No, never."

Soneri said nothing for a few moments. He was trying to understand, but the whole matter was beyond him.

"In your opinion, why did it happen?"

The man shrugged. "I don't know. You'll have to ask them."

Floriu's attitude had changed, and now he seemed keen to get away. Perhaps he was disappointed at the way the interview had gone.

"You do know why it all happened," Soneri insisted.

"I'm here to state that those boys had nothing to do with it, but if you don't believe me, I have nothing more to add." He stopped there. It seemed as though a shutter had been pulled down. The Romanian's grim expression was distrustful, so much so that when he had gone, Soneri felt he had not been up to the challenge. Perhaps subconsciously he had believed the case was all but closed and he had failed to pick up the signals the Romanian was giving him. He had not remained open to every possibility, as Sbarazza would have said.

"Juvara, do you remember that text relayed from the mast at Cortile San Martino, the one to Nina saying that everything was ready?"

"Yes, from the stolen mobile."

"What do you think it meant?"

"I haven't a clue," the inspector said. "On the other hand we have found something interesting among Soncini's papers."

"What's that?"

"There was money deposited in a current account in Iliescu's name at the Savings Bank."

"What's so extraordinary about that?"

"That she had 750,000 euros in that account."

"Do you think the money was hers?"

"No. Aimi has access to the account as well."

"The accountant?"

"Commissario, if there's one thing in this whole story I just don't get, it's the bomb at Golden. Everything up to that point has a logic of its own, but not that explosion. And now there's this account."

"I know. If only these Romanians would talk. The guy who came today seemed to want to tell me something."

"They're releasing the two teenagers. This morning they were let out of the Young Offenders prison and now they're with Marcotti at the magistrate's office."

Soneri jumped to his feet at once, as though his desk was

on fire. Juvara watched him walk briskly across the courtyard in the direction of Via Repubblica and disappear through the gate.

Ten minutes later he was in the investigating magistrate's office. The young men had the same hostile expression as before.

"Commissario, don't waste your breath. These two have made up their minds not to speak. They must have been ordered on pain of death to keep their mouths shut," Marcotti said.

The commissario pulled up a chair and sat facing them. "We know you didn't kill the girl, and we know the B.M.W. was stolen by other people, in fact by the four men arrested at Suzzara," he began.

The two exchanged glances and for a moment it seemed their hostility softened a little. "You'll be out in a short while. All I want to know is why you took the car when you knew that the men who had stolen it planned to send it to Romania bit by bit to make some money on it. You knew that you risked being stopped and that would wreck the whole scheme."

The two said nothing, staring straight ahead with the same impassive expression.

"Isn't it odd?" Soneri said to Marcotti. "There's a car which is really hot and two boys with no licence take it out for a ride. They say they were framed, but they framed themselves. A right pair of idiots, amateurs."

The last words struck home with the pair, who were apparently unwilling to be taken as fools in what they considered their line of work.

"That car no stolen," the older of the two burst out. "That car given."

Soneri continued to look at Marcotti. "Given by whom?"

"By Italian man. No know name."

"Soncini?"

"No know name," the Romanian repeated, raising his voice slightly.

The peremptory tone indicated that there would be no further dialogue. After a few minutes more, Marcotti cut proceedings short. "Let's take it slowly," she said, handing the two boys over to the officers who would take them back to the Suzzara camp.

"Commissario, you should be pleased," the magistrate said. "You've learned one important thing. It seems the car was not stolen as Soncini claimed."

"Do you think they're telling the truth?"

"Do you think someone who does my job could risk putting her hand in the fire? But if you really want my opinion, I do believe it," she said, winking at Soneri. "Why should they make up a story? People only do that when they have some reason for it, but in this case they've nothing to fear, don't you agree?"

The commissario nodded. "That means the Romas and Soncini were in business together."

"Cocaine?"

"I thought of that," the commissario said. "But in that case, what are we to make of the bomb at Golden?"

"Maybe it was directed at Soncini."

"If you're in business with somebody, you know nearly all about them. Anybody doing business with Soncini must have known that he and his wife wielded quite different levels of economic power," Soneri said.

"And who's to say, in spite of that, that they were not united when it came to business?"

He was about to reply, but he stopped himself. Marcotti's hypothesis suddenly shed a new light on the case.

"Who knows? You might be right."

When he emerged from the magistrate's office, night was falling and he had still not seen Medioli. He was grateful for the fact that this man who had lived in exile from the world had been caught up in the whirlwind of events. "Our infiltrator", Soneri had called him as he took his leave from Marcotti.

"I'd put my money on him," she had replied, winking at him once more.

2 0

AS HE DROVE along Via Mantova in the direction of the prison, he felt like Fabrizio del Dongo fleeing towards the Po, on the same road and perhaps in the same state of mind. His instinct was that this was the final round and there would be no second chance, whatever Sbarazza might think. Capuozzo had made him a lengthy speech, in his customary woolly style, strewn with vague suggestions. The murderer was behind bars, the motive was clear enough, Nina's relatives would soon forget and public opinion was pacified. Why waste more time? There was no shortage of work in the questura, and anyway digging too deep often resulted in bringing to the surface questions no-one really wanted spend even more time confronting.

Nonetheless, Soneri pressed on. He was aghast at the prospect of dealing with bureaucratic matters, signing papers or pursuing half-witted drug addicts who had held up tobacconists with a dirty syringe. And of contemplating life without Angela. The reasons for deciding to persevere with Medioli were professional pride and curiosity, but also vanity with regard to Angela. For some days, his name had been on the front pages of the papers she read. It was his way of keeping his profile up, even if there was only one reader who interested him.

*

He was escorted through a dozen doors and gates before he got to the interview room. Nothing had changed – same rattling locks, same low ceiling, same stifling atmosphere, same off-white paint. However, Medioli appeared in better shape, more healthy and more at peace with himself than when they had last met.

"I've been expecting you," was his promising opening. "But I was beginning to think that you didn't care anymore to hear what I had to say. As the days went by, I was more and more convinced that the law wasn't interested in probing too far beneath the surface. I presumed that extended to me. I thought of sending a message to the magistrate saying that I was ready to cooperate, but I never got round to it. I'm fine here. I've a good relationship with everybody and I've been teaching these unfortunate lads in here how to fix engines. I gave them hope and I've found a purpose in life. That helps, doesn't it?"

Soneri nodded gravely, but he preferred to get away from this subject. "I should have come sooner. I had the explanation to so many things within reach."

"I don't know about 'so many', but some, yes. From what I read in the papers, you're already very well informed."

"No, not 'very'. For instance, I don't know what kind of deal the Romas and Soncini had with each other."

"Soncini?" Medioli started to snigger, but immediately pulled himself together. "You know that in a camp there are all kinds, honest and dishonest, the same as anywhere else. But you must also know that the Romas have a weakness for gold."

Several different thoughts coalesced in Soneri's mind to form one unbroken thread – Golden, Soncini's deals, the

Romas' gold and Marcotti's idea that Nina's murderer and Soncini's wife were partners in business and not only to keep up appearances.

"Are you saying that Golden used gold stolen by the Romas and that Soncini was the go-between?"

"You're missing one item: Nina Iliescu."

"She was an intermediary?"

"What I reckon is that at the beginning she was put under pressure by her fellow countrymen, used as a means of recycling all that gold. With the Romas as with everybody else, nothing is like it used to be. They're as greedy for money as the next man. There was a gang in the camp who could never get enough to keep them satisfied. They even started robbing churches, and that's when the friction broke out. There are some things you just don't touch, and in their world tradition still counts. That's why the Romanians moved out, because the feuding was turning into an ethnic war."

"So Iliescu was caught in a web?" Soneri said. He still clung to the belief that Nina was a victim of the clan.

"In my opinion, yes. Don't forget that her family was related to the Romas."

"In the end they hated her. Maybe she had managed to crawl out of the dunghill?"

"Maybe that's what happened, maybe she was already condemned, but from the night of the accident, when you arrested me, I don't know anything more."

"What about Mariotto? Why did they beat him up?"

"Because in spite of the alcohol, he'd seen what really happened. The B.M.W., I mean. Without that information, you'd have had a hard job of it, wouldn't you?"

"Razzini's B.M.W., the same model as Soncini's," the commissario said, as though talking to himself.

"I don't know who this Razzini is," Medioli said. "What

I do know is that Soncini dumped the body there that night because it was the safest place. Nobody ever climbs down the slope beside an autostrada, and the Romas were there to guard it. But with all he'd been up to beforehand, it all back-fired on him."

"But Nina really was one of them . . . ?"

"You said it yourself. In the final stages they hated her. There were nasty rumours circulating about her."

"Why?"

"I think she'd breached some code. Or as you were imply-ing, probably she wanted to get out, which in the eyes of the community came to the same thing. I believe the Romas had agreed to eliminate her, and I wouldn't be at all surprised if one of them was there on the night of the murder. Business was going well with Soncini, if you see what I mean. Nina was a loose cannon and knew too much."

"So it wasn't just about the baby?"

"That was a matter for her lover's wife, but Signora Martini herself didn't do too badly out of the arrangement: access to cheap gold, you understand? And if Soncini hadn't been such a brainless cocaine addict, it'd all have gone smoothly. Mariotto was beaten up because he blurted every-thing out and that was no good to anybody, but it was really meant as a warning to Manservisi. He hates the Romanians like poison and told you what Mariotto had seen. He wanted to give you a tip-off, but he couldn't say too much because he was afraid."

"But then Soncini, when he reported the theft of his car, tried to double-cross the Romanians . . ."

"No, not at all! As I just said, Soncini is a moron who fucked up even his own swindles. His wife used to pass him the cash to pay off the Romas for the gold, but he pocketed it to feed his cocaine habit. When they came looking for their money, he had to hand over his car to keep them quiet. Then his wife found out, and I suppose she went crazy. She ordered him to report the theft to the police. Just imagine what would've happened if a B.M.W., property of Golden, had turned up in a Roma camp with no report submitted! That car was hot! So a deal was struck with the Romas. The vehicle would be theirs, but they would make it disappear when the time was right, perhaps by taking it apart. And that's not all. Soncini, to keep up appearances, got hold of another car of the same kind from some friend he'd made while they were snorting together. So you see, Soncini was the weak link in the whole chain."

"In other words, Soncini had no wish to put the blame on the Romanians. He did use that car for the murder, but he'd been driving about in it for a while, and he was doing so so as not to arouse suspicions about his gold deals," the commissario reflected, thinking that once again the coincidences were multiplying.

"Apart from anything else, it's a very fashionable car in their world. He would never have had the guts to dupe the Romanians. He's too much of a coward. You're attributing to him a bigger brain than he has. He simply got himself entangled in his own lies, in the games a prick like him gets up to and in his craving for cocaine. When you act like that, you're on a slippery slide and there's no way back."

When Medioli fell silent, he and the commissario sat staring at each other. "You don't look convinced," Medioli said.

"I see everything from a new perspective. I'd better get used to that."

"Reality has many faces. We get accustomed to one and think that's all there is to it. Maybe it's just laziness, but the others seem unbelievable. It happened to me when I entered the Roma world, and my previous life just melted away."

"Now I too . . ." the commissario began, but he stopped because he was beginning to think about Angela again.

"What a shit heap!" Medioli said. "Get out while you can, or you'll end up stinking as well."

"I'm more likely to go mad," Soneri corrected him as he was about to leave.

"Commissario, do you think what I've told you will be enough to get me some time off my sentence?"

"I'll do my best," he assured him.

It was only when he was walking to his car, in the centre of a square covered with a mist which made the lamplights seem to quiver slightly, that he realised how utterly he had lost his bearings. Reality kept losing its outlines in spite of all his efforts to impose some shape on it. Soncini was unquestionably a killer, but he was also a victim – his wife appeared to be in charge, but she was overwhelmed by unhappiness. The Romas suffered a life of exploitation while searching for prosperity; Nina's lovers seemed to be winners but ended up losers; and Nina? She was the only one who had lost everything, dead in her early twenties while pursuing the dream of a normal life.

As he drove, he gripped the steering wheel tightly and trembled with rage. To calm himself down, he took out his mobile and dialled Marcotti's number.

"That Martini woman is in it up to her neck," he said. "She was turning out jewellery and sacred vessels with gold stolen, even from churches, by a gang of Romas."

For a few moments the investigating magistrate made no reply, and the commissario imagined her shaking her blonde mane in indignation.

"We'll have to pay a visit to the Signora," she said finally.

"It won't be easy to find anything at this late stage, but it's worth a try."

His next call was to Juvara. "Get in touch with Musumeci. Organise a search at Golden. Maybe Martini will move from being a plaster-cast saint to a she-devil."

"What are we looking for there?"

"They'll have got rid of anything compromising. Get hold of balance sheets, order forms, movements into and out of the warehouse, and pay special attention to deliveries to the various curias."

Juvara tried to say something, but Soneri cut him off. "See if you can find a member of staff who's willing to speak. There might be an employee who's got a grudge against Martini, somebody who got sacked. Talk to the trade union. With a temperament like hers, she must have made a fair number of enemies."

All of a sudden he felt tired and a little afraid. He would have liked to stop and end the investigation there because he feared he had not yet got to the bottom of it. Every probe took him one more step further down.

He drove aimlessly around the city streets without knowing where he wanted to go, but when he was advised that the search was already under way he made for Lemignano. He avoided Signora Martini, fuming with rage inside Musumeci's car together with her daughter, who was just back from her honeymoon and was in all probability, after the clamour of recent days, facing an early divorce. It was unlikely in the extreme that the Dall'Argine dynasty would tolerate their new daughter-in-law figuring so prominently in such a scandal.

He went into the now familiar office and found Juvara

standing under the portrait of the Pope. The inspector was examining the sacred vessels one by one. Soneri joined him, and when he saw him pick up a chalice, he smiled contentedly.

"Commissario, I noticed this one because it seemed so out of place. When I took a closer look, it reminded me of something."

"You're improving all the time," the commissario told him, still smiling. "I'd have started from there myself. Very often clues are so obvious that it's easy to overlook them."

"No, I'm being serious. This chalice reminds me of an object I saw in the office on a website featuring reproductions of stolen goods. You see the engraved image of Christ? It's strange because it's a clean-shaven Christ, whereas normally he has long hair and a beard."

Soneri turned serious. "Where was it stolen from?"

"From the parish church at Pedrignano."

"Is there a parish priest there still?"

"No, but an aunt of mine who lives nearby says that the priest from Sorbolo goes there to say mass."

"Bring the chalice. We'll go now."

They drove again through the mist, with Juvara clutching his seat belt, scared out of his wits by Soneri's carefree driving and by all the plane trees looming suddenly and menacingly out of the mist.

The parish priest, Don Mario Baldini, was having dinner, and the housekeeper was taken aback when the two men told her they were police officers. The priest himself, a napkin still tucked into his collar, came to the kitchen door.

"We've got something for you," Soneri said, handing him the chalice.

Don Mario took it in his hand with respectful delicacy, walked over to a sideboard and put on his glasses to examine the object. After a very few moments examining it, he said: "It's the one that was stolen."

The commissario and Juvara let out a sigh of relief. A priest had just handed down a sentence on the Martinis, mother and daughter. Perhaps the prison chaplain would give them absolution.

On his return, Soneri called Marcotti and told her about the chalice and its identification.

"See if you can get in touch with Musumeci," he suggested. "He can carry out the arrests."

"This story's got everything, hasn't it? The only thing missing was a chalice used for holy Mass but manufactured in mortal sin," the magistrate chortled.

"For once I'm going to take Capuozzo's advice. I'm going no further with this case."

"We'll have to see about that, Commissario. Don't forget that I'm the one who makes the decisions on investigations."

Soneri drove Juvara back to the office, and decided he had done enough for the day. Hunger was calling him to the wine bar. Bruno laid out a mixed plate of *torta fritta, spalla cotta, coppa* and *prosciutto*, together with shavings of Parmesan and a bottle of Bonarda. This was his psycho-medicine of choice, and he was confident he would feel a new man after downing such delicacies. When his feelings of euphoria were at their height and the wine had quite gone to his head, his mobile rang.

"Commissario . . ."

"Angela!"

The tone of both voices was already reconciliation enough.

"If you're calling to give me bad news, you couldn't have

chosen a better moment. I've still got half a bottle of Bonarda on the table in front of me . . ." Soneri babbled.

"I can't say if it's good or bad news, but I was wondering if you'd like to come round."

The commissario hesitated.

"Assuming you've no other commitments, work or whatever . . ." Angela went on.

"You can't be serious."

"No, never more serious. But you'd be fully entitled to . . ."

"I'll be there in ten minutes."

He left half his meal on the table and ran out. Bruno, unaware of what was happening, shouted after him: "Man labours for food, but if man doesn't eat . . ." But Soneri was well on his way and did not hear him.

Once they were face to face, they gazed at each other intensely. Neither knew where to start, both deeply embarrassed, Angela restrained by a sense of guilt and Soneri by a feeling of insecurity. The relationship they hoped to rekindle appeared to both of them fragile, and each feared rupturing it with an ill-judged word or move. As often happened between them, they communicated by looks while their rambling words served to ease tension.

"You've done brilliantly," Angela said.

The commissario picked up in her tone of voice something more than a compliment. They were indirectly exchanging words of love, while pretending to speak of other things.

"The poor girl!" Soneri said. "All she wanted was to enjoy life like anyone else. She wanted a partner to spend her life with, but all she found were wealthy men on the prowl."

Angela looked at him affectionately and tenderly. "Are you sure that's the way it was?" she asked, laughing warmly as she spoke. "If there's one thing I like about you and have never found in any other man, it's that you manage to combine the naivety of a boy with the cynical pessimism of an old man."

"Everyone has their contradictions."

She shook her head. "That's not the point. You see the vilest aspects of this world and you accept them with pragmatic resignation, but you never give up thinking like a dreamer. Or a child. In spite of everything, there is a spring of hope in you. It's this quality that makes me love you."

Soneri was thoroughly confused. Angela had left him naked to the point where he had no idea what to say. He felt defenceless but happy to be so in front of this woman who, he now felt sure, was deeply attached to him.

"And that's why you're so wrong about Iliescu," Angela said.

He might have succeeded in finding the culprits, but he had not understood anything. He felt inept. His partner's words were both wounding and confusing.

"Are you determined to extinguish the hope that remains in me?"

"No. I've just said it's the thing I most admire in you. But that girl really was a pernicious person."

"How do you know?"

"You won't lose your temper if I tell you?"

The commissario shook his head.

"The other man, the one . . ."

"I understand."

"Well, he's defending Candiani . . ."

". . . who can now say anything he likes."

"No, there's only one version. The other man knows all about the cocaine deals."

"And what does all this have to do with Nina?"

"Quite a lot," Angela assured him. "The other man convinced Candiani to come clean, and in a couple of days he's going to hand over a memorandum to his defence team in which he'll detail all the various moves in the cocaine trade. Nina was more than a pawn."

Everything was falling apart around Soneri. His reality was evaporating into the mists.

"She worked for Aimi, and the Cerreto club was one of the distribution centres for 'snow' in Parma. She even had an account which was used to transfer the money raised by the drug deals. She took a percentage on the quantities ordered and she got a cut on any new clients she recruited."

Soneri turned a quizzical look on her, while the outlines of the affair shifted yet again, sinking to ever lower depths.

"Franco, it's the truth!" she smiled. "Iliescu was no more than a whore − a high-class whore, if you like, but a whore nevertheless. Her role was to seduce men who had money to burn. Or bored, empty-minded people searching for excitement. She had a real gift for that. Once she'd ensnared them, she talked them into taking a little of the stuff until she made them users. And you thought she was a victim?"

"She was. After all, she was murdered," Soneri insisted.

"She went too far. The Romas saw her as a traitor because she bowed out of the gold deals. They probably threatened her, and she thought she was in a stronger position than she actually was. She most likely threatened to blow the whistle, and so the Romas, Soncini and his wife decided to do away with her. But even with Aimi, according to Candiani, she carried on raising the stakes. She was pretty, she had them all at her feet, but there was no satisfying her. Greed is so often a factor."

"All this could well stand up, but what about the baby?" Soneri objected, thinking of his dead wife and his own sorrows. These were matters which had perhaps confused him all throughout the investigation.

"You have no idea what some women are like. Passion can go hand in hand with cynicism and calculation with emotion. Just possibly Iliescu really was in love with Soncini, maybe she did want to have that baby. She wanted the lot, but when you no longer experience hunger, you risk contracting indigestion. She wanted money and a comfortable life as well as a man and children. She never had time to bring all her hopes together and put them in order. She wanted them all, right away, in one go."

"I could go along with that as an investigator, but I'm still a very poor psychologist."

"That's not the point," Angela said. "It's that you are a better person than the people you have to deal with. And I'm not just talking about down-and-out criminals, but about the wealthy middle class of this city. That's where you find *real* criminals."

"You're speaking like a woman in love." Soneri tried to make light of the situation, but Angela took him seriously and nodded.

"Yes, I am," she said.

They embraced with raw urgency, like two old comrades-in-arms.

"I had given you up for lost, but now you're back," Soneri whispered. "I don't know how this has happened."

"I needed time to reflect. I knew I was hurting you badly, because I know you love me, but there were a lot of things going on. Let's say it's all down to Providence," Angela said with a touch of irony.

"You're not the first person to be lecturing me about that. I've been stumbling over it for some time now."

"We all trip over it. We try to make plans, but often

something turns up that blows us off course, like scraps of paper in the wind."

"And what blew you off course?"

"Life with you was too routine, that was the first thing. Then the other man came along and made me feel desired once again."

"You liked him, that's all there was to it. And perhaps you still do."

Angela did not deny it. "I never considered leaving you. Maybe if it had all worked out with the other man, I'd have had to choose. But, I don't know how to say this . . ."

"In what way did it not work out? Tell me who I have to thank?"

"Chance, providence," Angela said with a laugh. "A couple of days ago I bumped into a colleague I hadn't seen for ages. It just so happened that both of us were due to have trials before different courts, but both trials collapsed. What sort of coincidence was that? We found ourselves having a coffee in the same bar. In the course of the conversation, gossiping about mutual friends, the talk turned to the other man. She didn't know what had been going on between me and him, but she let slip that last month he had been courting her insistently. In other words, he was trying it on with both of us at the same time."

"So I should send a bouquet to your colleague."

"Maybe it would all have ended in any case," Angela said, without much conviction.

"I doubt it. You were fond of him, and if he hadn't slipped up, which you found out about by pure chance, you'd be with him still and you'd have left me," Soneri groaned.

"At some stage, I'd have had to make up my mind."

"You'd have chosen him. He excited you, you were elated."

"He made me feel important."

Soneri fell silent. He was gripped by anxiety over what might have been. "You had effectively left me. You were about to tell me so when something made you turn back. I was already an ex."

"But now we're here," she said.

"By pure chance."

"We are light, unbearably light, made of nothing. We can only seize the moment, but we can't claim there is any continuity in what we are, nor can we make plans that are anything more than vague desires. In a flash something can change the unstable formula of our attachments. It's an infinite round of waltz steps. Life produces saints and killers, monks and pimps, thieves and honest men."

"Now it has produced the two of us, and has allowed us once more to walk a little way together. It's no good thinking too far ahead," Angela said.

"Alright. Let's take full advantage of this opportunity your other man has offered us," Soneri said, taking out his mobile to call the investigating magistrate.

"Dottoressa, do you have a moment? It appears to be the case that Nina was a link in a chain for the distribution of cocaine, centred on the Cerreto club. In the next couple of days, you'll have in your hands a memorandum written by Candiani for his defence. That Aimi needs more attention as well."

As they spoke he could hear in her voice annoyance and disappointment over that human betrayal of his. "But, forgive me, why are you telling me this? I entrusted the case to you."

"We're talking about drugs now, something for the narcotics squad to look into. For the rest, no need to look any further than Musumeci, who took care of Candiani."

"Look here, and I'm saying this for your sake, it seems

they want to take the case out of your hands. I don't get it," she said.

"Capuozzo was right. It's as well to stop at a certain point. I have no desire to sink any deeper into this shit."

VALERIO VARESI is a journalist with *La Repubblica*. *Gold, Frankincense and Dust* is the third in a series of thrillers featuring Commissario Soneri, now the protagonist of one of Italy's most popular television dramas. The earlier novels, *River of Shadows* and *The Dark Valley*, were both shortlisted for the Crime Writers' Association International Dagger.

JOSEPH FARRELL is professor of Italian at the University of Strathclyde. He is the distinguished translator of novels by Leonardo Sciascia and Vincenzo Consolo, and plays by the Nobel Laureate Dario Fo.